Advances in Extracorporeal Membrane Oxygenation - Volume 3

Edited by Michael S. Firstenberg

Published in London, United Kingdom

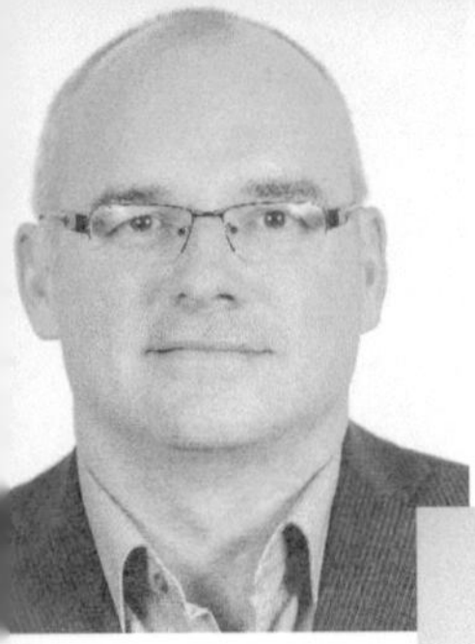
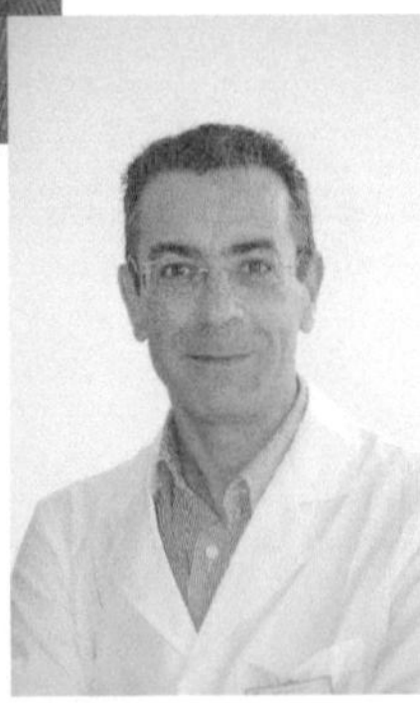
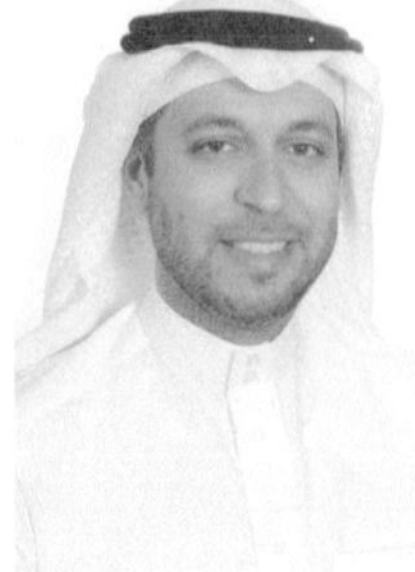
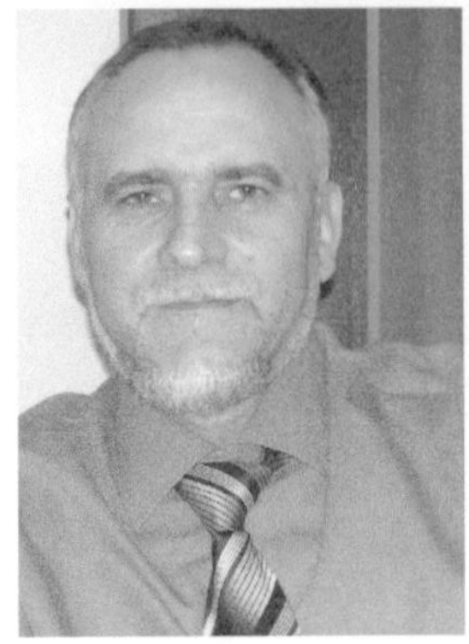
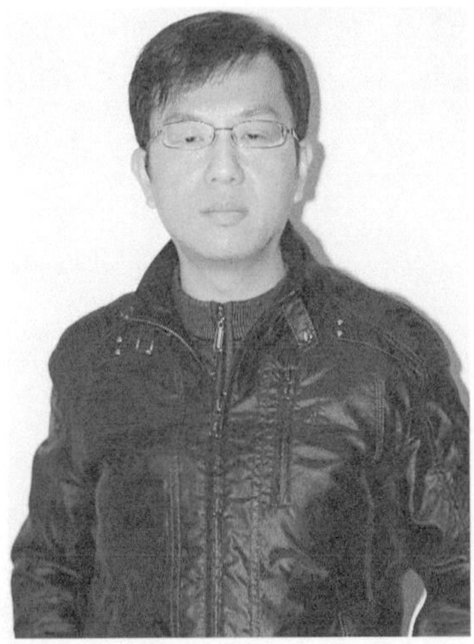
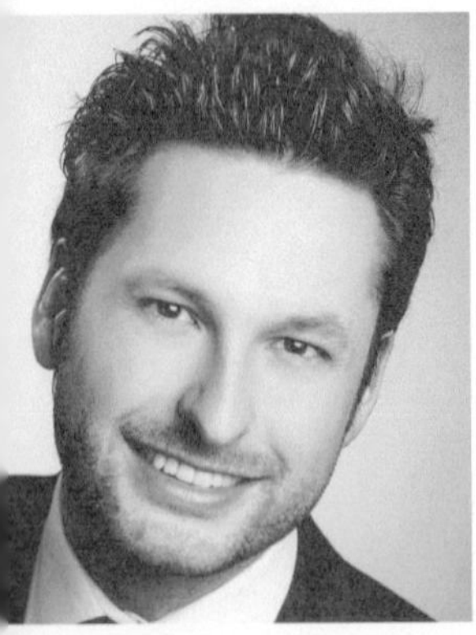
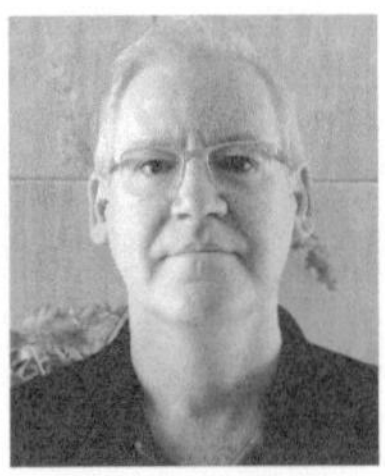

IntechOpen

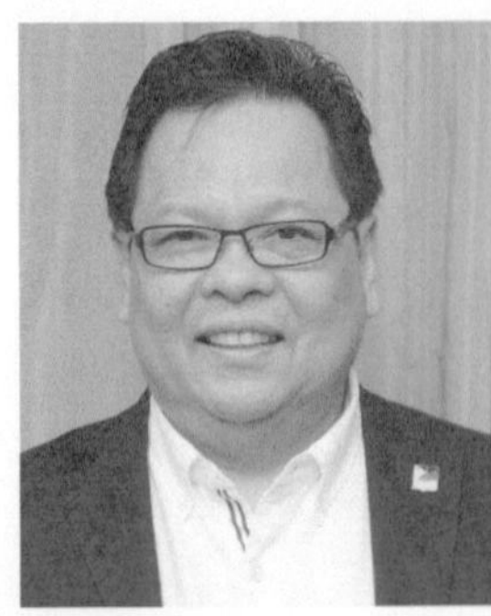
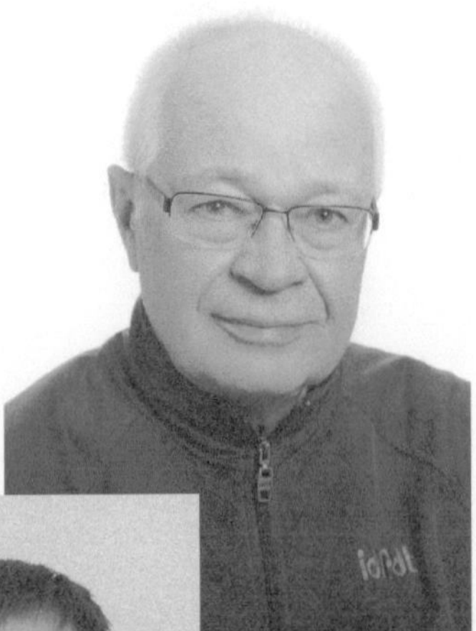
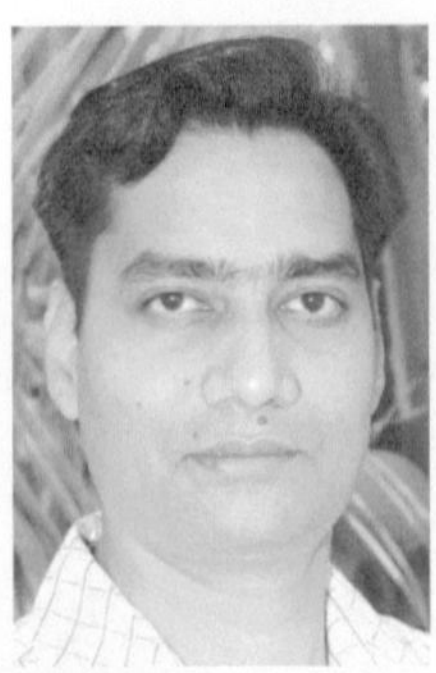
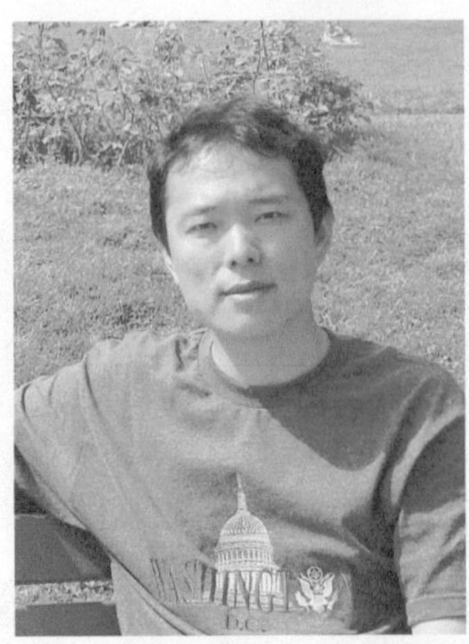
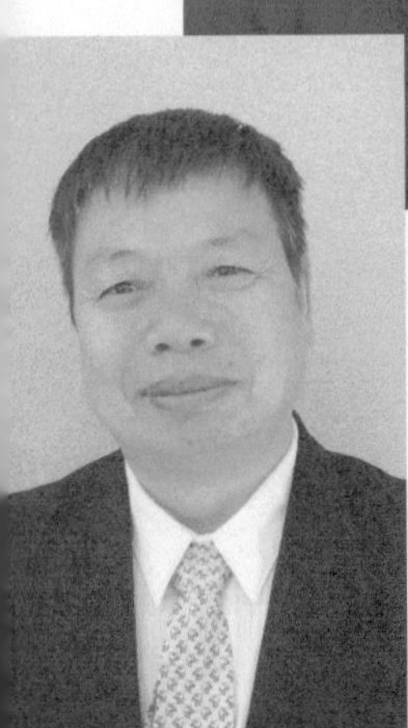
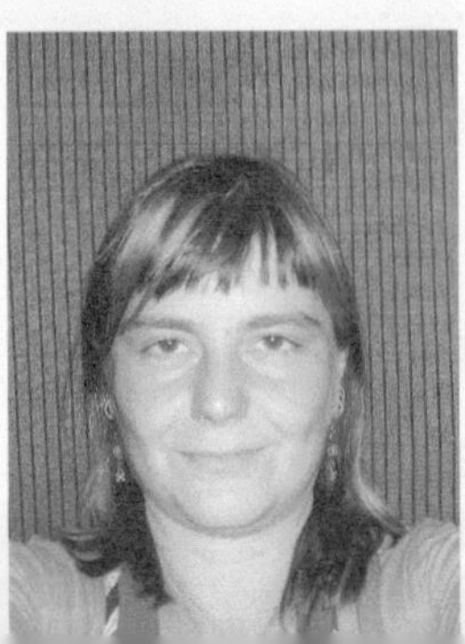

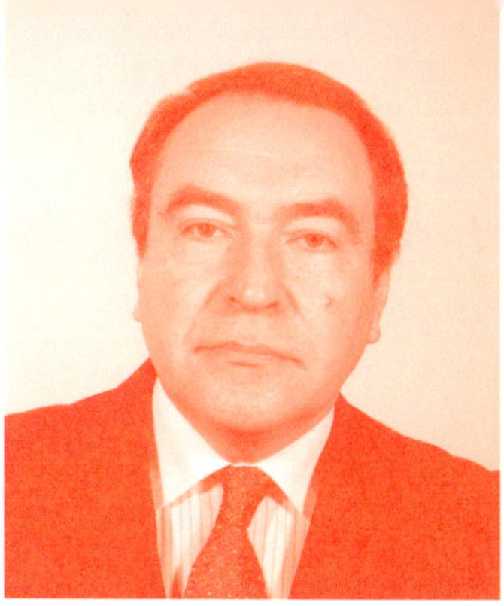
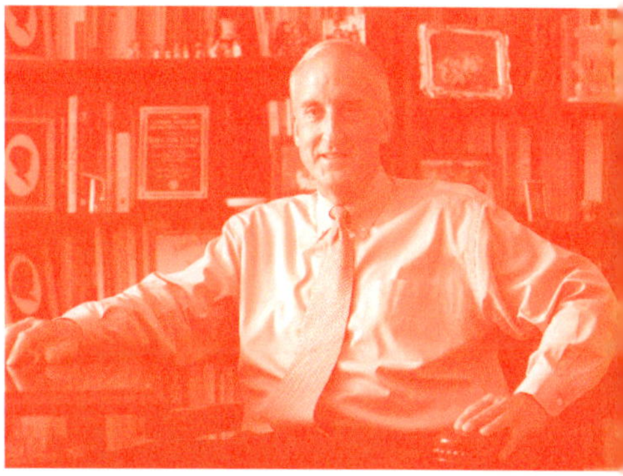
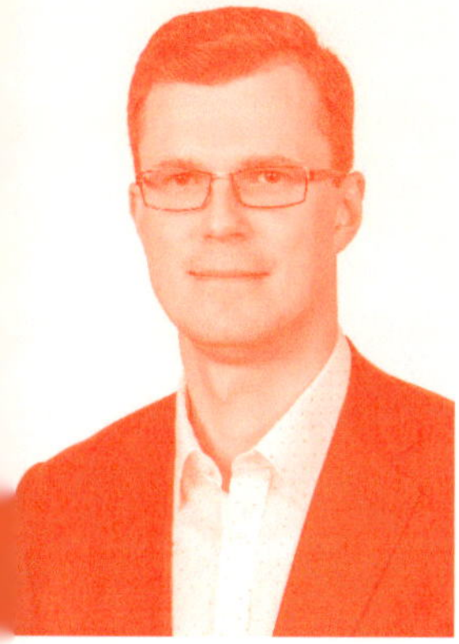
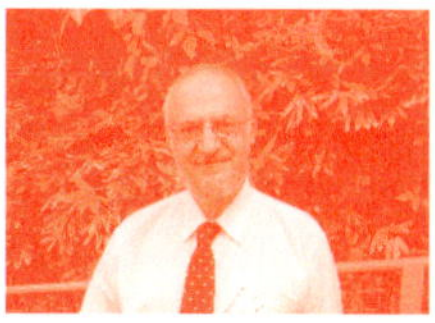
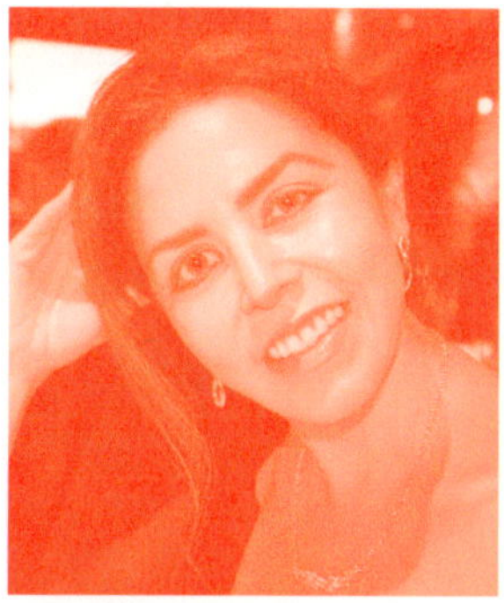

Supporting open minds since 2005

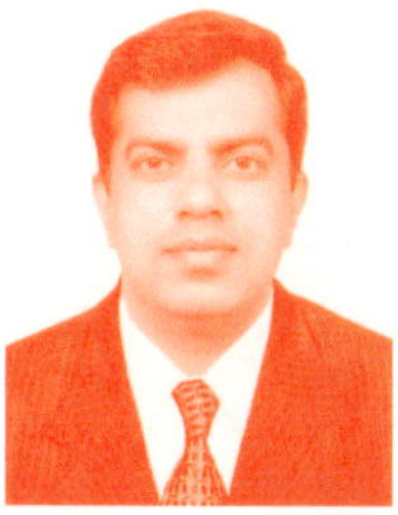
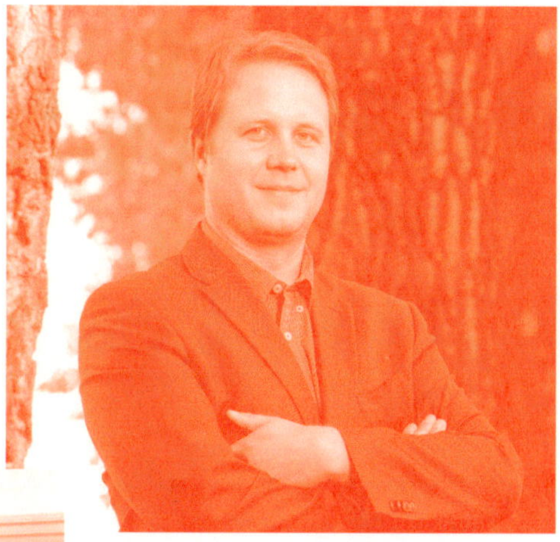
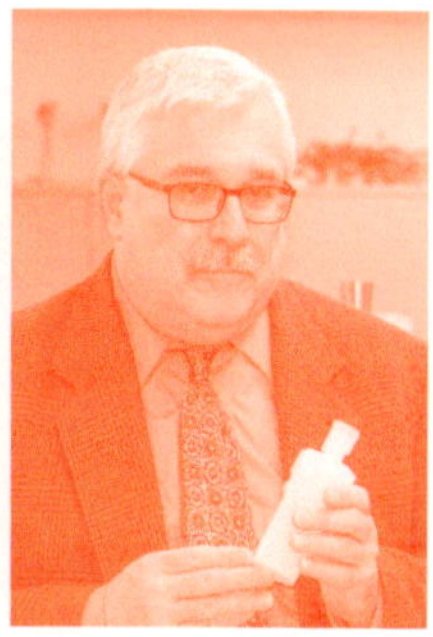
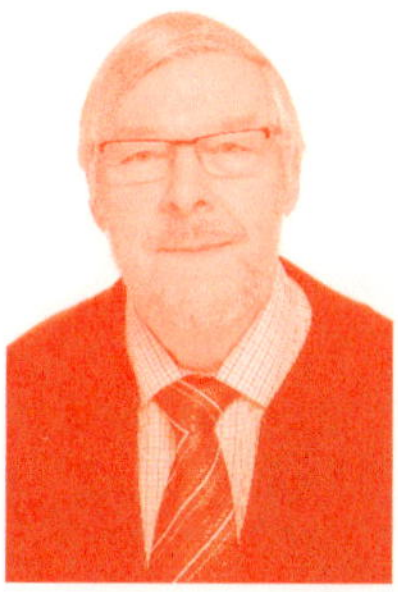
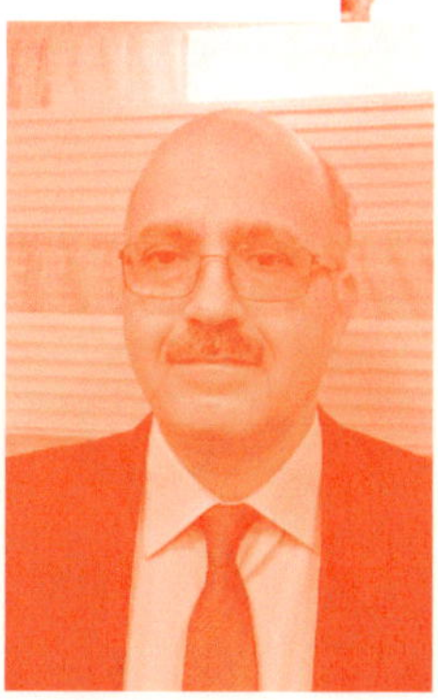
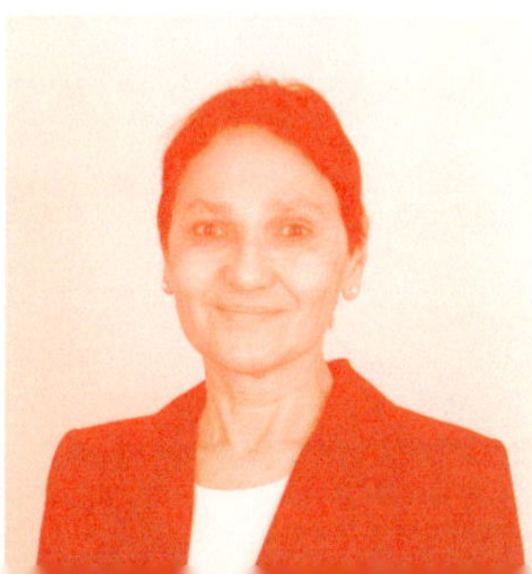
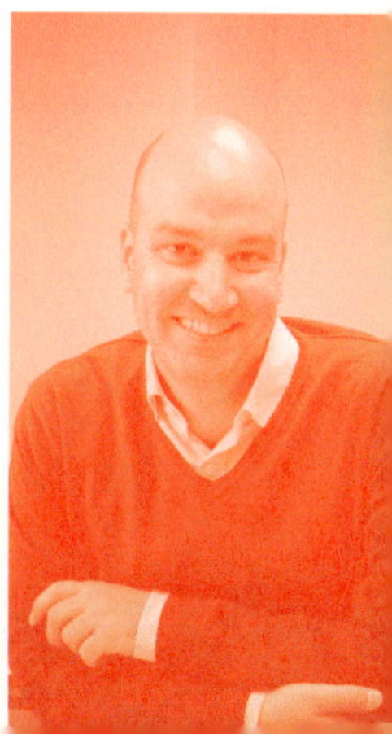

Advances in Extracorporeal Membrane Oxygenation - Volume 3
http://dx.doi.org/10.5772/intechopen.77697
Edited by Michael S. Firstenberg

Contributors
Venessa Pinto, Abdelaziz Farhat, Lakshmi Raman, Cindy Darnell-Bowens, Ravi Thiagarajan, Suresh Keshavamurthy, Yoshiya Toyoda, Michael Mazzei, Jamie Weller, Ali McMichael, Ayesha Zia, Michael S. S Firstenberg, Dianne McCallister, Linda Pilon, Nandini Nair, Enrique Gongora, Luis Morales-Quinteros, Antonio Artigas, Luigi Tritapepe, Ernesto Greco, Carlo Gaudio, Prashant Mohite, Andre Simon, Constantino Fondevila, Amelia Hessheimer, Jorge Silva Enciso, Kimberly N Hong, Julie M. Aultman, Alexander Botsch

First published in London, United Kingdom, 2019 by IntechOpen
IntechOpen is the global imprint of INTECHOPEN LIMITED, registered in England and Wales, registration number: 11086078, 7th floor, 10 Lower Thames Street, London, EC3R 6AF, United Kingdom
Printed in Croatia

British Library Cataloguing-in-Publication Data
A catalogue record for this book is available from the British Library

Additional hard and PDF copies can be obtained from orders@intechopen.com

Advances in Extracorporeal Membrane Oxygenation - Volume 3
Edited by Michael S. Firstenberg
p. cm.
Print ISBN 978-1-78923-923-2
Online ISBN 978-1-78923-924-9
eBook (PDF) ISBN 978-1-78984-397-2

For EU product safety concerns:
IN TECH d.o.o., Prolaz Marije Krucifikse Kozulić 3, 51000 Rijeka, Croatia, info@intechopen.com or visit our website at intechopen.com.

Meet the editor

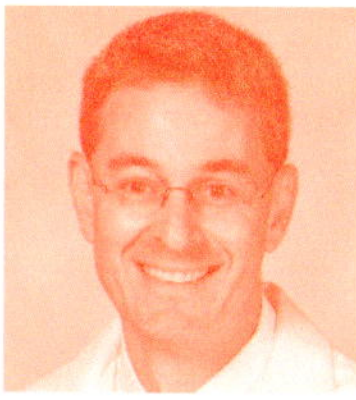

Dr. Michael S. Firstenberg is a board-certified thoracic surgeon practicing adult cardiac surgery at the Medical Center of Aurora (Colorado, USA) where he serves at the Chief of Cardiothoracic and Vascular Surgery. He currently holds adjunct appointments in the Colleges of Medicine and Graduate Studies at Northeast Ohio Medical University and serves on the teaching faculty at the Rocky Vista University. He attended Case Western Reserve University Medical School, received his general surgery training at university hospitals in Cleveland, and completed a fellowship in thoracic surgery at the Ohio State University. He also obtained advanced training in heart failure surgical therapies at the Cleveland Clinic. He is an active member of the Society of Thoracic Surgeons, American Association of Thoracic Surgeons, American College of Cardiology, and American College of Academic International Medicine (for which he is a founding fellow). He currently serves as Chair of the American College of Cardiology Credentialing and Member Services Committee as well as being active on several other national society committees. He is the author of more than 200 peer-reviewed manuscripts, abstracts, and book chapters. He has edited several textbooks on topics ranging from medical leadership, patient safety, endocarditis, and extra-corporeal membrane oxygenation—all of which include topics that he has lectured on worldwide.

Contents

Preface

Extracorporeal life support or extracorporeal membrane oxygenation (ECMO), as it is often known, continues to evolve into an effective therapy for managing patients who present, regardless of etiology, with acute severe cardiogenic shock and/or respiratory therapy. Previously, ECMO was thought to be a salvage therapy to be considered when all other conventional therapies had failed. However, with evolving guidelines, protocols, experiences, and tools to assist in patient selection, management, and various aspects of clinical (and administrative) decision making, ECMO has evolved into a mainstream therapy. With this evolution, outcomes have improved and overall, teams have become much more effective and efficient with regard to developing a structured "ECMO program." However, with thousands of cases being performed each year and with rapidly evolving technology along with an exponential growth of knowledge in this field, it is clear that there is still much to learn and understand. The technology is costly, not always readily available, and often very resource intensive—typically requiring very advanced specialty training of all involved providers. It is promising that there has also been an evolution of case reports, case series, large institutional experiences, meta-analyses, and even randomized trials in this area to help support clinical application and decision making. Hopefully, this text—along with the previous volumes in this area—will continue to add to the literature on this topic in a meaningful way to help programs grow and outcomes improve.

As experience grows, one thing that remains clear is that therapy must be initiated early, and having a well-structured and integrated clinical management team is critical to program success and good outcomes. Starting therapy before the development of irreversible end-organ damage is paramount. With a better understanding of the nuances of patient selection and management, protocols can be developed to aid those physicians and providers who are often faced with major decisions in which time is of the essence. Ethical (and social) implications cannot be overstated. While ECMO is often considered, along with many other therapies in healthcare currently, as a salvage option to potentially provide some hope for an actively dying patient, the concepts of futility, palliative care, and end-of-life must be considered. ECMO must not be considered as a "bridge to nowhere"—implying a final major intervention to avoid difficult conversations regarding the reality that everyone at some point will die.

Without doubt, as this text will hopefully illustrate and educate, ECMO continues to evolve into an extremely important, powerful, and effective clinical tool, and much like every other powerful tool at our disposal, we have a great responsibility to make sure that we continue to use it appropriately and safely.

Michael S. Firstenberg, MD FACC FAIM
Chief, Cardiothoracic and Vascular Surgery,
Director, Adult ECMO Program,
Associate Professor of Surgery and Integrative Medicine (Adjunct),
Graduate Adjunct Faculty,
College of Graduate Studies,
Northeast Ohio Medical Universities,
Rootstown, Ohio, USA

Teaching Faculty,
The Rocky Vista University,
Parker, Colorado, USA

The Medical Center of Aurora and Rose Hospitals,
Aurora, CO, USA

Section 1

Introduction

Chapter 1

Introductory Chapter: ECMO – Rapidly Evolving Technology, Expanding Indications, and Growing Challenges

Michael S. Firstenberg and Jennifer M. Hanna

1. Introduction

This text is now the third volume in a series of books focused on extracorporeal membrane oxygenation (ECMO) and extracorporeal life support (ECLS) [1]. With each volume, it becomes clearer that there has been a rapid evolution in the technology and the applications of it with regard to indications, management, outcomes, and the challenges in offering a very resource-intensive (and expensive) therapy in which the overall benefits are still questioned. Nevertheless, without a doubt, there has been an ongoing evolution of the use of ECMO as a salvage therapy offered only in extreme and potentially inherently futile cases, to now a mainstream therapy that can be routinely offered in well-defined cases of acute cardiac and respiratory failure. Early experiences resulted in few survivors and poor outcomes, but the reasons for this were clearly complex and multifactorial etiologies [2]. The development of more advanced pumps and circuits, better resources and guidelines for patient selection and management, and a broader understanding of the complex interactions between humans and an extracorporeal pump circuit for longer periods of time all have contributed to the advances in ECMO as an appropriate and reasonable therapy—even, as some would debate, standard of care for acute respiratory failure and/or cardiogenic shock. As these three volumes illustrate, over the years, there has been tireless improvements in all aspects of the use of ECMO. However, as the chapters in this text clearly illustrate, there is still much to be learned and understood. Challenges remain as clinicians continue to push the envelope of this technology to better define a patient population that might benefit from ECMO and how to apply and manage a very complex therapy to optimize outcomes [3].

As the indications for therapy evolve, there continues to be unusual and challenging clinical situations that deserve special attention for many reasons. For example, the chapter by Professor Nandini highlights the very complex issue that is becoming more common—the role of ECMO as a bridge to transplant. It was only a few years ago (and illustrated in the previous texts in this series) that the concept of ECMO as bridge to transplant was discouraged and difficult to justify due to the risks, concerns of limited resource allocation, and technical difficulties to a concept and management pathway that is routinely considered and offered to selected patients.

Additional chapters focus on the growing literature and experiences in other specific disease state or clinical situations for which ECMO might be considered.

One area that is particularly challenging is incorporating ECMO into the management of patients who develop acute cardiopulmonary collapse. ECMO-assisted CPR (eCPR) is one of the fastest growing uses of ECMO, and many rapid response/code teams are increasingly using ECMO in the management of patients who develop cardiac arrest. The data, experiences, and outcomes in this very complex area are rapidly evolving, and the controversies are substantial. The chapter by Dr. Lakshmi illustrates the current state of the art in this area and how patients can be selected and managed, with a focus on illustrating the improved outcomes in a patient population that was historically considered unsalvageable. Other similar unique applications for ECMO discussed in this text include a chapter on carbon dioxide removal by Dr. Morales-Quinteros. The very unusual role of normothermic regional perfusion in the setting of solid organ transplantation is discussed by Dr. Constantino.

A major focus of this volume is the specific management challenges that complicate the use of ECMO, especially in high-risk patient populations. Despite a greater awareness, peripheral cannulation techniques that are often used are associated with high rates of limb complications including amputation. Such concerns are discussed in the chapter by Dr. Prashant. Imaging of patients on ECMO, with an emphasis on assessing for cardiac recovery and prognosis, is especially important and discussed by Dr. Luigi, while the actual techniques, concepts, and applications of various weaning strategies are the focus of another chapter. Meanwhile, Dr. Weller's chapter on anticoagulation in the pediatric patient and Dr. Pinto's chapter on neurologic complications and monitoring revisit some of the difficult topics addressed in the previous editions and emphasize the growing experiences and literature in these complex topics [4, 5]. As some aspects of these topics have been addressed in the earlier books in this series, the contemporary experiences highlight that there remains much to understand and learn about many of these topics.

Again, it is also clear that to successfully offer ECMO as a viable therapy—and especially to strive for reasonable outcomes—there must be alignment of all key stakeholders. Without a doubt, ECMO requires an extensive team of providers at all levels working together in a manner that respects professionalism, competencies, compassion, and strict attention to details. The substantial and tireless efforts of the entire team must be recognized and appreciated by all and at all levels [6].

A frequently asked question is "how do we start an ECMO program?" Offering ECMO as a therapy involves so much more than just purchasing capital equipment and some disposable supplies. The chapter on program development emphasizes the many administrative aspects that must be considered within an appropriate framework to establish a program. This chapter considers the importance of physician, nursing, and administrative leadership and collaboration as a foundation for a successful program. While a great deal has been written on the extensive medical and surgical aspects of the management of a patient on ECMO, the chapter by Mr. Botsch and colleagues reviews the many aspects of the nursing bedside care. Of course, these topics continue to illustrate the importance of teamwork which cannot be overemphasized.

As discussed in the previous editions, a highly functioning "ECMO team" is a cornerstone in building a successful program. The ability to initiate therapy at any time and place is increasingly considered an important component of a well-organized team. While the makeup of an ECMO team can vary across institutions; each requires a champion to provide leadership and help with structure and organization. A fundamental principle is effective communication and a multidisciplinary approach to all aspects of management. Just as importantly, all members of the team—regardless of experiences, education, training, degrees, and titles—need to have respect and trust and place value on all aspects of the contributions of all members. This is the basis of crew resource management (CRM). The key concept of CRM is that every team member has input and that each voice is valued and respected. Every member of the team needs to be empowered to speak up, particularly when there are concerns about safety. The different disciplines that are represented in an ECMO Team, as mentioned, can vary from program to program, but given the complexities of patient selection and management—including, the least of which are the technical aspects of cannulation and cannula management—membership must be comprehensive with regard to surgical and medical expertise. Membership should include, but clearly, not be limited to:

Physicians

- Surgeons (cardiothoracic, general, trauma, emergency medicine)
- Critical care intensivists (pulmonary, surgical)
- Medical specialists (infectious disease, neurology, cardiology, nephrology)

Advanced providers

- Nursing (bedside, advanced practice providers)
- Pharmacists
- Perfusionists
- Respiratory therapists
- Social workers/case management

Palliative care

- Often physician or advance practice nurses

Hospital leadership and administration

- C-suite executives (chief executive, financial, operating, and other officers)
- Quality managers
- Marketing

It is critical that even with dedicated, hardworking, and engaged clinical teams, there must be support and encouragement from hospital leadership and administration (**Figure 1**) [7].

Many of the chapters in these volumes discuss the various indications for ECMO (veno-venous and venoarterial) support and special patient populations and circumstances. However, a critical component of any program remains the role of striving for optimal clinical outcomes. Regardless of the indications and populations, outcomes and clinical complications (e.g., renal failure, limb complications,

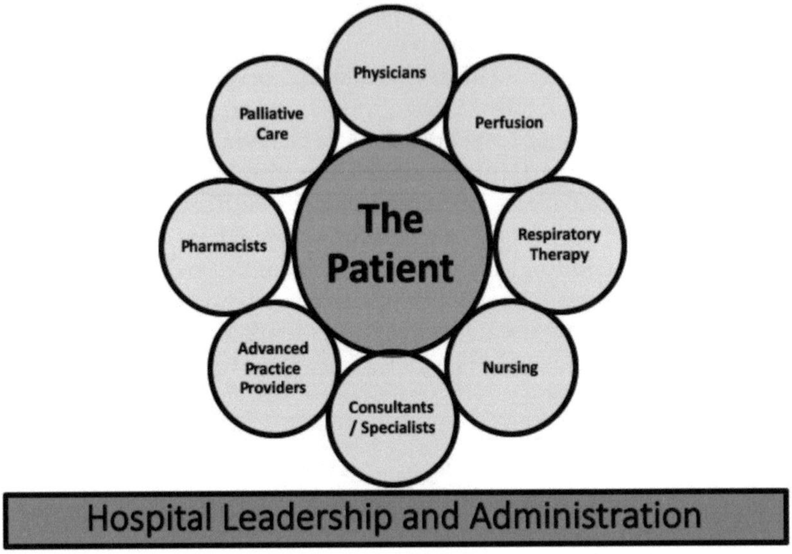

Figure 1.
ECMO "team". Adopted from reference intro chapter in Volume 1 [1].

transfusion rates, etc.) must be tracked and compared to published benchmarks. Quality conferences in which cases are discussed can help a team and program formally recognize their successes while looking for opportunities for collective improvement. As discussed previously in the introductions (and various chapters) of the previous volumes, outcomes still remain less than ideal with survival rates that range from 60 to 70% for veno-venous respiratory support and 25–35% for venoarterial cardiopulmonary support and eCPR [8, 9]. These less-than-ideal success rates should improve over time as programs gain experience and implement guidelines and protocols, teams learn to function more effectively and efficiently, and patient selection and management improve. However, poor outcomes must also be tempered by the concerns that outcomes that are potentially "too good" might suggest that potentially salvageable but higher risk patients might not be offered therapy out of fear of experiencing a bad outcome. Nevertheless, it becomes the priority of a program to develop a "culture" of how aggressive they want to be with regard to offering therapy to high-risk (or low-risk) patients. Fortunately, scoring systems for venoarterial and veno-venous support indications can assist in patient selection. Again, outcomes and quality metrics must be benchmarked against similar programs, like institutions and established registries. Membership in the Extracorporeal Life Support Organization (ELSO: https://www.elso.org) is an important component of tracking outcomes and can play a key role in documenting program progress and success. In addition, membership can provide an opportunity to establish relationships with other programs to exchange ideas, share protocols, and have access to important and timely developments and technological innovations.

While the advances in the field of ECMO are rapid and there has been an equally rapid worldwide growth in programs and the number of patients supported, a key aspect of ECMO therapy is the ethical component of a highly invasive, resource-intensive, and complex intervention. Because ECMO is still associated with less than ideal outcomes, relatively high complication rates (including neurologic complications), and high resource intensivity (not to mention expensive, depending on the reimbursement circumstances which can vary dramatically), a fundamental question remains regarding not on whether we can offer and continue support, but within an ethical and moral framework should we offer support. The chapter by Dr. Aultman on the ethics of ECMO therapy explores many of the difficult decisions and circumstances that providers often face when considering offering or continuing therapy in patients who would most likely immediately die if support is neither offered nor continued.

2. Conclusions

Experiences in the selection and management of patients with acute cardiac and respiratory failure who are treated with ECMO continue to grow. Recent trials continue to help demonstrate the effectiveness and role of ECMO as outcomes continue to slowly improve [10, 11]. Even though many patients treated with ECMO still die even in the best of circumstances, it remains important for everyone to continue to search for opportunities for improvement. Good outcomes must be embraced and shared with the entire team, as they can provide hope while also inspiring and motivating a team—even when there are concerns of futility (**Figure 2**). The goal of this volume is to offer further insights, experiences, and discussions of the current state of the art regarding many topics that challenge those who believed in the tremendous potential benefits of ECMO [12].

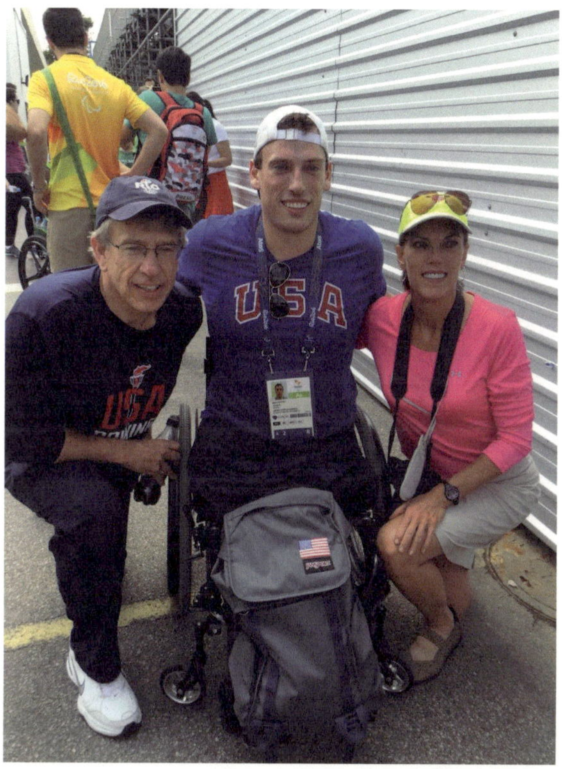

Figure 2.
BH (center in wheelchair) with his parents after qualifying for the finals in the single-scull, arms and shoulder only, rowing competition in the 2016 Paralympics in Rio de Janeiro. BH, a five-time US national champion in the event, represented the USA in Rio as a member of the Olympic team. In 2016, he was selected US rowing "rower of the year." several years prior, BH lost both legs to complications of a necrotizing soft tissue infection and required cardiopulmonary support with venoarterial ECMO due to overwhelming septic shock. Picture used by permission by all represented [11, 12] and adopted from volume 2 [13].

Author details

Michael S. Firstenberg* and Jennifer M. Hanna
Cardiothoracic and Thoracic Surgery, The Medical Center of Aurora, Aurora, CO, United States

*Address all correspondence to: msfirst@gmail.com

References

[1] Firstenberg MS. Introductory chapter: Evolution of ECMO from salvage to mainstream supportive and resuscitative therapy, extracorporeal membrane oxygenation. IntechOpen; 2016. DOI: 10.5772/64345. Available from: https://www.intechopen.com/books/extracorporeal-membrane-oxygenation-advances-in-therapy/introductory-chapter-evolution-of-ecmo-from-salvage-to-mainstream-supportive-and-resuscitative-thera

[2] Zapol WM, Snider MT, Hill JD, Fallat RJ, Bartlett RH, Edmunds LH, et al. Extracorporeal membrane oxygenation in severe acute respiratory failure. A randomized prospective study. Journal of the American Medical Association. 1979;**242**(20):2193-2196

[3] Bartlett RH, Roloff DW, Custer JR, Younger JG, Hirschl RB. Extracorporeal life support: The University of Michigan experience. Journal of the American Medical Association. 2000;**283**(7):904-908

[4] Bowling SM, Gomes J, Firstenberg MS. Neurologic issues in patients receiving extracorporeal membrane oxygenation support, extracorporeal membrane oxygenation. Advances in Therapy, IntechOpen. 2016. DOI: 10.5772/64269. Available from: https://www.intechopen.com/books/extracorporeal-membrane-oxygenation-advances-in-therapy/neurologic-issues-in-patients-receiving-extracorporeal-membrane-oxygenation-support

[5] Maul TM, Patricia Massicotte M, Wearden PD. ECMO biocompatibility: Surface coatings, anticoagulation, and coagulation monitoring, extracorporeal membrane oxygenation. Advances in Therapy, IntechOpen. 2016. DOI: 10.5772/63888. Available from: https://www.intechopen.com/books/extracorporeal-membrane-oxygenation-advances-in-therapy/ecmo-biocompatibility-surface-coatings-anticoagulation-and-coagulation-monitoring

[6] Australia and New Zealand Extracorporeal Membrane Oxygenation (ANZ ECMO) Influenza Investigators, Davies A, Jones D, Bailey M, Beca J, Bellomo R, et al. Extracorporeal membrane oxygenation for 2009 influenza a(H1N1) acute respiratory distress syndrome. Journal of the American Medical Association. 2009;**302**(17):1888-1895. Epub 2009 Oct 12

[7] Firstenberg MS, Swaminath D. Left ventricular failure—Extra-corporeal membrane oxygenation: An update. World Society of Cardiothoracic Surgeons Journal. 2016;**1**(1):12-14

[8] Rastan AJ, Dege A, Mohr M, Doll N, Falk V, Walther T, et al. Early and late outcomes of 517 consecutive adult patients treated with extracorporeal membrane oxygenation for refractory postcardiotomy cardiogenic shock. The Journal of Thoracic and Cardiovascular Surgery. 2010;**139**(2):302-311, 311.e1

[9] Peek GJ, Mugford M, Tiruvoipati R, Wilson A, Allen E, Thalanany MM, et al., CESAR Trial Collaboration. Efficacy and economic assessment of conventional ventilatory support versus extracorporeal membrane oxygenation for severe adult respiratory failure (CESAR): A multicentre randomised controlled trial. Lancet. 2009;**374**(9698):1351-1363

[10] Combes A, Hajage D, Capellier G, Demoule A, Lavoué S, Guervilly C, et al. Extracorporeal membrane oxygenation for severe acute respiratory distress syndrome. New England Journal of Medicine. 2018;**378**(21):1965-1975

[11] Schmid C, Philipp A, Hilker M, Rupprecht L, Arlt M, Keyser A, et al. Venovenous extracorporeal membrane oxygenation for acute lung failure in adults. The Journal of Heart and Lung Transplantation. 2012;**31**(1):9-15

[12] Tulman DB, Stawicki SPA, Whitson BA, Gupta SC, Tripathi RS, Firstenberg MS, et al. Veno-venous ECMO: A synopsis of nine key potential challenges, considerations, and controversies. BMC: Anesthesiology. 2014;**14**:65

[13] Firstenberg MS, Hanna JM. Introductory chapter: ECMO-growing indications, applications, and understanding of a complex supportive therapy. Advances in Extra-Corporeal Perfusion Therapies, IntechOpen. 2018. DOI: 10.5772/intechopen.81777. Available from: https://www.intechopen.com/books/advances-in-extra-corporeal-perfusion-therapies/introductory-chapter-ecmo-growing-indications-applications-and-understanding-of-a-complex-supportive

Section 2

ECMO Program Structure

Chapter 2

Nursing Implications in the ECMO Patient

Alex Botsch, Elizabeth Protain, Amanda R. Smith and Ryan Szilagyi

Abstract

Effective care and positive outcomes of the extracorporeal membrane oxygenation (ECMO) patient necessitate optimal interdisciplinary management from the healthcare team, including expert care from specially trained registered nurses (RNs). It is incumbent upon the RN caring for the ECMO patient to excel in both time management and assessment skills, as this population often demands care delivery at the pinnacle of intensive care unit (ICU) acuity. Astute and nuanced monitoring of neurological status, bleeding risk with potential (often massive) transfusions, poor hemodynamics, and integrity of the ECMO pump itself are only the few specialized areas of focus that must share priority with traditional nursing considerations involving the critically ill, such as prevention of pressure injuries and bloodstream infections. These high-intensity medical foci must be balanced with ethical considerations, as the ultimate goal of returning the patient to their normal life is not always possible. These demands highlight the dynamic proficiency of the RN caring for the ECMO patient. The following chapter will highlight the importance of specialized nursing care in the critically ill patient supported with ECMO.

Keywords: ECMO patient necessitates, interdisciplinary management, importance of specialized nursing care

1. Introduction

The patient requiring extracorporeal membrane oxygenation (ECMO) for any etiology is almost always managed in the intensive care unit (ICU) and requires care around the clock, which is delivered by a collaboration of physicians, nurses (RNs), respiratory therapists, perfusionists, and many others. Close collaboration between care providers is crucial, particularly between the RN managing hemodynamic medication infusions and the ECMO specialist managing the pump. RNs provide extensive, holistic care for ICU patients and their families, much of it geared toward traditional, clinical care with the additional implications of ECMO therapy, which requires additional specialized training. Acuity, unpredictability, and heavy resource requirements of the ECMO patient, especially when initiating therapy, can necessitate unusual and innovative staffing models, which rely on flexibility and often extra hours and shifts to accommodate individual patient and unit needs.

RNs are essential to the delivery of optimal healthcare and play an integral role in the care of patients admitted to the ICU, so it is important that, when staffed well, RNs reduce the risk of inhospital mortality anywhere from 14 to 36% [10, 29].

A recent expert consensus suggests RN-to-ECMO patient ratios should be at least 1:1 or 1:2 to deliver safe and quality patient care [33]. A recent survey found that RNs were allocated 1:1 in nearly 60% of ECMO centers internationally when also monitoring and intervening on the ECMO circuit [9]. This chapter will further discuss the nursing implications involved in the care of the ECMO patient, the RN's role in prevention of associated complications, and the importance of the holistic approach required at the bedside.

2. Nursing implications for cannula site management

Nursing care should include monitoring of the ECMO circuit as nurses and associated staff, such as respiratory therapists and perfusionists, are at the bedside with the patient continually. ECMO cannulae require the same, if not more, attention that any peripheral or central venous catheter would, including assessment for erythema, purulence, adequacy of securement, and dressing integrity. It is significantly important to monitor for fixation of the ECMO cannulae. Initial placement of ECMO cannulae is usually confirmed by echocardiography and the position reaffirmed by radiographs [19]. Thus, ensuring the securement and stability of the cannulae by routine and repeated physical assessment is integral, as misplaced cannulae, loose sutures, or distant lashing straps can lead to specific complications such as inadequate flows or cannula dislodgment [28]. Ideal placement of lashing straps and appropriate securement of cannulae can be seen in **Figure 1**.

It is particularly important for the nurse and other bedside clinicians to be mindful of the integrity of the pump, as mispositioning of cannulae or hypovolemia can result in end-organ injury [11]. Suction events involve disruption of flow secondary to venous collapse onto the drainage cannula and can result in thrombus formation [11]. The occurrence of thrombi in the pump or oxygenator can be recognized by a visible thrombus, an increasing pressure decrease across the oxygenator, or a low post-oxygenator pCO_2 [11].

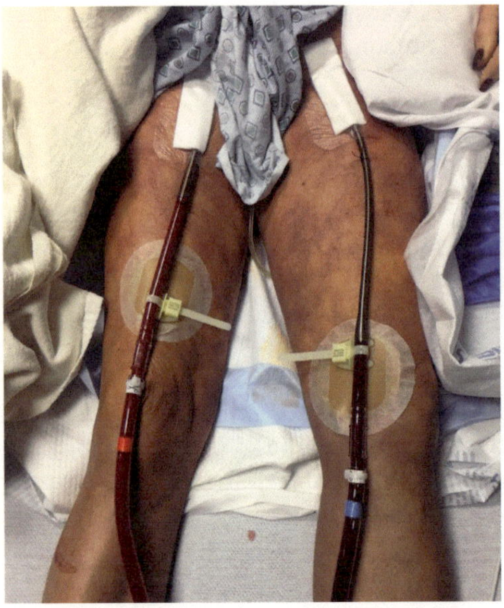

Figure 1.
Appropriate lashing strap distance demonstrating safe securement and appropriate tension on the ECMO cannulae.

There are additional considerations that the nurse caring for the ECMO patient will need to exercise specific to the therapy. Disruption of innate circulatory flow secondary to ECMO can result in limb ischemia. Thus, it is important to monitor limbs, especially those distal from cannulation sites. Clinical judgment, pulse palpation, and Doppler sonography of limb vessels are effective tools for this purpose [28]. Another modern tool for monitoring tissue oxygenation in lower extremities in ECMO patients is near-infrared spectroscopy [28]. The nurse may also note that clinicians will often place distal perfusion catheters to help prevent or treat distal limb ischemia, as demonstrated in **Figure 2** [28]. Harlequin syndrome can present in patients with venoarterial (VA) cannulation, where the heart has recovered but the lungs are still poorly functioning. The hallmark assessment finding for this is upper extremity cyanosis [28].

Vessel perforation may take place on insertion; but, symptoms may not present immediately [28]. The most serious complication is a large retroperitoneal hematoma; but, considerable local bleeding at the insertion site is also possible, and site assessment, as well as assessment of the abdomen, flanks, and inguinal areas for ecchymosis, hypotension, and acutely worsening anemia, is necessary [28]. Additional assessment findings may include bulging or swelling at the insertion site, most consistent with pseudoaneurysm. Mild insertional hematomas may be mitigated and controlled by application of manual pressure, with subsequent monitoring of flows and distal pulses, both of which are imperative for clinical safety.

Infection is an associated risk of ECMO therapy as well and linked to greater likelihood of mortality. In one study, patients on ECMO experienced an overall mortality of 68.3:75.6% in patients with infections and 67.1% in patients without infections [30]. The use of steroids in acute respiratory distress syndrome (ARDS) or adrenal insufficiency, body temperature control, and multiple blood transfusions after cardiac operations for coagulopathy during ECMO can interfere with the presentation of infection in patients undergoing ECMO [30]. Thus, routine inspection and care of all invasive lines, including ECMO catheters, become integral. Implementing standard decolonization practices set forth by the nurse's institution is appropriate for ECMO catheters, such as antimicrobial scrubs and occlusive dressings.

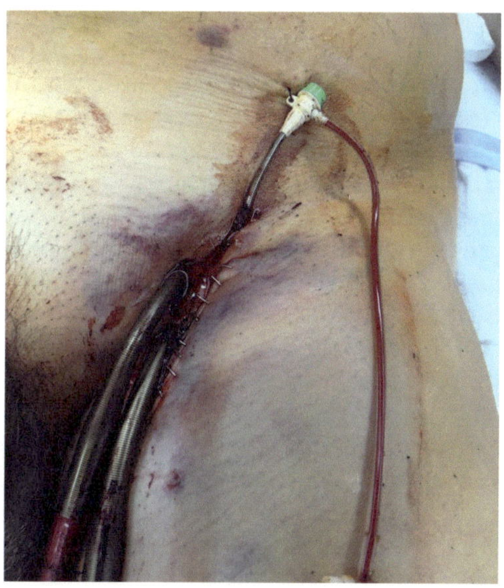

Figure 2.
Left femoral artery perfusion catheter in place providing flow from the arterial ECMO cannula to the left lower extremity.

3. Skin integrity implications in ECMO patients

Hospital-acquired pressure ulcers (HAPUs) are seen often in the intensive care setting and continue to be a significant financial burden within the healthcare system. The costs range anywhere from $500 to $70,000 per pressure ulcer and can cause length of stay (LOS) to increase by as much as 11 days [26]. While incidence of pressure ulcer development ranges per hospital and patient population, in a database of 710,626 patients, an estimated 3.6% of all patients within the adult critical care and step-down units developed a HAPU [31]. In the acute care setting, a range from 0.4 to 12% has been found [31]. Within the cardiac surgery patients which comprise a portion of patients on ECMO, pressure ulcer incidence as high as 29.5% occurs [26]. The consequences of these pressure ulcers often include infection leading to sepsis, increased pain, further disability, and sometimes death [26]. Although general risk factors such as age, immobility, poor nutritional status, altered sensory perception, moisture, diabetes mellitus, vascular disease, and other comorbidities have been identified, patients receiving ECMO support are also at an increased risk for pressure ulcer development due to multiple factors unique to this population [7, 26]. If patients do undergo cardiothoracic surgery, factors that increase the likelihood of a HAPU include cardiopulmonary bypass time, vasopressor therapy, and body temperature while in the operating room [26]. While on ECMO support, hemodynamic instability related to turning can inhibit appropriate prevention measures, leading to higher incidence of skin breakdown. Nurses can experience apprehension related to routine turning due to the potential of accidental decannulation or risk of worsening hemodynamic instability. High doses of multiple vasopressors that are utilized in patients newly placed on ECMO can lead to decreased peripheral perfusion and have also been shown to increase risk of HAPU. These risk factors make it essential to establish a dedicated skin care regimen for patients receiving ECMO support to prevent HAPU.

Skin care goals for patients receiving ECMO support should largely be similar to any patient that is in the intensive care setting. "At-risk" patients are identified by using a standardized risk screening tool such as the Braden Scale score and treated with stratified skin care interventions implemented based on severity of risk. Patients with a Braden Scale score of 14 or less (moderate to high risk) receive maximum interventions [31]. Patients need to be turned and repositioned every 2 h as tolerated. Turns should be scheduled and require a multidisciplinary team to ensure patient safety (perfusionist or respiratory therapist to hold ECMO cannulas, nurse for lines, etc.). For patients who do not tolerate a full turn, such as those who are hemodynamically unstable on ECMO, specialty beds have been shown to be very effective in reducing HAPU [20]. These rotation and pressure redistribution beds can be set to rotate every 30 min to different ranges as patients tolerate. Even subtle and small frequent position changes have been shown to reduce HAPUs [7]. Many facilities also use fluidized repositioning devices to offload pressure [31]. Silicone gel adhesive dressings should be utilized when possible and can be applied on the sacrum, elbows, and heels. Specialized heel-protective boots can also be used if available. Nutritional status also has a significant impact on the body's ability to repair wounds. This makes dietitians an essential part of the treatment team to ensure these patients receive adequate nutrition in order to prevent skin breakdown and promote healing.

There are multiple factors all contributing to this patient population's increased risk of HAPU. Staff education, awareness, and motivation are essential in delivering the proper skin care measures in ECMO patients. When possible, a multidisciplinary skin care team can address each of the challenges present in this population to ensure that adequate prevention measures are being implemented.

4. Early mobility in ECMO

Early physical rehabilitation and mobility implemented in patients receiving ECMO support have been shown to significantly improve patient outcomes, including decreased LOS in the ICU and hospital, decreased rate of delirium, shorter durations of mechanical ventilation, decreased time to ambulation, increased function, and increased likelihood of returning home to family versus a rehabilitation facility [1, 36]. In spite of the obvious importance of early mobility in ECMO patients, there are limitations to this, particularly hemodynamic instability. The first 24–48 h after the initiation of ECMO are typically the most critical and often do not allow for aggressive physical therapy regardless of the type of ECMO. Most patients during this time are requiring the maximum amount of ventilatory and circulatory support. Eligibility for physical therapy is based upon hemodynamic stability and degree of mechanical and pharmacological support and is specific to each patient case.

Historically, a dual-lumen ECMO catheter would occupy one vessel, usually the internal jugular vein, and provide veno-venous (VV)-ECMO through one cannulation site, allowing bridge-to-transplant patients to participate in early mobility more easily. This was optimal for ambulation because both lower extremities were free and the patients were seen as less high risk for accidental decannulation. However, recently there has been a significant push to mobilize all types of ECMO patients whether they are bridge-to-transplant patients or bridge-to-recovery patients, despite the location and type of cannulation. Whatever the level of physical therapy the patient can tolerate, whether this is passive range of motion or ambulation in the hallway has been shown to improve patient outcomes [1]. Typically, VV-ECMO patients are more stable than VA-ECMO patients, and thus bedside nurses are more comfortable with early mobility in these patients. Patients on VA-ECMO with bi-femoral cannulation are some of the most difficult to ambulate. Fear of accidental decannulation, risk of hemodynamic instability, and lack of training in the physical rehabilitation of these patients have all been barriers to early mobilization. However, the study at the University of Maryland demonstrates that physical mobility is safely possible regardless of the type of ECMO or cannulation site [36].

Many institutions who have an established ECMO program have developed a dedicated multidisciplinary team highly trained in the initiation of physical therapy for ECMO patients [36]. These teams typically include a physical therapist, one to two critical care nurses, a perfusionist or respiratory therapist, and a critical care attending physician. When assessing for eligibility, it is helpful to have a standardized screening tool [36]. The University of Maryland developed a protocol for the initiation of ECMO physical therapy [36]. The initial screening was composed of two parts: a medical screening and a physical therapy assessment [36]. The medical screening criteria included hemodynamic stability specific for each patient, coagulopathy: no bleeding at the cannulation site, stable ECMO flows with RN activities, a RASS goal of −1 to 0 with a range (−2 to +2), and stability of cannulation position [36]. The physical therapy assessment included vital signs, assessment of mental status, ECMO flow remaining stable (hip flexion with femoral cannulated lower extremities), and documented ECMO cannulation position [36]. If both of these screens were passed, then the patient met the criteria for further rehabilitation as tolerated [36]. The common physical therapy progression included bed activities/bed mobility such as passive range of motion and resistive training [36]. If that was well tolerated, then patients progressed to the edge of bed activities including balance training and pre-transfer activities [36]. Following this were sit-to-stand transfers, standing and pre-gait activities, and lastly ambulation [36]. Stabilization devices to secure the ECMO cannulas are recommended before physical therapy is initiated [1]. Adjustments on the sweep gas flow rates and increased oxygenation settings can be used during physical therapy based on clinician assessment [1].

In the aforementioned study, 167 of the 254 patients supported on ECMO received physical therapy [36]. One hundred and thirty-four of those patients had at least one femoral cannula, while 66 patients had two, 44 of which were on VA-ECMO and 39 of whom were on VA-ECMO with bi-femoral cannulas. Only five patients had a dual-lumen catheter. Only three minor events were recorded during physical therapy: one episode of hypotension and two episodes of arrhythmias. Of the patients who received physical therapy, 109 patients survived hospital discharge, and 26 of those patients were discharged home. The patients who received physical therapy while on ECMO scored higher on their ICU mobility scale (IMS) than the ones who only received physical therapy after decannulation [36]. It is important to note that this was only possible due to a dedicated team of individuals specifically trained for the initiation and completion of physical therapy and mobility in ECMO patients and that the resources necessary to develop this type of team may not exist at all institutions who utilize ECMO support [36].

The Society of Critical Care Medicine developed the ABCDEF (**A**ssess, prevent, and manage pain; **B**oth spontaneous awakening and breathing trials; **C**hoice of analgesia and Sedation; **D**elirium assess, prevent, and manage; **E**arly mobility and exercise; **F**amily engagement/empowerment) bundle as an ICU Liberation Collaborative [25]. A recent study measured the success of this bundle on over 15,000 patients spread across 68 academic, community and federal intensive care units. Patients who received more of the ABCDEF bundle each day showed lower delirium rates, less use of physical restraints, decreased length of mechanical ventilation, avoidance of ICU readmission, increased instances of being discharged to home, and ultimately decreased mortality rates [25]. The significance of this bundle is that it can be applied to every ICU patient regardless of their diagnosis, including the ECMO patient population. Implementing the ABCDEF bundle on ECMO patients potentially increases the likelihood of returning to their baseline function sooner.

5. Nursing implications for detection and prevention of systemic complications related to ECMO

The use of ECMO is accompanied by a myriad of potential complications across multiple body systems that are considered calculated risks upon initiation of therapy; however, without it, mortality may increase in conditions like severe acute heart failure [32]. A recent, international, randomized controlled trial (RCT) also suggests a potential mortality benefit with the use of ECMO in severe acute respiratory distress syndrome (ARDS); however, it was found to not be statistically significant [8]. There is abundant literature surrounding the complications of ECMO; but, despite these risks, survival to hospital discharge is greater than 50% [4, 12]. In one recent meta-analysis, the most frequently reported complications associated with ECMO include acute kidney injury (AKI), bleeding, and infection [6]. Specialized RNs have knowledge and understanding of potential complications related to ECMO therapy and can assist with early detection through critical thinking, performing frequent assessments, and reporting them through an open dialog with the team of providers involved.

5.1 Renal and other intraabdominal complications

The incidence of acute kidney injury (AKI) has been reported as high as 80% of ECMO patients and is associated with a quadrupled mortality risk [13, 34]. Severe fluid overload is one of the major reasons that renal replacement therapy (RRT) is initiated in this population and is often performed through the ECMO circuit but can also be performed after the pump, which could lower the risk of air embolism not trapped by the oxygenator [34]. Fluid overload is independently associated with increased mortality, prolonged LOS, prolonged ventilator time, and prolonged ECMO time [13, 34].

This consideration can lead providers to assume earlier RRT for therapeutic fluid removal would reduce these comorbidities; however, there is little data to suggest the efficacy of this. In fact, studies suggest increased mortality in ECMO patients who require RRT during their time on pump [16, 37]. Of ECMO patients who suffer AKI, an estimated 46% of survivors require RRT after ECMO is completed [6]. The bedside RN can assist in early identification of AKI by monitoring urine output; measuring strict fluid intake and output; assessing serial serum chemistry values, particularly serum creatinine and trends of electrolyte dyscrasias; and identifying physical exam findings consistent with fluid overload.

Abdominal compartment syndrome (ACS) is a known complication of ECMO [3]. This can be caused by massive fluid overload, which can be necessary to keep ECMO flows appropriate (read aforementioned suction events) [3]. This significantly positive fluid balance is associated with generalized edema, pleural effusions, and ascites, all of which are known to be causes of ACS. ACS can also compress femoral cannulas, thus diminishing the effectiveness of the ECMO therapy [28]. Clinical assessments significant for the monitoring of abdominal compartment syndrome include physical monitoring of abdomen for tension, distention (diameter), discoloration, and, if the technology is readily available, measurement of intraabdominal pressure.

5.2 Hematological complications

Bleeding is the most frequent complication associated with ECMO and affects approximately 30% of the patients receiving the therapy [2]. Bleeding may occur secondary to primary injury such as trauma and surgery or as a result of ECMO itself. Disruption of the red blood cell membrane leads to hemolysis, which is a common complication of patients on ECMO [11]. SIRS and contact between the patient's blood and the ECMO circuit lead to activation of the coagulation cascade, affecting fibrinolysis, thrombin formation, and platelet function [2].

Large amounts of bleeding will cause losses and consumption of coagulation factors and platelets, leading providers to believe that a heparin overdose may be occurring, thus decreasing the heparin, leading to acute thrombosis of the ECMO circuit or in other places where blood flow may be stagnant [22]. Thrombosis is mainly associated with VA-ECMO and can occur in the atria, ventricles, upper and lower extremity deep vein thrombosis (DVT), pulmonary vasculature, brain, or the ECMO circuit [22]. Unfractionated heparin (UFH) is well known, easily monitored, and easily reversible, allowing its frequent use managing hypercoagulability in the ECMO patient. Institutional guidelines vary; but, systemic anticoagulation with UFH infusion to target aPTT between 50 and 70, with some variations [2]. Despite ease of use, UFH can be associated with complications such as heparin-induced thrombocytopenia (HIT), further contributing to bleeding [22]. Alternatives such as warfarin, lepirudin, or argatroban may also be used in lieu of UFH for anticoagulation in the event of HIT [2]. The ECMO patient provides a unique challenge for providers, who must balance hypercoagulability with coagulopathy with careful but aggressive, administration of blood product transfusions and anticoagulants.

It is clear that there is a litany of reasons the patient on ECMO may experience bleeding and bleeding often results in the need for transfusion. Adult patients on ECMO may require 2–3 units of packed red blood cells (PRBCs) and up to 14 units of plasma or cryoprecipitate daily [11]. Additionally, platelet counts of 45,000–60,000 count/μL are associated with mild to moderate bleeding [11]. Demands on bedside clinicians can be burdensome, as transfusion requirements have been reported to average 45 units of packed red blood cells transfused per adult ECMO patient [11].

Large transfusion volumes are independently associated with increased mortality [11]; despite this, anticoagulation remains the standard practice in patients undergoing ECMO due to thrombotic complications [2]. With the significant risk for bleeding and the subsequent need for anticoagulation, nursing can expect regular and repeated blood draws, transfusions, and anticoagulant titration to be a part of their daily practice in the care of the ECMO patient.

5.3 Infectious complications

A prospective, 1-day study identified approximately 50% of adult patients in over 1200 ICUs internationally whom were thought to have some form of infection, increasing ICU, and hospital mortality rates by over double that of patients without infection [35]. The literature suggests that from anywhere 13–26% of reported nosocomial infection rate in adults receiving ECMO (particularly VA-ECMO) is significantly associated with infection before initiation of ECMO, prolonged LOS, ECMO duration (particularly >10 days), and prolonged ventilator days [5, 14, 15, 30]. In the ICU patient, respiratory infections are most common; however, with the addition of ECMO, blood stream infections become most prominent [17, 35]. Other reported nosocomial events in ECMO patients include respiratory, urinary, and surgical site infections [17].

Care provided by the specialized RN remains inherently important in the prevention of infection, particularly when caring for lines and their cannulation sites with thorough hand, cannulation site, and patient hygiene and the application of impermeable site dressings. Protocols preventing ventilator-acquired pneumonia (VAP) are common practice and include interventions like hand hygiene, meticulous oral care with chlorhexidine gluconate solution, endotracheal tube cuff pressure control, and control of sedation [27]. Further management of routine line and cannulation site management are further discussed earlier in this chapter under Section 2.

5.4 Cardiopulmonary complications

Cardiopulmonary complications are often resultant of high left ventricular (LV) afterload, especially on prolonged ECMO (particularly VA-ECMO), which can lead to pulmonary edema [21]. Other cardiac sequelae include aortic valve regurgitation, biventricular failure, and LV thrombus which have been treated with a variety of modalities including intra-aortic balloon pump (IABP) and other percutaneous and surgical procedures to shunt elevated LV pressures [24]. Additional lung complications significantly associated with ECMO include pulmonary hemorrhage, hemorrhagic pulmonary infarct, pulmonary calcifications, and fibrinous pleuritis [18]. The bedside RN can assist with early detection of these complications by close assessment of vasopressor and inotrope requirements, endotracheal secretions, monitoring the ventilator for peak and plateau pressures, and ensuring daily chest radiographs and frequent echocardiograms which are ordered to monitor progression of cardiopulmonary disease.

5.5 Neurological complications

A study reviewing nearly 24,000 patients on ECMO revealed 10.9% of incidence of nearly equal prevalence of seizure, stroke, or intracranial hemorrhage (ICH) [23].

These patients who suffered ICH while on ECMO had increased mortality, while strokes and ICH alike both demonstrated increased LOS and increased likelihood of requiring placement in a skilled nursing facility (SNF) or long-term acute care hospital (LTACH) upon discharge [23]. Other sources suggest up to 50% of patients on ECMO demonstrate severe neurological sequelae [19]. Intracranial hemorrhage has been identified in as high as 40% of non-survivors of ECMO, and thrombotic events have been identified in approximately 15% of ECMO courses [2].

The clinical suspicion for stroke may be obscured in ECMO patients given the multitude of other systemic or metabolic derangements usually encountered in ICU patients [19]. The bedside RN becomes integral to monitoring subtle neurologic indicators such as pupilometer and bi-spectral index, which can read zero in the event of catastrophic neurologic injury.

6. Nursing implications in ethics and ECMO withdrawal

With the advent of advancing ECMO technology comes an expanded library for indications of use. VA and VV support are commonly being utilized for bridge-to-transplant and respiratory or cardiac failure. Additionally, ECMO therapy is being utilized as bridge to support the body through a medical emergency in the form of extracorporeal cardiopulmonary resuscitation (ECPR). With the introduction of high-tech innovation, critical care nursing frequently encounters stressors due to resource scarcity, increased workloads, and moral distress related to carrying out aggressive life-sustaining treatments that may conflict with the patient's best interests or maybe even personal preferences.

ECMO is a costly, resource-intensive therapy requiring commitment from the patient, family, and multiple disciplines. The impact of caring for an ECMO patient puts a mental and physical strain, not only on the patient and family but the entire medical team involved in the patient's care. Providing the intense, complex nursing care impacts not only the nursing staff or ECMO provider but the entire nursing unit caring for the patient. Institutions employing the use of ECMO in treating complex, critically ill patients as one of their only means of survival must have a process that addresses the moral and ethical dilemmas that arise from caring for the critically ill. Common questions are "Who receives ECMO treatment?", "When should support cease?", and "What is the goal of therapy, *quantity* or *quality* of life?"

Allocation of nursing resources has become undoubtedly one of the most challenging aspects in caring for patients and families. Nursing staff ratios, complexity of patients, and the mental and physical impact on the bedside nurse become compounded when one critically ill patient draws a majority of a unit's resources. ECMO patients can begin their treatment with significantly unstable hemodynamic parameters requiring multiple blood transfusions, circulatory support with several vasoactive medications, and frequent lab draws pulling a majority of the nursing unit's resources for the care of one patient. This places an enormous burden on the nursing staff to be creative and flexible with patient care assignments. RN:patient ratios may be less than desirable, ultimately impacting the care provided to other patients on the unit as well. Everyone, from the unit manger to housekeeping, plays a hands-on role in supporting the entire unit as well as the ECMO care team.

How do we reduce some of the ethical or moral dilemmas nurses experience caring for complex, critically ill patients? Communication is the key in healthcare. An integral part of communication is developing and maintaining a team not isolated to healthcare workers but also including the patient and family. Early involvement of the palliative care team and social work is crucial to providing consistent support to the patient and family. Interdisciplinary daily rounds including the bedside nurse, family members, palliative care team, and social work are integral to find commonalities for all regarding goals of care. If conflict arises about treatment benefits or burden and the patient's best interest is no longer being served, support from the ethics committee can be beneficial to the family and healthcare team. These are just the foundation. In critical care nursing, it is important that the nursing staff's voice be heard. It is vital to recognize the nursing assessment of not just the patient but the situation and to be included in the decision-making that nurses are ultimately responsible for performing.

6.1 Withdrawal of ECMO therapy

Unfortunately, despite a team's best efforts, an ECMO patient may continue to decline, with multiple organ systems failing or a devastating systemic event. In such cases, withdrawing care may be imminent, and the question must be asked of the patient and family should be "is the patient's preference *quantity* or *quality* of life?" Can the patient make their wishes known? In the case of bridge-to-transplant, patients may be able to make their wishes known to their families and healthcare team. For the critically ill patient who is dependent on their family or the healthcare team for their medical decisions, is this truly representative of what the patient's wishes would be? Does conflict arise between the healthcare team and family regarding withdrawal of care? These questions are applicable in any situation involving ECMO; however, they cannot be answered algorithmically or methodically, as they need to be answered uniquely to each situation.

Nurses are in a unique position in healthcare. They are at the bedside for 8- or 12-hour shifts as most consistent patient advocate. They support and inform family members and build personal and emotional bonds with them. Although valuable, this rapport can be morally taxing to the bedside RN. As nurses witness a patient and families suffering during clinical decline, they begin to question the continued aggressiveness of care that likely will not benefit from treatment, thus causing moral distress to the nursing staff. Sadness, frustration, and anxiety felt by the nursing staff for prolonged periods of time can lead to staff burnout, job dissatisfaction, and decreased staff retention.

7. Conclusion

The ECMO patient is often the most critically ill within the hospital at any given moment, prompting highly trained bedside RNs as well as other healthcare providers, familiar with the therapy, to be readily available to provide the multifaceted care this population requires. In addition to routine ICU care, the ECMO patient necessitates additional monitoring due to associated risk factors assumed when being placed on pump. Medical, ethical, and emotional considerations exist and must be addressed regularly in order to provide the best care of this unique patient population. Despite high mortality associated with ECMO, the survivability continues to increase as time progresses and the bedside RN will continue to be responsible for vital functions in continuing that trend.

Author details

Alex Botsch*, Elizabeth Protain, Amanda R. Smith and Ryan Szilagyi
Summa Health, Akron, Ohio, United States

*Address all correspondence to: alexander.botsch@gmail.com

References

[1] Abrams D, Javidfar J, Farrand E, et al. Early mobilization of patients receiving extracorporeal membrane oxygenation: A retrospective cohort study. Critical Care. 2014;**18**:R38

[2] Aubron C, DePuydt J, Belon F, Bailey M, Schmidt M, Sheldrake J, et al. Predictive factors of bleeding events in adults undergoing extracorporeal membrane oxygenation. Intensive Care. 2016;**6**(97):1-10

[3] Augustin P, Lasocki S, Dufour G, Rode J, Karsenti A, Al-Attar N, et al. Abdomoinal compartment syndrome due to extracorporeal membrane oxygenation in adults. The Annals of Thoracic Surgery. 2010;**90**:e40-e41

[4] Zangrillo A, Landoni G, Biondi-Zoccai G, Greco M, Greco T, Frati G, et al. A meta-analysis of complications and mortality of extracorporeal membrane oxygenation. Critical Care and Resuscitation. 2013;**15**:172-178

[5] Bizzarro M, Conrad S, Kaufman D, Rycus P. Infections acquired during extracorporeal membrane oxygenation in neonates, children, and adults. Pediatric Critical Care Medicine. 2011;**12**:277-281

[6] Cheng R, Hachamovitch R, Kittleson M, Patel J, Arabia F, Moriguchi J, et al. Complications of extracorporeal membrane oxygenation for treatment of cardiogenic shock and cardiac arrest: A meta-analysis of 1,866 adult patients. Annals of Thoracic Surgery. 2014;**97**:610-616

[7] Clements L, Moore M, Tribble T, Blake J. Reducing skin breakdown in patients receiving extracorporeal membranous oxygenation. The Nursing Clinics of North America. 2014;**49**(1):61-68

[8] Combes A, Hajage D, Capellier G, Demoule A, Lavoué S, Guervilly C, et al. Extracorporeal membrane oxygenation for severe acute respiratory distress syndrome. New England Journal of Medicine. 2018;**378**:1965-1975

[9] Daly K, Camporota L, Barrett N. An international survey: The role of specialist nurses in adult respiratory extracorporeal membrane oxygenation. Nursing in Critical Care. 2017;**22**:305-311

[10] Driscoll A, Grant M, Carroll D, Dalton S, Deaton C, Jones I, et al. The effect of nurse-to-patient ratios on nurse-sensitive patient outcomes in acute specialist units: A systematic review and meta-analysis. European Journal of Cardiovascular Nursing. 2018;**17**:6-22

[11] Esper SA, Levy JH, Waters JH, Welsby IJ. Extracorporeal membrane oxygenation in the adult: A review of anticoagulation monitoring and transfusion. Anesthesia and Analgesia. 2014;**18**(4):731-743

[12] Extracorporeal Life Support Organization. ECLS Registry Report—International Summary. Ann Arbor: ECLS; 2018

[13] Hamdi T, Palmer BF. Review of extracorporeal membrane oxygenation and dialysis-based liver support devices for the use of nephrologists. American Journal of Nephrology. 2017;**46**:139-149

[14] Hsu M, Chiu K, Huang Y, Kao K, Chu S, Liao C. Risk factors for nosocomial infection during extracorporeal membrane oxygenation. Journal of Hospital Infection. 2009;**73**:210-216

[15] Juthani B, Macfarlan J, Wu J, Misselbeck T. Incidence of nosocomial infections in adult patients undergoing extracorporeal membrane oxygenation.

The Journal of Acute and Critical Care. 2018;**47**:626-630

[16] Kielstein JT, Heiden AM, Beutel G, Gottlieb J, Wiesner O, Hafer C, et al. Renal function and survival in 200 patients undergoing ECMO therapy. Nephrology, Dialysis, Transplantation. 2013;**28**:86-90

[17] Kim G, Lee K, Park C, Kang S, Kim D, Oh S, et al. Nosocomial infection in adult patients undergoing veno-arterial extracorporeal membrane oxygenation. Journal of Korean Medical Science. 2017;**32**:593-598

[18] Lee HE, Yi ES, Rabatin JT, Bohman JK, Roden AC. Histopathologic findings in lungs of patients treated with extracorporeal membrane oxygenation. Chest. 2018;**153**:825-833

[19] Lee S, Chaturvedi A. Imaging adults on extracorporeal membrane oxygenation (ECMO). Insights Imaging. 2014;**5**:731-742

[20] Logue B. Focus on eliminating pressure ulcers in patients undergoing extracorporeal membrane oxygenation. Critical Care Nurse. 2015;**35**(2):31

[21] Mehta H, Eisen HJ, Cleveland JC. Indications and complications for VA-ECMO for cardiac failure. American College of Cardiology. 2015. Retrieved from: https://www.acc.org/latest-in-cardiology/articles/2015/07/14/09/27/indications-and-complications-for-va-ecmo-for-cardiac-failure

[22] Mulder M, Fawzy I, Lance M. ECMO and anticoagulation: A comprehensive review. Netherlands Journal of Critical Care. 2017;**26**:6-13

[23] Nasr DM, Rabinstein AA. Neurologic complications of extracorporeal membrane oxygenation. Journal of Clinical Neurology. 2015;**11**:383-389

[24] Ong CS, Hibino N. Left heart decompression in patients supported with extracorporeal membrane oxygenation for cardiac disease. Postepy Kardiol Interwencyjenj. 2017;**13**:1-2

[25] Pun BT, Balas MC, Barnes-Daly MA, et al. Caring for critically ill patients with the ABCDEF bundle: Results for the ICU liberation collaborative in over 15,000 adults. Critical Care Medicine. Published online ahead of print October 18. 2018;**47**:3-14. DOI: 10.1097/CCM.0000000000003482

[26] Rao AD, Preston AM, Strauss R, Stamm R, Zalman DC. Risk factors associated with pressure ulcer formation in critically ill cardiac surgery patients: A systematic review. Journal of Wound, Ostomy, and Continence Nursing. 2016;**43**(3):242-247

[27] Rello J, Afonso E, Lisboa T, Ricart M, Balsera B, Rovira A, et al. A care bundle approach for prevention of ventilator-associated pneumonia. Clinical Microbiology and Infection. 2012;**19**:363-369

[28] Rupprecht L, Lunz D, Philipp A, Lubnow M, Schmid C. Pitfalls in percutaneous ECMO cannulation. Heart, Lung and Vessels. 2015;**7**(4):320-326

[29] Sakr Y, Moreira C, Rhodes A, Ferguson N, Kleinpell R, Pickkers P, et al. The impact of hospital and ICU organizational factors on outcome in critically ill patients: Results from the extended prevalence of infection in intensive care study. Journal of Critical Care Medicine. 2015;**43**:519-526

[30] Sun H, Ko W, Tsai P, Sun C, Chang Y, Lee C, et al. Infections occurring during extracorporeal membrane oxygenation use in adult patients. The Journal of Thoracic and Cardiovascular Surgery. 2010;**140**:1125-1132

[31] Swafford K, Culpepper R, Dunn C. Use of a comprehensive program to reduce the incidence of hospital-acquired pressure ulcers in an intensive care unit. American Journal of Critical Care. 2016;**25**(2):152-155

[32] Tang G, Malekan R, Kai M, Lansman S, Spielvogel D. Peripheral venoarterial extracorporeal membrane oxygenation improves survival in myocardial infarction with cardiogenic shock. The Journal of Thoracic and Cardiovascular Surgery. 2013;**145**:e32-e33

[33] The International ECMO Network [ECMONet]. Position paper for the organization of extracorporeal membrane oxygenation programs for acute respiratory failure in adult patients. American Journal of Respiratory and Critical Care Medicine. 2014;**190**:488-496

[34] Villa G, Katz N, Ronco C. Extracorporeal membrane oxygenation and the kidney. CardioRenal Medicine. 2016;**6**:50-60

[35] Vincent J, Rello J, Marshall J, Silva E, Anzueto A, Martin C, et al. International study of the prevalence and outcomes of infection in intensive care units. JAMA. 2009;**302**:2323-2329

[36] Wells CL, Forrester J, Vogel J, Rector R, Tabatabai A, Herr D. Safety and feasibility of early physical therapy for patients on extracorporeal membrane oxygenator: University of Maryland Medical Center experience. Critical Care Medicine. 2018;**46**:53-59

[37] Wolf MJ, Chanani NK, Heard ML, Kanter KR, Mahle WT. Early renal replacement therapy during pediatric cardiac extracorporeal support increases mortality. Annals of Thoracic Surgery. 2013;**96**:917-922

Chapter 3

Clinical and Administrative Steps to the ECMO Program Development

Dianne McCallister, Linda Pilon, Joseph Forrester, Samer Alsaleem, Chakradhar Kotaru, Jennifer Hanna, Gregory Hickey, Rachele Roberts, Erica Douglass, Matthew Libby and Michael S. Firstenberg

Abstract

Extra-corporeal membrane oxygenation (ECMO) is a rapidly evolving therapy for acute lung and/or heart failure. ECMO, from a technical standpoint, is conceptually simple—however, it can be very challenging to implement therapy at the individual patient level as well as at hospital (or healthcare system) level. ECMO program development involves engagement of key stake-holders including physicians, nursing, and administrative leadership. The goal of this chapter is to outline some of the crucial steps in developing a successful ECMO program including highlighting the necessary resources, team members and structure, and basic program structure and function.

Keywords: ECMO, administration, leadership, development, guidelines

1. Introduction

Extra-corporeal membrane oxygenation (ECMO) or extra-corporeal life support (ECLS) is quickly becoming a well-established form of therapy for patients presenting in severe respiratory failure and/or cardiogenic shock. The fundamentals of therapy, while technically challenging and involving a complex dynamic human-artificial circuit system, also requires a huge reliance on a multi-disciplinary team and an institutional infrastructure with robust administrative support at all levels to function effectively. While the medical and technical aspects of therapy are covered extensively in this text—and the others in this series [1, 2], a common fundamental question that is often asked is "how do we start and develop a program?" The development of an ECMO/ECLS program is far more complex than organizing a small group of interested providers and acquiring the hardware necessary for support—as such, the goal of this chapter is to outline those steps necessary to help establish a foundation for a successful institutional program.

2. Background

Acute respiratory failure—regardless of the etiology—remains a complex and difficult problem to treat. Management focuses on treating the primary problem and allowing lung healing via lung protective ventilation strategies, while maintaining adequate oxygenation and ventilation [3]. Unfortunately, morbidity and mortality remain high in patients with severe lung injury, despite implementing standard lung protective strategies. Even for those patients who survive, quality of life can be severely impacted for many years after their initial illness [4]. Acute cardiac failure, or cardiogenic shock, also presents a difficult clinical problem for which even contemporary outcomes are less than ideal. While the most common cause of cardiogenic shock remains pump failure after an acute myocardial infarction, other mechanical problems such as acute papillary rupture (with acute mitral regurgitation), ventricular septal rupture, and myocarditis [5] must be considered [6]. While the use of ECMO for either acute respiratory failure or cardiogenic shock (or often a combination of both) is well-described, in part due to more comprehensive reviews of these topics elsewhere in this text, their incidence and challenges—regardless of the circumstances—serve as a foundation for why there is a substantial interest in developing and growing ECMO programs.

There is growing evidence to support the role of ECMO in the management of these very difficult problems. ECMO has been shown to be an important tool in the armamentarium of any program that serves as a tertiary or referral center for complex cardio-pulmonary pathologies. In fact, excluding the survival benefit that has been demonstrated in patients who are supported with ECMO, there is also growing evidence to suggest that overall outcomes of patients with Adult Respiratory Distress Syndrome (ARDS) or cardiogenic shock treated at "ECMO Program Centers" are better regardless of whether they are treated with ECMO. In other words, the multi-disciplinary and administrative commitment to take care of patients (both adults and children) with complex and difficult cardiac and pulmonary problems can lead to improved outcomes independent of the actual use of ECMO [7–10].

Two randomized clinical trials in patients with severe ARDS support the implementation and increased utilization of ECMO therapy [11, 12]. These randomized trials—again, topics that will be discussed elsewhere in this text—despite their controversies, have demonstrated a clinical benefit of ECMO in the setting of ARDS. These well-conducted randomized trials, in addition to the extensive body of literature (case series, single center reports, and Extracorporeal Life Support Organization (ELSO) registry reviews—far too numerous to reference) combined with growing society guidelines and position papers, serve as a solid foundation of medical science to support the development of ECMO programs worldwide [13].

3. Implementation process

The clinicians and administrators first determine the need and support for an ECMO program. This multidisciplinary group then operationalizes the care team that needs to be assembled and trained. The team includes clinical, administrative, ancillary, and other stakeholders, which are required to care for the patient and support the infrastructure, while moving the program to implementation.

3.1 Physician members

Physicians from Cardiothoracic Surgery, Pulmonary/Critical Care, and Cardiology form the foundation of physician support for veno-veno and veno-arterial ECMO patient identification, insertion, and management. In addition to the core physician team, there is a need to engage neurologists and infectious disease specialists to understand the therapy and the unique patient care challenges and complications associated with ECMO support. Vascular surgeons often will get involved with cannulation if others are not available or comfortable with placing large bore cannulas—likewise, there is a growing interest by general and trauma surgeons [14].

In addition, the Palliative Care team must be involved from the very beginning of program's development and some will advocate, especially in pediatric programs (while the focus of this chapter is on adult program development), Palliative Care providers are automatically involved and consulted on every ECMO case. As such, their understanding of the risks and benefits of ECMO are critical given the marginal outcomes associated with ECMO, even in the best of circumstances [15].

Inclusion of emergency physicians in the team can assist with early identification of patients on presentation to the emergency room, and implementation of protocols in the emergency room for cardiogenic shock and respiratory failure [16].

3.2 Administrative stakeholders

Administrators from the executive team should be engaged early to help support the creation of structures to accelerate implementation, project management, and assurance of adequate capital and personnel resources for a sustainable program. Financial models, which obviously vary from system (and country) to system, must be considered—and given the amount of resources required to establish and maintain an ECMO program, it is wise to have someone to monitor the financial implications.

3.3 Ancillary services

Respiratory therapists assist with identifying possible candidates and work closely with the team ensuring the implementation of lung protective strategies. The growth of electronic medical records can allow for daily (if not more frequent) reports of those patients who might be considered for ECMO based upon ventilator settings and arterial blood case results.

Perfusionists must be engaged to help with setup, oversight of the ongoing treatment and for their skill sets in understanding the complexities of the machines and testing required.

Finally, there are implications for laboratory department around testing and blood bank needs; as well as coordinating and consulting with case management, ethics, and chaplains in regard to complex shared decision-making to implement, care for, and remove therapy; and the rehabilitation needs for patients post-ECMO removal.

3.4 Nursing

In addition to leadership described previously, executive nursing leadership, departmental nursing leadership, nursing advanced practice providers (APP), and frontline nursing engagement are fundamental and are essential to assure the success of the program. This includes communication, input and collaboration with policy, procedures and evidence-based protocols, education and competency training of high performing clinical staff, and provision of surveillance and care of patients. Frontline nursing from outside the ICU are often engaged in patient flow and early identification of decompensating acute care patients, who may need to be considered for ECLS. Since patients might require ECMO at any time, day or night, and given the amount of resources required to initiate and care for such patients, nursing administration must be involved to help develop protocols to organize "phone tree" lines of communication and specialized competent staff schedules to help recruit and arrange appropriate resources on very short notice.

3.5 Critical care transport

As the program grows beyond supporting the host hospital, it is necessary to engage Critical Care Transport to organize a system to transport patients from outside the facility with appropriate support and skill sets. This engagement is discussed more fully later in the chapter.

3.6 Nonclinical support

The IT department can help with order set development and the Medical Staff office will need to support the development of privileging requirements to assure consistent skill sets for new team members.

3.7 Establishing relationships with other tertiary centers

Especially in the situations with VA-ECMO use, long-term myocardial support may be needed. It is essential to build relationships with centers that can provide bridge to long-term LVAD support or transplant.

Additionally, the marketing and public relations departments engage to help in creating materials to help outlying hospitals and physicians have awareness of the program, with knowledge of how to identify patients and when to transport to higher levels of care for consideration of ECMO support.

4. Rapid change management

4.1 Triad leadership structure

A rapid pace for implementation is best served by a strong triad leadership: experienced physician leaders and champions who are experts in ECMO; nursing leadership; and hospital executives. All need experience in change management and are given support and authority to use project tools and cross-functional influence to fast track project goals across a wide span of departments. These members then must communicate progress within the executive team.

4.2 Change management approach

Following Kotter's change management theory, a small group of physicians, nursing leadership, and administrators gather to set a vision, determine the feasibility and challenges of the project, then create a shared project plan for the organization, structure, and timeline for implementation of the program [17]. The creation of a Gantt chart with key requirements and milestones is helpful in the early stages of program development—also useful in a sense of accomplishment and motivation of the team. Regular recurrent frequent meetings with agendas driven by a project management tool to assure progress is made on key deadlines, accountability to the individuals and team, and to create a shared message and plan for continued communication. Initial work should focus on best practice, research-based literature review, professional organization review of standards and data, then develop a gap analysis of clinical guidelines, equipment, skill sets, and organizational readiness. This small group should include Cardiothoracic surgeon(s), Pulmonologists, a "C" level executive, the cardiovascular service line, and Intensive Care nursing leadership. A small tactical group allows for more rapid progress through the initial stages and supports creation of a shared vision to accelerate momentum when the inevitable resistance to change surfaces—as well as working through team dynamics, comfort level, and building relationships. This group must strive to produce early wins, however small, to enable the organization to "feel the progress" as more difficult hurdles are faced. These can include shared clinical guidelines, order sets, and eventually patients that lived thanks to the program—as a true connect to purpose for all involved.

Putting screening guidelines in place and educating the teams on the benefits of ECMO to patients who would otherwise be terminal are very compelling when used in a story format.

Finally, change in management requires vigilance to newly implemented care processes, or the tendency of the organization will slide back to previous status quo. Tools and strategies that assist in holding on to new skills are most effectively done through audits, constructive timely feedback, continuous process improvement discussions, and accountability to the process. While education can assist in reminding staff of the "why", it is not a sticky tool in terms of cementing new behaviors into a culture.

Once the ECMO program is up and running, collaboration with the quality abstractionist and review of registry data at regular intervals generates quality improvement projects to assure new practice and clinical referral patterns producing the optimal outcomes. It is also a way of preventing politics and rumors from gaining momentum as the facts are reviewed and discussed in larger quality forums. These forums are ideally multi-disciplinary and followed up with tangible action items that have due dates and closed-loop communication back to the CQI team, as the action items are completed.

5. Equipment

5.1 Hardware

The obvious hardware required for the program is the ECMO machine. The variables needed to make the correct choice for the program include need for portability of transport between facilities, as well as within the host organization, ease of use, skill sets of those responsible for managing the process, and the capital budget of the organization.

5.2 Disposables

In addition to the perfusion/ECMO machine, there is a need for a readily available stock of cannulas in various sizes, as well as for the variety of approaches that may need to be used. In addition, a well-stocked cart that allows the necessary equipment for sterile fields, cut-down, suturing, and possible complications of the cannulation procedures should be available to take to the patient's location, as often the patient is not stable to transport to the OR for the procedure. As these are tools routinely used by perfusionists and cardiothoracic surgeons, they need to be engaged in selecting the appropriate sizes, manufacturers, connectors, introducers, wires and par levels. Many programs, as a function of the need to initiate ECMO therapy on short notice and in many different clinical areas, will create an "ECMO cart" which consist of all the key disposable equipment and tools needed to cannulate anywhere at any time (**Table 1** and **Figure 1**).

Supplies	Size	Ref #	Qty
Cannulae:			
Medtronic bio-medicus single stage venous	23Fr	CB96605-023	×1
	21Fr	CB96605-021	×1
Medtronic bio-medicus multi-stage venous	25Fr	96880-025	×1
	21Fr	96880-021	×1
Maquet avalon	31Fr	10031	×1
	27Fr	10027	×1
Medtronic bio-medicus arterial	15Fr	96530-015	×1
Medtronic bio-medicus nexgen arterial	17Fr	96570-117	×1
	19Fr	96570-119	×1
	21Fr	96570-121	×1
Wires/dilators/introducer kits:			
Medtronic arterial introducer kit		96552	×1
Medtronic venous introducter kit		96551	×1
Lunderquist extra stiff		G31453	×1
Amplatz super stiff		M0066401080	×1
Sorrin dilator kit			×1
4Fr micro puncture			×4
4Fr introducer			×1
6Fr introducer			×2
8Fr Introducer			×1
Packs:			
Basic pack			×1
Angiography pack			×1
Suture:			
Pledgets			
2-0 Prolene SH			×4
2-0 Prolene MH			×4
3-0 Prolene SH			×4
3-0 Prolene RB-1			×4
4-0 Prolene SH			×12
4-0 Prolene RB-1			×12
4-0 Prolene large needle pledget			×12
4-0 Prolene small needle pledget			×12
5-0 Prolene C-1			×4
6-0 Prolene BV-1			×4
6-0 Prolene C-1			×4
7-0 Prolene BV-1			×4

Supplies	Size	Ref #	Qty
#1 Sofsilk			×6
0 Silk popoffs CT-1			×4
1 Vicryl CTX			×2
0 Vicryl CTX			×2
0 Vicryl CT-1			×2
2-0 Vicryl CT-1			×4
3-0 Vicryl SH			×2
4-0 Vicryl PS-1			×2
4-0 Monocryl PS-2			×2
3-0 Ethibond SH			×6
Heavy silk ties			×4
2-0 Silk ties			×4
3-0 Silk ties			×4
4-0 Vicryl ties			×4
2-0 Ethicon pacing wires			×2
Orange pacing wires			×4
Blue pacing wires			×2
#6 Sternal wires			×2
Double wires			×2
Prep:			
Chloraprep			×5
Duraprep			×1
Alcohol bottles			×2
PVP			×2
CHG surgical scrub brush			×5
Blades:			
#10			×10
#11			×10
#15			×10
Stryker sternal blade			×4
Hall redo blade			×2
Umbilical tapes			×8
Tourniquet 4 packs			×6
Red vessel loops			×2
White vessel loops			×4
Shods 10 pack			×2
Small yellow clip racks Qty 4			×5
Small red clip racks Qty 4			×5

Supplies	Size	Ref #	Qty
Small automatic clip applier			×1
Large automatic clip applier			×1
Asepto			×2
Suction tubing			×3
Cell Saver tubing			×2
Yankauer tip			×3
Poole tip			×2
Bovie pencil			×2
Bovie pad			×2
Long bovie tips			
Short bovie tips			
Eye cautery			×2
Snake clamp inserts			×1
86 mm inserts			×2
61 mm inserts			×2
33 mm inserts			×2
Hemostatics:			
Bone wax			×6
Felt 4×4			×1
Felt 6×6			×1
GelFoam			×1
Fibrillar			×5
Snow			×2
Nu-Knit			×1
Laps			×9
Baby laps			×5
Raytec			×5
Gowns			×7
Towel packs			×4
Gloves			
Drapes:			
Split sheets			×2
3/4 Sheets			×6
Bi-Lat split sheet			×1

Supplies	Size	Ref #	Qty
Cardiac drape			×1
Tegaderms			
4×4s			×5
Esmark			×1
Prineo			×1
Stapler			×1
Dermabond mini			×5
Hollister horizontal tube attachment device			×2
18 Ga Hypo			×4
Hep/blunt tip hypo			×4
60 cc syringe			×2
20 cc syringe			×2
10 cc syringe			×2
5 cc syringe			×2
Defib pads			×1
Pacing cables			×2
Decanters			×2
Plasmalyte 1 L			×2

Table 1. *ECMO cart supplies (sample).*

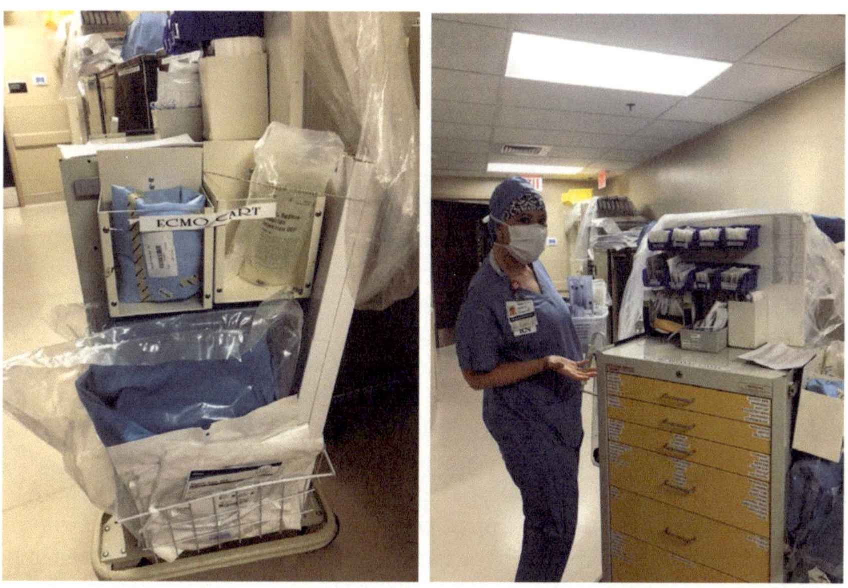

(a) (b)

Figure 1.
(a and b): Portable ECMO cart that contains all the disposable tools needed for initiating therapy.

6. People

6.1 Structure and team building

The ECMO team skill set crosses a variety of normal reporting structures within the hospital, as well as contracted services used in hospitals, including surgical services, nursing, laboratory, perfusion, physicians—employed and independent. Hence, thought must be placed into creating a strong team-based culture among a group of individuals who may have primary team affiliation across multiple departments.

The use of multidisciplinary teams to develop project goals can serve as the first team building structure. Recognition of the team publicly can serve to bond the team more closely, and debriefings can prevent "silo formation" as individuals must often integrate in and out of the ECMO team due to patient volume and clinical needs. To cement this sense of team, the leaders of the departments that support the ECMO program should have regular meetings to discuss issues that arise, including productivity and interpersonal issues. Finally, the executive champion of the program should assure that there is accountability from all parties to the success of the program through goals and metrics, periodic meetings of the entire group of stakeholders, and shared public recognition of the successes of the program.

6.2 Who watches the patients?

Early in the development of any ECMO program, there must be a strategy for establishing "who watches what"—specifically, while nursing will always have bedside management of the patient, there must be consideration given as who has dedicated responsibility for the ECMO pump and circuit. As with any technology or "machine" that is directly connected to a patient—and provides critical life-saving support—there must be institutional guidelines and protocols regarding who monitors the functional status of the pump and circuit assuring safe and continuous functionality. In addition, the specific roles and responsibilities of this individual also need to be clearly defined. Various staffing models exist as described below.

6.2.1 Perfusionist based

Perfusionist is ideal bedside ECMO care providers, while initiating an ECMO program. Their advantages are considerable experiences in managing patients requiring extra-corporeal support as a function of their primary job responsibilities in the operating room supporting cardiac surgery procedures. Their training, credentialing, and licensure will often include formal experiences in managing patients requiring short-term mechanical circulatory support, including ECMO, outside of the operating room environment. A perfusionist-based model is appealing, however there are resource and financial limitations of this model. Perfusionists are usually limited in number (especially if they are also supporting an active clinical cardiothoracic surgical program) and their perspective is from a different care model which is focused around staffing limited time intervals in the operating room rather than 24/7 ICU-based ECMO care management. They are also an expensive resource for 24/7 daily ECMO use in the ICU. Given their availability and cost (and depending on how a program "employs" perfusionists—salary, per diem, hourly, contract employees, etc.), other care models are preferred for providing bedside ECMO support, particularly for veno-veno ECMO patients.

6.2.2 Nursing/respiratory therapy (RN/RT) based

RN/RT ECMO specialist staffing models are becoming widely accepted and utilized in programs nationally—these programs and the combination structure of RT and RN staffing pools are mainly volume dependent to maintain competence. RNs have many advantages with regards to their inherent familiarity with the complexities and challenges in managing sick patients who require various life-support therapies. For example, in many programs, nurses manage renal replacement therapy technologies, wean and manage ventilators directly, and even have ownership in the management of both short- and long-term cardiac/ventricular support therapies. An additional advantage is, as a function such nurses are often extremely experienced in the management and assessment of critically-ill patients, they can serve as a valuable resource in other areas of immediate patient care—and potentially with volume and competence that become a primary care model for the more stable ECMO patient. Although respiratory therapists (RT) often have extensive experience in the management—and independent assessment—of patients requiring mechanical ventilatory support, it has only been relatively recently that their experiences and training in pulmonary mechanics and respiratory physiology, have they as a profession, been engaged as ECMO specialists. In theory, since most busy intensive care units are often staffed with a high volume of RNs and RTs, who are clinically high performing and engaged, the addition of monitoring ECMO pumps and circuits might not require a substantial investment in human resources and expanding staffing models. As such, using RNs and RTs might be viewed as being potentially less expensive—it is important to recognize that prior to using this human resource to monitor ECMO patients, a substantial investment in extensive ongoing education and training to maintain competence is needed. There are many courses offered by large ECMO programs, professional societies, and ELSO (see below) that can assist in the training of bedside ECMO specialists. Significant advantages in the ECMO specialist staffing model, already described as financially fiscal, also include continuity of nursing-based care provided by hospital staff who have an investment in the organization and unit, as well as the patients they serve.

6.2.3 Hybrid models

Another attractive option is a combination of various specialists—often as a function of the acuity of the patient and the needs of the program at any given time. Such a model takes advantage of the strengths of each type of healthcare professional. Even though such models can be difficult to implement as protocols defining individual roles and when and how handoffs can occur, nevertheless, with a strong collaborative team, a hybrid model can be successful. For example, for "routine" (if such exists) veno-veno cases of isolated respiratory failure in an otherwise hemodynamically stable patient, a perfusionist might help initiate therapy, provide the first 24 hours of support, and once the patient is deemed stable on ECMO, care is handed off to a RT or RN ECMO specialist. On-call perfusion support for technical questions and issues can then be easily provided from home and might not require immediate bedside support. Veno-arterial cases, especially in post-cardiotomy patients, might be more complex, and therefore might require more direct involvement of perfusionists given their experiences of managing such patients in the operating room. The challenge in a hybrid model is to determine either objectively or subjectively—the clinical parameters that would allow for an appropriate hand-off between one type (or level) of provider to another (i.e. perfusionist to RN/RT ECMO Specialist).

Regardless of the care model provided, there must be collaboration between the team members to build evidence-based standardized protocols, as well as strong physician buy-in in terms of supporting the individuals who manage the patient and pump at the bedside. Availability for immediate communication, using current technology, should be established between the ECMO specialist and/or perfusionist and the in-house physician. In addition, a strong and collaborative relationship between the ECMO specialist, perfusionist, and the bedside nurse must exist. Everyone must work together—inter-personality or professional conflicts cannot be tolerated and only get in the way of safe and effective patient care. Strong provider leadership, such as a perfusionist team leader, can be extremely effective in helping mentor other providers and serving as a resource for some of the day to day challenges in the management of an ECMO pump and circuit that might involve various disciplines, each of which have various levels of training and experiences.

In addition, while current ECMO pumps and circuits are much more reliable than previous technologies, they will often have more advanced monitoring options. Each specialist involved in the care of the patient must have extensive training and a sound understanding of the functionality and troubleshooting of the entire circuit. Simulation training, as discussed in other chapters, plays a critical role in education and maintaining proficiency and, therefore, should be a key component—when feasible—of every ECMO program.

7. Guidelines for therapy and patient selection

7.1 Access center/system

In a multiple hospital system of care, there is not generally a need for more than one ECMO center for the system to accommodate the needs for non-CT surgery-related ECMO support. A helpful resource to assure patients have rapid transfer to the ECMO program from other hospitals, it is useful to set up a access center process to assure a standardized approach to hand-offs, transport, and tracking of patient movement. Call system personnel trained in the indications for ECMO can assist critical access and other facilities in routing possible ECMO patients for evaluation at the Center of Excellence. Early coordination with the call center leadership will allow them time to develop protocols, education, and coordination with transport services to assure smooth operations when the first patient call is received (**Figure 2**).

7.2 Where is ECMO initiated

A question that is often asked early in the development of any ECMO program is "where the patients should be cannulated?" While each institution must identify the ideal location for ideal cases, it is critical to recognize the nature of ECMO often dictates therapy must be able to be initiated anywhere within the hospital, including, but not limited to the following locations:

- Emergency department
- Operating rooms (cardiac and non-cardiac)
- Catheterization labs
- Obstetric labor and delivery suites
- Intensive care units (medical, cardiac, surgical, neuro, etc.)

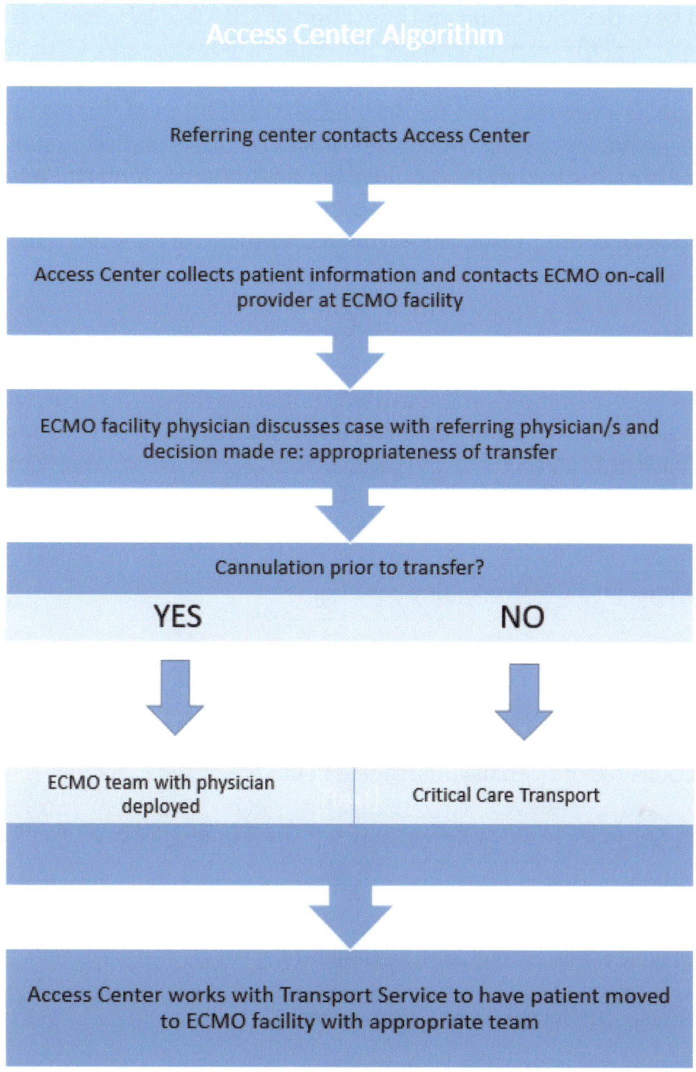

Figure 2.
Patient access/call center flow.

In fact, depending on the resources available and the resilience of the team, some centers will often consider initiating therapy in unusual out-of-hospital locations with the extreme example being the recent initiation of ECMO in the Louvre Museum in Paris, France [18].

Prior to considering the ideal location for initiating therapy, it is critical to outline those technologies that might be required. As discussed above, while it is important to have an "ECMO Cart" that contains, in a single location, all the key disposables that might be required, there might be a need for less portable equipment. For example, for cannulation, physicians might need immediate access to fluoroscopy and/or transesophageal echocardiography. Such technology might only be readily available in an operating room or catheterization lab. As many operating rooms, especially major trauma centers, and cardiac catheterization laboratories that support STEMI programs will often have access to advanced imaging, the exact ideal location often is dictated not only by physician preference, but also by potential administrative considerations. Such administrative considerations include the availability of a team to support cannulation, how disruptive emergency ECMO cases would be to the scheduling and allocation of OR/Cath lab resources, and often "how comfortable" the team is with the procedures. For example, Cath lab teams who are more comfortable with the catheter and wire-base procedures than surgical team might be a better option for peripheral cannulation of ECMO (arterial and venous)—while operating room teams might be better skilled at assisting with central cannulation (especially if the chest is already open). Nevertheless, a core "ECMO team" of providers beyond physicians and perfusions must be identified and included in all communications so that therapy can be initiated efficiently and safely anywhere needed.

7.3 Order sets

Order sets provide a rapid, standardized, initiation for ECMO. The order set should include guidance for the perfusion team and nursing team to appropriately care for the patient in a variety of settings, as well as give parameters for physician notification to address changes in patient status quickly.

Order set elements should include:

- Instructions for ECMO machine priming
- ECMO circuit settings
- ECMO daily parameters
- Instructions for the perfusionist/nurse in charge of the machine
- Instructions to leave all catheters in if not functioning and notify physician
- Ventilatory settings
- Blood products and transfusion parameters
- Massive transfusion protocol parameters
- Post-cannulation radiology studies
    - AP abdomen post-cannulation
    - AP chest post-cannulation
- Radiology ◦studies
    - Echocardiogram for symptoms
    - Daily and routine laboratory studies
- Anticoagulation and associated laboratory monitoring and adjustments
- Triggers for notification of the ECMO physician/nurse practitioner
- Other
    - Nursing care
    - Sedation medications

- Physical therapy
    - Occupational therapy
    - Case management
    - Routine ICU parameters

8. ECMO transports

Critically ill patients requiring ECMO can be transported by ground, helicopter, and fixed wing aircraft. Considerations in choice of transport include distance, number of team members required, equipment, electrical and oxygen needs, and cost. Ideally, patients can be identified and transported prior to initiation of ECMO therapy, however there are models of care with good results in which the team goes to the patient and initiates ECMO, and then the patient is transported to the ECMO center.

8.1 Team members for transport

Per the 2015 ELSO guidelines, team members will vary depending on the need to cannulate the patient [19]. An ECMO specialist physician is required in either case, as is an ECMO specialist and a transport RN/RT. If cannulation is required, and the ECMO specialist physician is unable to perform this, there may be the need to add a cannulating physician and a surgical assistant to the team. Each team member has specific roles that should be delineated and understood prior to deployment to the outlying facility.

A checklist, should include all the needed equipment for the return trip with the patient, and should be verified prior to departure.

The equipment recommended by ELSO includes [20]:

1. Suitable blood pump, centrifugal, or roller
2. Membrane oxygenator, appropriate for the patient size
3. Device(s) for heating and regulating circuit blood temperature (less critical for adult transports)
4. Medical gas tanks, regulators, hoses, connectors, flow meters, and blenders for provision and adjustment of blended sweep gas to the oxygenator
5. Venous and arterial pressure monitoring device(s), according to center-specific practices
6. Point-of-care anticoagulation monitoring equipment (e.g., activated clotting time)
7. Emergency pump or manual control mechanism in the event of primary pump failure or power failure
8. Uninterruptible power source(s) capable of meeting the electrical power needs of all equipment during transfer between vehicles and in the event of vehicle power source failure.
9. Portable ultrasound machine, if not provided by the referring facility

Method of transport	Advantages	Disadvantages	Distance for transport
Ground	1. Lowest cost 2. Least noise 3. Number of team embers 4. Ease of loading equipment 5. Unlimited weight	1. Shortest ideal distance for transport	Up to 300 miles
Helicopter	1. Speed 2. Ease of loading equipment 3. Limited weight	1. Least number of team members 2. Noise 3. Higher cost	Up to 450 miles
Fixed wing	1. Speed 2. Number of team members 3. Limited weight	1. Costly 2. Can be difficult to load equipment 3. Noise	Unlimited

Table 2.
Decision-making for ECMO transport options.

Additional equipment recommended by 2015 ELSO to improve safety includes:

1. System for servo-regulation of flow to balance venous drainage rate from the patient and blood return to the patient

2. Blood flow rate monitor (may be internal or external to the blood circuit)

3. Monitor(s) for circuit blood temperature, blood gas, oxygen saturation, and hemoglobin (may be internal or external to the blood circuit)

4. Capacitance "bladder" incorporated into the circuit

5. Bubble detector with or without automatic pump regulation function

Of note, the requirements for voltage, current, and power for all equipment should be verified for the transport vehicle prior to departure and monitored throughout transport. An adequate oxygen source must also be available with sufficient reserve to support high-flow 100% oxygen delivery for the duration of the transport. Provisions must be made to adequately secure the equipment during transport—brackets, holders, straps, etc. should be tested prior to first-time transport and should be compliance with appropriate regulatory guidelines (i.e., Federal Aviation Administration for the United States) (**Table 2**).

No patient should be transported without a means of manually providing circuit flow in the event of an electrical pump failure or malfunction.

9. Quality and outcomes

As with all areas of medicine, the optimization of patient outcomes must be a priority. This concept is especially important in the context of developing and maintaining an ECMO/ECLS program. Many other disease therapies have an infrastructure for monitoring clinical outcomes and benchmarking them against peer groups, national, and even international programs. These infrastructures typically are in the form of voluntary registries and databases (although some might argue that participation is becoming less and less voluntary and more and more a requirement—especially are payor sources are starting link payments to participation and eventually outcomes in such programs). Examples of these types of programs include the Society for Thoracic Surgeons (STS) Outcomes database (https://www.sts.org/registries-research-center/sts-national-database) and the American College of Cardiology National Cardiovascular Data Registry (ACC NCDR: https://cvquality.acc.org/NCDR-Home). Both organizations also for submission of patient characteristic data, comorbidities, therapies performed, and outcomes with the goal of providing program (and sometimes provider) specific outcome data—often risk adjusted, therapy specific, and benchmarked against other programs with provided summaries that can allow for continuous quality improvement initiatives.

9.1 Role of ELSO

Currently, the Extracorporeal Life Support Organization (ELSO) provides a mechanism for tracking and benchmarking outcomes for ECMO programs (https://www.elso.org/Home.aspx). The organization was founded in 1989 and is headquartered in Ann Arbor, Michigan, USA. While the organization serves many roles to assist ECMO providers and programs—voluntary membership allows for the submission of clinical program outcome data and in return, summary data are provided. The organization also provides access to clinical guidelines, discussion forums, announcements for relevant meetings, links to key publications and references, and overall serves as a hub for ECMO/ECLS-related activities. Membership is strongly encouraged and the organization claims international membership and helps coordinate worldwide activities.

9.2 Interval reviews

In addition to submitting clinical patient and outcome data for benchmarking to ELSO, programs should also establish a formal case presentation and review process. Much like traditional surgical "morbidity and mortality" reviews, given the high-acuity and resource intensive nature of ECMO, similar periodic reviews of institutional ECMO outcomes should also be reviewed. While the focus should not be in individual practices or decision-making, ideally, each case should be reviewed by the team in a non-judgmental fashion to explore for potential areas of opportunity. Likewise, while good outcomes should be discussion in the context of "what went right"—such cases should also serve as team learning opportunity for growth and improvement. Depending on the number of cases performed, such meetings should be held in a timely manner (monthly, quarterly, etc.) so that real-time assessments can be performed and the nuances of each case might still be relatively fresh in the minds of the providers. While the structure of such meetings can be variable, many "quality" meetings typically will only involve key stakeholders—both providers (i.e. physicians, ECMO specialists, perfusionists, etc.) and appropriate administrators. The benefit of having meetings limited is that there is then the opportunity for open, honest, and transparent conversations—either on a case-by-case basis or from a programmatic standpoint—in a manner that can and should be protected from legal disclosure under the umbrella of a formal peer-review or quality improvement initiative. Appropriate protections of patient data and provider involvement must be maintained and established from the onset.

Likewise, summary data of program outcomes—such as the number of cases, types of cases, and overall outcomes should be actively tracked in real-time and made available to institutional leadership as a gauge of program growth and success. Institutional leadership/administration should also be able to provide financial data as profit/loss margins must be tracked in the context of program growth and success. Additional benchmarking information should also be considered and tracked in real-time to help monitor the evolution of a program—and should include, but not necessarily be limited to:

(1) Patient demographics (i.e., age, gender, and major comorbidities)

(2) Primary indications for support and etiologies of respiratory failure and/or cardiogenic shock

(3) Type of support (VV, VA, eCPR, and cannulation)

(4) Duration of support

(5) Blood and blood product utilization

(6) Outcomes

- Successful weaning from support
- Death on support
- Death despite successful weaning
- Major factors contributing to patient death (i.e., multi-organ failure, neurologic, etc.)

Such summary data should be in addition to the extensive amount of clinical and circuit data that is collected and tracked in the ELSO registry (see above).

9.3 Continuous quality improvement (CQI)

As discussed above, the tracking of outcome data should be a key component to helping measure program growth and success. Such initiatives must be established from the onset and involve the program champions—both clinical and administrative leaders to be successful. While it is important to review cases in the context of

Topics for review	Potential desired outcome
Anticoagulation protocol	Reduction in bleeding and bleeding related complication. Reduction in blood product utilization
Antibiotic utilization	Integration in an antibiotic stewardship program Reduction in multi-drug resistant infections Reduction in opportunistic infections
Time from admission/intubation to initiation of ECMO support	Potential impact on improving weaning and survival outcomes
Mortality despite successful weaning from ECMO	Improving overall outcomes and survival to discharge.
Medication utilization	Opportunities for potential cost savings
Family/patient satisfaction scores	Opportunities to improve communication with families, Improved satisfaction metrics

Table 3.
Suggested topics for continuous quality initiatives

tracking outcomes—both good and bad—from a programmatic standpoint, it is also important to examine outcome summary data with the focus of exploring potential opportunity for improvement. It should be a primary objective of the ECMO team to consider periodic continuous quality improvement (CQI) activities. The activities should be viewed as opportunities to review best practices, current literature on various topics, and metrics with the focused goal of improving outcome metrics—while the primary focus should always be on improving patient survival, other metrics, program practices, and guidelines should also be considered as topics for review. Key topics can be identified, champions identified, and a timeline established for review and the development of potential action plans. While the specific details of how to develop and implement CQI is out of the scope of this topic—it does emphasize the importance of engaged administrative leadership individuals and team who have established experiences with these programmatic and institutional activities. By no means, comprehensive, various CQI topics are listed in **Table 3**.

10. Miscellaneous topics

10.1 Referral sources engagement

Once the complex set of internal processes, personnel, and patient care skills are established, the ECMO program has the potential to serve patients in a wide area around the ECMO center. To assure that other hospitals and emergency facilities have the information to know of the resources available, and when to engage them, the primary facility should engage a multi-pronged approach to raise awareness and clinical decision-making skills of potential patient care partners. As with all endeavors, this should be done in the WIIFM (What's In It For Me) with the patient and practitioner at the outlying facilities interests' in mind. A good place to begin this is to address the benefits to the patient, the current science that supports the need for ECMO, the parameters for consideration of ECMO support, the process to easily move the patient, and the resources to enhance education of the topic. This is accomplished by marketing informational materials, individual outreach to create awareness, an education program that includes lectures, publication of successes, a plan for follow-up communication to the referring institution to help them understand the results of their referrals, and finally, by creating branding that helps the referral sources easily retain a connection to the program.

10.2 Marketing

Marketing materials should ideally be created to reflect the ECMO program as a larger system of care around ARDS and shock. In addition to the organization housing the ECMO program, clear guidance on referral processes (see Call Center Section), there should also be some succinct explanation of the use of VV and VA ECMO, parameters for initiation of referral, as well as references to studies supporting the decision. Consideration should be given to having two sets of guidance; one for critical access lower acuity facilities/ER's and one geared toward facilities with ICU care directed by intensivists, as the threshold for referral will be different.

10.3 Outreach

The personal touch of a visit cannot be underestimated when establishing trusted referral center status for complex procedures such as ECMO. It affords a chance to create personal trust, as well as allowing answers to questions are procedures and processes for transfer, and expectations for communication regarding patient status from the ECMO center. The outreach should be well versed on all of these processes, as well as having the ability to provide physician to physician conversations to answer any outstanding issues.

10.4 Education

Education is a valued commodity for referring physicians and clinicians when learning a new resource for their patients. The education can include multiple formats to meet the needs of the audience including lectures, educational brochures, webcasts, publications regarding outcomes and patient stories, and conferences at the ECMO center on topics related to ECMO such as current ARDS and shock therapies.

10.5 Follow-up communication

While clearly an avenue to enhance education, follow-up communication is also an important tool to create the interpersonal relationship that develops trust between the organizations. It is very important for referring provider to learn the "end of the story" regarding patients that were sent for therapy. In addition, this provides a transition of care so that appropriate ongoing care can be provided to the patient in their home medical community. This also establishes that trust of the referring providers that patients sent for a specific therapy will be sent back to the home community for the care that can be provided in that setting.

10.6 Branding

As the use of ECMO increases, the need to create a memorable brand for the program becomes a key component to establishing the reputation of the ECMO center that is distinguishable from other future programs. The program should ideally be branded as a part of the larger cardiothoracic-vascular/pulmonary/critical care program of the institution. This allows the halo of the organization's programs to create synergistic enhancement quality outcomes and growth opportunities.

11. Conclusions

The initiation of an ECMO program is a comprehensive multidisciplinary project, which must be based on the clinical needs of the patients served. It requires advanced clinical capabilities and decision-making, and clear pathways for patient care to make it high quality and financially sustainable. As such, strong leadership is needed from physician leaders, nursing leaders, and administrative leaders working in a triad professional leadership model.

Once the clinical case for implementation is made, a multidisciplinary team should be identified, and given the ability to work across multiple departments and stakeholders to assure all quality and operational details are aligned and accomplished. The team is encouraged to work using change management format and techniques supported with strong project guidelines to assure that the internal and external resources needed to support ECMO care are identified, captured as project goals, and systematically completed prior to initiation of ECMO patient care. Use of tools such as order sets, access center protocols, and education tools support clinical standardization across the team, and provides a consistency of clinical care.

Quality metrics are identified at project initiation and can be supported by ELSO tools allowing comparisons across programs internationally. The commitment to high quality and a relentless curiosity to find improvements that can be made, are critical to provide best practices to this high acuity population. The data and outcomes collected can help educate and encourage referrals from other programs that do not have ECMO capabilities, thus providing added advanced patient care options on regional basis.

The literature has previously benchmarked an 18 month ramp up to program initiation as rapid deployment. Using the tools provided by others in the literature, a strong triad leadership process, and a dedicated multidisciplinary team with strong project management support, it is possible to accomplish program initiation in a six-month period in a hospital with an established CV Surgical program. We believe this process is replicable, and provides tools and implementation models that can be used by other hospitals to add needed ECMO support to meet their community needs [8–10].

Author details

Dianne McCallister, Linda Pilon, Joseph Forrester, Samer Alsaleem, Chakradhar Kotaru, Jennifer Hanna, Gregory Hickey, Rachele Roberts, Erica Douglass, Matthew Libby and Michael S. Firstenberg*
The Medical Center of Aurora, Aurora, CO, USA

*Address all correspondence to: msfirst@gmail.com

References

[1] Firstenberg MS. Extracorporeal Membrane Oxygenation–Advances in Therapy. Rijeka, Croatia: InTech; 2016, 2016. p. 392. ISBN: 978-953-51-2553-2. Print ISBN: 978-953-51-2552-5. Under CC BY 3.0 license. DOI 10.5772/61536. http://www.intechopen.com/books/how-to-link/extracorporeal-membrane-oxygenation-advances-in-therapy

[2] Firstenberg MS, editor. Advances in Extra-corporeal Perfusion Therapies. London, UK: InTech Publishing Limited; 2019. ISBN: 978-1-78984-914-1. Print ISBN: 978-1-78984-913-4. https://www.intechopen.com/books/advances-in-extra-corporeal-perfusion-therapies

[3] Putensen C, Theuerkauf N, Zinserling J, Wrigge H, Pelosi P. Meta-analysis: Ventilation strategies and outcomes of the acute respiratory distress syndrome and acute lung injury. Annals of Internal Medicine. 2009;**151**(8):566-576

[4] Bernard G. Acute lung failure—Our evolving understanding of ARDS. The New England Journal of Medicine. 2017;**377**(6):507-509

[5] Van Diepen S, Katz JN, Albert NM, Henry TD, Jacobs AK, Kapur NK, et al. Contemporary management of cardiogenic shock: A scientific statement from the American Heart Association. Circulation. 17 Oct 2017;**136**(16):e232-e268

[6] Thiele H, Ohman EM, Desch S, Eitel I, de Waha S. Management of cardiogenic shock. European Heart Journal. 2015;**36**(20):1223-1230

[7] Combes A, Brodie D, Bartlett R, Brochard L, Brower R, Conrad S, et al. Position paper for the organization of extracorporeal membrane oxygenation programs for acute respiratory failure in adult patients. American Journal of Respiratory and Critical Care Medicine 2014;**190**(5):488-496

[8] Kattan J, Godoy L, Zavala A, Faunes M, Becker P, Estay A, et al. Improvement of survival in infants with congenital diaphragmatic hernia in recent years: Effect of ECMO availability and associated factors. Pediatric Surgery International. 2010;**26**(7):671-676

[9] Unai S, Tanaka D, Ruggiero N, Hirose H, Cavarocchi NC. Acute myocardial infarction complicated by cardiogenic shock: An algorithm-based extracorporeal membrane oxygenation program can improve clinical outcomes. Artificial Organs. Mar 2016;**40**(3):261-269

[10] Dalia AA, Ortoleva J, Fiedler A, Villavicencio M, Shelton K, Cudemus GD. ECMO is a team sport: Institutional survival benefits of a formalized ECMO Team. Journal of Cardiothoracic and Vascular Anesthesia. 2018

[11] Peek GJ, Mugford M, Tiruvoipati R, Wilson A, Allen E, Thalanany MM, et al. Efficacy and economic assessment of conventional ventilatory support versus extracorporeal membrane oxygenation for severe adult respiratory failure (CESAR): A multicentre randomised controlled trial. Lancet. 2009;**374**(9698):1351-1363

[12] Combes A, Hajage D, Capellier G, Demoule A, Lavoué S, Guervilly C, et al. Extracorporeal membrane oxygenation for severe acute respiratory distress syndrome. The New England Journal of Medicine 2018;**378**(21):1965-1975

[13] Extracorporeal Life Support Organization (ELSO). Guidelines for Adult Respiratory Failure. Ann Arbor Michigan, USA: Extracorporeal

Life Support Organization; August, 2017. https://www.elso.org/Portals/0/ELSO%20Guidelines%20For%20Adult%20Respiratory%20Failure%201_4.pdf. [Accessed on 05.05.2019]

[14] Bosarge PL, Raff LA, McGwin G Jr, Carroll SL, Bellot SC, Diaz-Guzman E, et al. Early initiation of extracorporeal membrane oxygenation improves survival in adult trauma patients with severe adult respiratory distress syndrome. Journal of Trauma and Acute Care Surgery. 2016;**81**(2):236-243

[15] Doorenbos AZ, Starks H, Bourget E, DM MM, Lewis-Newby M, Rue TC, et al. Examining palliative care team involvement in automatic consultations for children on extracorporeal life support in the pediatric intensive care unit. Journal of Palliative Medicine. 2013;**16**(5):492-495

[16] Joseph T, Selzman Craig H, Malin Michael P, Smith Brigham R, Youngquist Scott T, Antigoni K, et al. Development and implementation of a comprehensive, multidisciplinary emergency department extracorporeal membrane oxygenation program. Annals of Emergency Medicine. 2017;**70**(1):32-40

[17] Kotter J. Leading Change, Harvard Business School Press, © September 1, 1996

[18] Lamhaut L, Hutin A, Deutsch J, Raphalen JH, Jouffroy R, Orsini JP, et al. Extracorporeal cardiopulmonary resuscitation (ECPR) in the prehospital setting: An illustrative case of ECPR performed in the louvre museum. Prehospital Emergency Care. 2017;**21**(3):386-389

[19] Broman LM, Frenckner B. Transportation of critically Ill patients on extracorporeal membrane oxygenation. Frontiers in Pediatrics. 2016;**4**:63

[20] Dan D, Richard F, Chris H, Dirk L, Matthew B, Steve C, et al. Extracorporeal Life Support Organization (ELSO) Guidelines for ECMO Transport. Ann Arbor Michigan, USA: Extracorporeal Life Support Organization. 2015. https://www.elso.org/Portals/0/Files/ELSO%20GUIDELINES%20FOR%20ECMO%20TRANSPORT_May2015.pdf. [Accessed on 05.05.2019]

Chapter 4

Finding a Bridge to Somewhere: An Ethical Framework for Veno-Arterial Extracorporeal Membrane Oxygenation Decisions

Julie Aultman and Michael S. Firstenberg

Abstract

Extracorporeal membrane oxygenation (ECMO) is an established therapy for the management of acute cardiopulmonary failure. A substantial concern when considering ECMO therapy is whether the patient will recover enough function to be weaned from support and survive to discharge. The concept of "a bridge to nowhere" is where a patient is supported on a therapy for which there is no hope for recovery and would, by definition, immediately die if support is discontinued—a somewhat unique concept in clinical medicine, but often considered when considering short-term mechanical support for acute heart and/or lung failure. Much like initiating mechanical ventilator support in patients who have no chance of meaningful recovery, there are concerns about embarking on or continuing with ECMO support in patients in whom recovery is unlikely. The purpose of this chapter is to review the ethical foundation and principles to support the clinical decision-making process when there are concerns regarding the initiation, continuation, or withdrawal of this highly invasive, resource-intensive life-support technology. Specific attention will be given to well-established principles of the ethical application of advanced life support and how to appropriately limit offering or continuing therapies for which meaningful outcomes are unlikely or further support is considered futile.

Keywords: ethics, ECMO, ECLS, extra-corporeal membrane oxygenation, palliative care, morality, end-of-life, futility

1. Introduction

Veno-arterial extracorporeal membrane oxygenation (VA-ECMO) has been widely described as a bridge to recovery for acute reversible illnesses, transplantation, ventricular assist devices (VADs), or when the prognosis of patients with cardiorespiratory failure is uncertain [1–4]. Advancement of this technology has increased accessibility of ECMO and mobile ECMO teams, leading to several ethical issues of VA-ECMO. Few authors in the ethics literature delineate veno-arterial (VA) from veno-venous (VV) extracorporeal membrane oxygenation (ECMO) given the similarities among these technologies and related ethical issues (e.g., when to initiate or withdraw ECMO). However, for purposes of this chapter, the focus will be on ethical analyses particular to VA-ECMO situations, illustrated through cases and ethical dilemmas we have encountered in the clinical setting.

Because of the distinct feature of VA-ECMO in providing both gas exchange and circulatory support through central or peripheral cannulation, it bears inherent potential problems, including, but not limited to, "separate perfusion of the lower and upper part of the body (watershed phenomenon), distention of the left ventricle (LV), and resulting pulmonary edema due to increased afterload produced by ECMO" [5]. Although close monitoring, optimizing vasopressor and inotropic support, the use of multiple cannulas, fluid offloading, alternative circuit configurations [e.g., veno-venous-arterial (VVA)], and adherence to guidelines [e.g., extra-corporal life support organization (ELSO)], can be beneficial for minimizing risks and maximizing peripheral and central VA-ECMO support, patients are nonetheless more susceptible to clinical risks, which contribute to further ethical examination. Some studies (particularly in the pediatric literature), however, have shown no difference in complication rates between VA-ECMO and VV-ECMO [6].

Although, as Pavlushkov et al. [5] describe, the use of *central* VA-ECMO, is a particularly invasive approach for cardiorespiratory support that contributes to heightened risks of infection, injury, and bleeding as it requires chest opening (sometimes for days) for providing optimal perfusion flow. As the authors note, this type of ECMO is reserved for those patients, who will imminently die. Given the invasiveness and inherent levels of risk of central and peripheral VA-ECMO, it is critical for healthcare providers, patients, and families to engage in shared decision-making based on a clear understanding of the treatment goals, and the values and interests of the patient regarding advance care planning.

Thus, an ethics coherence framework, and not simply a set of guidelines, principles, or policies, is required for evaluating the complex ethical issues of ECMO, while guiding critical decisions in its initiation, management, and withdrawal of this technology, particularly given the potential for serious risks and unanticipated events. Specifically, we will be utilizing a theoretical model that builds upon the work of Nelson and others, known as the Wide Reflective Equilibrium (WRE), while appropriately integrating narrative approaches within this model that enhances the WRE and other ethical models for reflection and decision-making.

To begin, it is critical to identify and understand the ethics of ECMO as presented in the literature and based on real clinical scenarios. And while there is consistency among authors who have written about this subject matter, this is not to say the types of ethical issues and dilemmas presented are exhaustive; as ECMO technology, research, and clinical care becomes more widespread and advanced, it is likely we will encounter ethical issues unidentified by current experts. The WRE, however, will be a useful model for when new information needs to be considered for ethical decision-making. The flexibility and ability to accommodate new information makes the WRE an attractive model for ethicists and healthcare professionals alike. Following a brief review of the literature and descriptions of the WRE, we will analyze two scenarios based on actual clinical cases to illustrate the value of the WRE for enhancing communication and decision-making among healthcare teams, patients, and their families.

2. A bridge to nowhere

Although ECMO is better known and valued among healthcare teams as a beneficial stabilizing technology that is able to prolong artificial cardiac and respiratory support external to the body, allowing patients to heal, if not fully recover, from traumatic injuries and diseases, it can be beneficial for giving patients and families more time with each other and for collective decision-making. However, decision-making is at the heart of great ethical controversies from points of initiation to withdrawal of ECMO. Courtwright et al. [7] explain the most common ethical issues involving disagreements among and between healthcare teams, patients, family, and other surrogates, particularly when confronted with decisions about the continuation or withdrawal of ECMO.

When patients, who have started ECMO, are unable to be bridged to recovery, transplant, or destination device therapy, this "ethically challenging and emotionally charged situation is sometimes referred to as a 'bridge to nowhere', with obvious implications for the patient, his or her family, the caregivers, the hospital, and the healthcare system" [1]. These ethical issues are further exacerbated by a need for evidence-based scientific research taking into account patients' comorbidities and the use of ECMO, improved scoring systems for determinations of survivability, reliable and consistent brain death evaluation and neurological testing, comprehensive advanced care planning prior to initiating ECMO, and improved availability, accessibility, and management of ECMO resources, particularly for disadvantaged populations. Essentially, since patients can be kept "alive" almost indefinitely while on VA-ECMO (particularly, given the lack of key tools for medical decision-making—like determining brain death on ECMO), much emphasis is placed on determining those patients who have the greatest chance of survival, either being weaned or transitioned to transplant or a long-term support device. The primary goal of such scoring systems is not just to optimize the appropriate use of an expensive and resource intensive therapy, but to help decision-makers prevent initiation of therapy in those patients for whom there is fundamentally, no hope of meaningful survival. While such concepts can be vague and subjective, the approach is not all that much different than why certain therapies (i.e., major surgery) are not offered in patients with advanced cancers or end-stage heart disease. Basically, the progress is so poor, however, with ECMO, advances in therapy and experiences are occurring at such a rapid pace that such threshold is hard to define.

For example, Makdisi and Wang [2], citing Bartlett and Gattinoni [8] wrote "… some helpful and score systems have been presented to assess the probability of survival with extracorporeal life support, using multivariate analysis of comorbidity, the history of lung or cardiac failure, and additional organ dysfunction, unfortunately there is no definitive measure of heart or lung failure to identify 80% mortality risk." Without definitive measurements, these places undue burdens on healthcare teams when trying to communicate prognosis and treatment options, including when treatment is no longer beneficial to the patient's survivability. This lack of certainty has further implications for non-beneficial treatment policies, the process of informed consent, determinations of patient capacity for decision-making, palliative care resources, DNR orders, hospice care, and other spiritual, social, and emotional resources for patient and family and/or surrogate. Thus, the ethical issues are more complex than "simply" disagreements about continuing or stopping ECMO; there are several decisions to be made, and, in most cases, patients, family, and surrogates are not well-prepared for such decision-making due to several factors, including, but not limited to, poor advance care planning, miscommunication, and unexpected confounding issues (e.g., cardiac arrest, sepsis, etc.).

One of the greatest difficulties that families experience when faced with a loved one, who is doing poorly on ECMO, is helping healthcare providers understand what the limits of what care patient would want—how much they want to live. Providers try to remain objective and unbiased, but often their own experiences and insights help pave a direction. For example, in the context of facing truly imminent death of a loved one, and often someone, who was previously perceived to be relatively young and healthy (which is why ECMO might have been offered in the first place), familiar members must very quickly prepare and come to terms with the reality that their loved one might not even survive. If a patient is on ECMO, especially if they are experiencing complications (which are quite common), then conversations about leg and digit amputations and major disfiguring surgery often occur. Even discussions about temporary therapies as further bridges to what can be perceived as a long and difficult recovery are unclear and difficult, such as the need for dialysis, feeding tubes, tracheostomies, prolonged stays for recovery in long-term care facilities, or nursing homes. Without a doubt, such conversations, time-sensitive and emotionally charged, and often financially difficult, topics can be very difficult to process and reconcile.

And, while the ethical issues would be less complex when patients are alert, and able to make their own decisions, there are instances where the "bridge to nowhere," as Abrams et al. [1] describe, leave the patient in a type of limbo: without ECMO, they will not be able to interact with family and others with some quality of life at the end of life, yet ECMO is no longer beneficial for the patient's transition to transplantation, VADs, or recovery and survivability. The question, then, is when should ECMO be withdrawn?

For Abrams et al. [1], it would be cruel and unethical to withdraw ECMO without the consent of the patient. But what if the patient will not consent to its withdrawal? What are the implications of using ECMO when it has no direct clinical benefits, but acutely sustains the quality of one's life, as measured by human interactions and relationships, and the ability to buy more time to make end of life plans? While we agree with Abrams et al. [1], it would be cruel and unethical to simply withdraw ECMO in such cases where patients are alert, we also argue that the prolonged use of clinically non-beneficial ECMO does not always provide a quality of life or effectively aid the patient to make end of life preparations. When the patient is awake on non-beneficial ECMO, the reality is they are terminally ill, requiring pain management, and not necessarily in a position to make critical decisions. Furthermore, the patient's quality of life may be misunderstood by family/surrogates and healthcare professionals at the bedside; their perceptions are contrary to the actual experiences and values of the patient. Thus, it is imperative that hospitals and ECMO facilities utilize comprehensive resources for providing:

1. grief counseling for patients and families;

2. access to end of life preparations (e.g., funeral homes, burial sites, family legal representatives, etc.);

3. ongoing and direct communication about the prolonged physical, cognitive, and emotional effects of ECMO on the patient (and family/surrogate), financial costs, and the scarcity of ECMO technologies, and;

4. palliative and spiritual care, to ease social, physical, and emotional pain and suffering and to accommodate the cultural, religious, and spiritual needs of the patient.

However, this assumes that such resources are available and accessible. By having such resources, not only the burdens of prolonged non-beneficial ECMO (including financial costs, inability to serve other patients in need, etc.) are reduced, but healthcare teams can prepare patients and families/surrogates to withdraw support and accept death without fear or resistance. While it is difficult to determine the scope of this problem, what is clear is that as ECMO is being used more frequently—especially in extreme cases—there is a growing number of patients, who are awake and alert, but are being kept immediately alive by life support for which discontinuation would result in immediate death. Even patients who take themselves off of other forms of organ replacement therapies—such as dialysis and ventilators—can live for days (if not longer, depending on the circumstances) before slowly, and often painlessly, succumbing to the consequences of the lack of organ function. The facing of immediate death is what separates removing ECMO from removing other therapies such as dialysis or even medical therapies, like chemotherapy. While the literature is sparse in this area, many providers who are involved in the care of patients requiring long-term life support with mechanical cardiac support devices (i.e., ventricular assist devices) are intimately aware of cases in which patients clearly took themselves off of support, essentially committed suicide, by removing or not replacing the power sources that such devices are dependent upon.

2.1 When surrogates disagree with the healthcare team

Ramanathan et al. [9] wrote, "Potential conflicts occur when the next of kin or the patient's proxies and physician do not agree on treatment options, when options are scarce or unavailable, and when the options themselves are unclear because of uncertainties about the effectiveness or the duration of treatment" [9, 10]. While such events are common in medicine, in the context of ECMO, while therapy can continue for a long-term, often in the absence of clearly defined decision-making, often the decisions will be made by themselves—frankly, patients often will develop life-threatening (or ending) complications that will define an outcome regardless of objective decision-making. Massive bleeding, neurologic catastrophes, overwhelming sepsis, and infections are common in the context of ECMO and often lead to the obvious discussions of the fact that "nothing else can be done."

Howe [11], in considering what clinicians should do if patients and/or loved ones never agree to stop treatment, wrote, "hospital authorities would stop ECMO if patients, loved ones, and clinicians won't" and confirms our own experiences that "[P]ediatricians have told me than when children have ECMO, clinicians may have more discretion" [11]. Hospital authorities may be justified to intervene for purposes of fair resource allocation; ECMO is unavailable to patients in need due to continued use among patients, who are no longer benefiting from this limited resource. However, decision-making should not simply be about fair resource allocation. While children are often considered much more resilient than adults, the survival rates on ECMO are not that much different between adults and children, and there must be early discussions with families regarding this reality to help better manage expectations. Similar models of care and discussions are often held in the context of young children, who otherwise appear to be very much "alive," but who are, in fact, irreversibly neurologically devastated or even brain dead.

Makdisi and Makdisi [4] explain "It is important not to force the family into making decisions that are against their beliefs and to provide them with adequate psychological support through and after the process, it is also important to understand their emotional needs, and understand the program from their perspective" [1, 12]. However, Abrams et al. [1] argue, "a strong case can be made to discontinue the intervention, with appropriate concessions of timing to the surrogates. There is no issue of emotional or physical patient suffering in that case and it is even possible, if not probably that the patient would not want his or her life prolonged in such circumstances" [1]. So, while the healthcare team should not force decisions without support, there are limits to the extent ECMO should be used for patients, who are no longer benefitting clinically, socially, or otherwise, and are kept alive for the sake of the surrogate(s) own interests. Ongoing communication and a robust informed consent process with detailed information (e.g., harmful outcomes of prolonged ECMO use) can contribute to improved family or surrogate understanding and decision-making that is in the best interests of the patient. Unfortunately, such a comprehensive approach is not always beneficial. Shah et al. [12] suggest:

> *"Conversely, some may offer 'comprehensive' explanations inundated with technical points and statistical data incomprehensible to family members. Often, medical care in such acute situations may shift to a less desirable 'paternalistic model' in which the clinician is directing care rather than partnering with the patient or family acting on his behalf. These ethical dilemmas stem from the uncertainty of the outcome as well as lack of clarity on the intended treatment direction, whether bridge or lifetime support" [12].*

Meltzer and colleagues [13] describe a 40-year-old Hasidic Orthodox Jewish mother of four children, diagnosed with large B-cell lymphoma, which contributes to acute heart failure and the need for ECMO treatment. Prior to treatment, discussions surrounding the potential need to withdraw ECMO were discussed early on with the patient, her family, and their rabbi. The family agreed to stop ECMO when the need arises; however, when it became clear, ECMO was no longer providing beneficial treatment, the family refused to stop the treatment. In reflecting on this case, Howe [11] explains:

> *We do not know why the family changed their minds. Perhaps even they didn't know, but primarily responded to their fear the patient would die. That the family changed how they felt illustrates how unsure shared decision-making can be. The family's experiences convey the pain all those involved in deciding to stop ECMO may feel, whether clinicians decide on their own or share the decision-making [11].*

This and other similar situations reveal not only simple changes in a patient's story or a change of mind among family and surrogates, but also how the narrative continues and develops over time with decisions and courses of action that are informed by new experiences, moral thinking, clinical information, emerging feelings of hope, and so forth. Religious, racial, cultural, emotional, and ethnic themes are common in such conflicts and must be recognized very early in the discussions. In addition, every healthcare provider who needs to be involved with such critical family (and patient) conversations must acknowledge, and prepare, for the reality that thoughts about continuing life-sustaining therapies is very much different when one is dealing with the abstract (i.e., your mother might not survive therapy and we might need to stop support) versus the impending and immediate reality (i.e., your mother is not going to survive therapy and we must consider stopping support *right now*).

Furthermore, from the example illustrated by Howe [11], it is important to understand that the patient and her family are situated in different points of time with a new set of ethical considerations. A patient and family could be well-informed and prepared for future decision-making, however, that information does not necessarily carry any meaning until a critical decision is required. The life story of the patient merely continues and is not "re-written" and the family or surrogate is not simply "changing their minds," but are acquiring new information, i.e., the impending death of their loved one, which transforms their thoughts, emotions, and behaviors such that decisions to forgo or withdraw treatment can be difficult and any future hope for survival is lost. Early discussions, hypothetical scenarios, and some shared decision-making (e.g., DNR orders) might prepare some patients and families, but even with such preparations they are not—*at that time*—required to make life-altering decisions or give up hope. Certainly, it may be the case that shared decision-making might be "unsure" because the healthcare team and family did maintain ongoing communication or a mutual understanding of each other's values, thoughts, and overall interests.

However, even with the best communication, the moment treatment is no longer beneficial, it is the moment that family or surrogate decision-makers are receiving new information and expected to "do what is best or right" for the patient, despite their own emotional suffering and loss of hope. So, instead of thinking families and surrogates "change their minds," which can elicit feelings of frustration among healthcare providers, understanding they are simply confronted with new information and need further guidance and support in decision-making (e.g., discussions about quality life *now* versus then) can alleviate frustration and lead to better outcomes. Caring for the family [8] and recognizing the difficulty of their predicament can effectively lead to a mutually supported ethical decision to withdraw ECMO and provide comfort care measures, allowing for a peaceful death of a loved one.

2.2 Disagreements among healthcare professionals and institutions

Besides the ethical difficulties of decision-making among surrogates, healthcare professionals may also encounter ethical dilemmas, when there are disagreements among team members or at the institutional level (e.g., policy disagreements). While many ethics cases focus on disagreements between the healthcare team and patients and/or family members, where miscommunication, misunderstanding, and conflicting values and interests contribute to these disagreements, similar problems can arise among healthcare professionals and institutions, particularly when new technologies or new uses for technologies emerge with unanticipated ethical issues and problems, and a lack of standards, policies, or laws to provide guidance toward resolution. Such disagreements might be motivated by or directly lead to burnout, moral distress, lack of healthcare professional autonomy, and disregard of team-based practices. Disagreements among the healthcare team involving the initiation or withdrawal of ECMO might also be related to a general lack of institutional guidance (procedures, processes, and policies), conflicts of diagnostic and prognostic opinions, and misinterpretations of patients' cultural and moral values and interests. Ongoing communication, respect for healthcare team members, and collaborative contributions to the improvement of guidance measures (e.g., policy development), are essential for minimizing disagreements and those negative consequences that follow.

2.3 Extracorporeal CPR and DNR

Another ethical issue presented by Abrams et al. [1] involves VA-ECMO for extracorporeal CPR (ECPR), which is a more evasive and resource intensive intervention than traditional CPR that has the ability to cause undue suffering and harm to an already medically compromised patient. And ECMO, especially VA ECMO, "places the DNR order under severe conceptual strain both to the family and the physician" [9].

The prognosis for ECPR is uncertain during a cardiac arrest even when factors, such as the patient's condition, available resources, expertise, and past patient experience of the healthcare team are known. Because the concept and application of E-CPR (the focus of other areas of this book) are so rapidly evolving with large spectrums of potential outcomes based upon many complex circumstances, it is difficult to establish a timely and appropriate reference for objectively engaging in discussions about outcomes and prognosis. Abrams et al. [1] wrote "If the use of ECPR becomes even more widespread, there is a real concern that it would be an expected intervention for patients suffering acute cardiac arrest. If this occurs, physicians would need to incorporate ECPR into advance directive discussions, potentially requiring the development of a DNR with ECMO order." Regardless of infrequent or limited occurrences of ECPR, it is the opinion of these authors to incorporate ECPR into advance directive discussions whenever the situation arises, including education, training, and policies that require ECPR to be a part of DNR orders or Medical Order of Life Saving Treatment (MOLST) orders. It is perplexing why healthcare teams would not be doing this advance care planning already when such planning can be reasonably done. Nevertheless, the rapid growth of the utilization of ECPR must prompt such conversations—especially, since it is a therapy that is currently not available widely, yet.

2.4 Organ preserving ECMO

Another set of ethical issues arise for those healthcare teams, who are using ECMO to preserve organs. Organ preserving extracorporeal membrane oxygenation (OP-ECMO) may be used for patients, who are already on ECMO and who become brain dead. In such cases, vital organs can be preserved for transplantation, which have obvious benefits to others who are in need of organs for survival. Dalle Ave and authors wrote, "Organ-preserving extracorporeal membrane oxygenation can benefit society by fulfilling the wishes of those who wish to donate, by making more organs available for transplantation and by saving the lives of patients in need of organs." [14]. From a utilitarian perspective, saving several people with the viable organs of an individual, who no longer has quality of life and has irreversible loss of brain function, is a valid ethical justification.

Dalle Ave et al. [14] suggest that OP-ECMO is analogous to the continuation of mechanical ventilator for purposes of procurement. However, as these authors have also pointed out, there are challenges, similar to patients supported by ventilator, in determining brain death. Such determinations may be even more difficult given that the oxygenation process of ECMO can compromise neurological testing. Nonetheless, despite its uncertainty, a declaration of brain death holds great ethical (and legal) value in ensuring that organs are not being procured from patients who categorically are still living. However, this leads to deeper philosophical discussions as to what counts as "living" and whether brain death criteria should be used for purposes of organ procurement from patients, let alone ECMO patients. Furthermore, there is evidence in the past decade or so that patients, who were initially declared brain dead based on neurological standards, narrowly "escaped" organ harvesting by waking up prior to or during operating room preparations [15–19] or had reversible "brain death" determinations [15, 19, 20]. Although these "narrow escape" cases are few, they should give healthcare professionals pause in relying on existing brain death criteria and neurological testing. Furthermore, Dalle Ave et al. [14] have explained that ECMO can increase the potential risks of intracranial bleeding, causing undue suffering among individuals, who may have some undetected brain activity and can hasten death [14].

Given the uncertainty of determining brain death among ECMO patients, the risks of the aforementioned issues may not adequately outweigh the potential benefits of having viable organs for procurement (and this is assuming the organs will, in fact, be viable upon procurement). With further scientific data to validate clinical tests used with any brain-injured patient, as well as those specifically on ECMO for both acute and prolonged periods of time, as well as more consistency among medical professionals in determining brain death, the threshold of uncertainty may be reduced, thus minimizing, if not eliminating, potential direct harms to patients, and subsequent emotional, social, and financial harms to their families and potential organ recipients. Nguyen [15] also adds that there have been logical and scientific inconsistencies when reasoning brain death at the bedside, as well as a general lack of understanding of the pathophysiology of the brain, where an absence of evidence of brain functions is not necessarily the equivalent to irreversible loss or death of the brain.

Furthermore, in his brief ethical assessment of care for the patient with (possible) brain death, Nguyen [15] emphasizes the importance of the physician's moral attitudes and subsequent actions to reflect caring for the patient, motivated by the inherent value of the patient as person, and not by a set of ethical rules or principles. However, Nguyen, a Catholic physician, who is guided by non-secular ethics, also argues that brain death cannot be equated with the biological death of the person; harvesting organs from brain death donors, thus, "brings about their true and premature death." His attentiveness to the inconsistencies and inadequacies of brain death determination are valuable, as is his personal moral perspective, which aligns with the teachings of Catholicism. However, for those patients for whom we can identify as brain dead (or in the future with improved research, testing, and technologies), the definition and meaning of death should be left up to the healthcare team and surviving family; hence, the need to have advance care planning and conversations much earlier, if possible, prior to the urgency of patient care, and often, subsequent paternalistic decision-making. Further challenging this concept is the very concept that "brain death" is "death" and that any continuation of medical care is medically, ethically, and legally inappropriate. Even patients who have been appropriately declared "brain death" are often kept on support for prolonged periods of time for family members to completely understand the scope of the circumstances, and even waiting for a family member to come from out of town in a few days to "buy time" is not appropriate. Such events are not uncommon and are very dependent on experienced healthcare providers appropriately managing expectations and having open, honest, and transparent conversations with families from the onset of therapy.

3. Toward an integrated approach: the wide reflective equilibrium

Bein et al. [21] wrote, "At the end of the day, we are left alone with our own 'common moral.' However, there should be a method of finding a solution for the individual patient and for his dignity in a sensible and faithful way if we understand that the medical perspective is not the only one that needs to come to a decision." Howe [11] in reflecting on Meltzer and colleagues [22], places importance on shared decision-making among healthcare professionals, patients, and their loved ones when the withdrawal of ECMO results in the patient's death despite the fact some clinicians believe such decisions are theirs alone. Reasons why clinicians may want to make the decision to stop ECMO include "from wanting to spare patients and families the exceptional pain of making the decision to reasons that are less altruistic" such as alleviating suspected guilt among family and alleviating the burdens of decision-making, assuming family may simply want the physician to decide [11].

Nevertheless, the concept of shared decision-making, making sure that patients and families have an increased sense of ownership and responsibility to make their own medical decisions that will ultimately impact both the quality and quantity of life, is becoming more common. This is especially true in area of medicine in which it is unclear of what the "best" or most appropriate decision should be and the responsibility is then placed in the hands of the patient. Nevertheless, as discussed above, some patients and families become completely paralyzed by the inability to sometimes even make basic medical decisions and will often defer to the concept of "do everything" or "do whatever you think it best."

Such authors suggest an integrated approach, however, they do not provide one that might appropriately guide ethical decision-making, while taking into account the complex values of the healthcare team, patient, and family, as well as, the healthcare organization or system. Thus, we propose using the Wide Reflective Equilibrium (WRE), a theoretical model that builds upon contemporary philosophical theories and considerations, including narrative ethics. In the discussion of two case studies (based on features of existing clinical cases), we apply this model and illustrate its benefits in guiding pragmatic and ethical decisions prior to and during the use of VA-ECMO technology for patient care.

3.1 The wide reflective equilibrium (WRE)

The WRE is a theoretical model developed by Nielsen [23, 24] by extending the work of Norman Daniels and political philosopher Rawls [25]. This method consists of working back and forth among our judgments about particular situations, beliefs about those principles or rules that guide them, and additional considerations and beliefs relevant to the situation. The aim to find coherence by testing our beliefs against other systems of belief, moral theories, and non-moral views, revising and refining them, in a process of moral deliberation. The WRE as a model for practical ethics can be a way to recognize the value of multiple, methodologies in ethics (e.g., principlism, casuistry, and narrative) such that specific cases, theories, principles, and context (of stories or situations) matter and can contribute to the interplay of the WRE framework.

By using the WRE with an ethical situation, we work back and forth between three elements, including our initial moral judgment, background beliefs, and theories (e.g., social theory, clinical information, and legal laws), and ethical theories and principles to achieve coherence. WRE is then continually rewoven in light of new knowledge or circumstances, which may alter any or all elements of the WRE. Beauchamp and Childress [26] explain that "No matter how wide the pool of beliefs, we have no reason to anticipate that the process of pruning, adjusting, and rendering coherent will either come to an end or be perfected" ([27], p. 66). Joan McCarthy writes, "On this understanding, the processes of moral deliberation are akin to scientific processes: they involve the setting up of hypotheses that are tested and modified or rejected on the basis of reasoning and experience. In turn, the aim of unifying one's moral beliefs and background commitments is analogous to the scientific goal of achieving theoretical consistency and unity" [27].

While McCarthy shows the value of the WRE that incorporates principles into ethical decision-making, she also identifies the benefits of a narrative ethic, which draws upon "narrative concepts and methodologies drawn from literary criticism and philosophy as tools of moral understanding and assessment," [27] and is formulated through various approaches such that individual stories are closely read, or compared to, even woven within, other stories, giving context to existing moral theories and models, serving as a theory in and of itself, or promoting the emergence of new ethical thought. McCarthy suggests that one can test various personal narratives against various criteria similar to the way moral rules or principles are tested through the process of reflective equilibrium, and, thus, proposes a Narrative Reflective Equilibrium (NRE) to challenge and modify first person narratives. This narrative approach can be particularly useful for end of life decision-making, especially when healthcare professionals, surrogates, and others try to make sense of an incompetent patient's life story, which can reveal multiple courses of actions that are compatible with and would be "meaningful and consistent with the patient's self-conception" if she were the one deciding [27].

McCarthy shows that both principlism and narrative ethics provide important, often overlapping, ethical skills that can reinforce each other through deliberative, reflective processes that aim to achieve coherence and shared understanding [27]. Yet, the NRE is unnecessary unless we give primacy to a narrative approach over other ethical approaches under consideration. That is, the WRE is able to be a valuable model that incorporates principlism, narrative ethics, among other methodologies without be reductive to one approach or another; thus, it is unnecessary to have such a coherence model distinct from WRE. The other elements of WRE, including initial moral judgments and background beliefs and theories, including clinical and scientific facts, legal laws and policies, religious and spiritual beliefs and perceptions, and so forth are significant for not only further understanding the context of patients', caregivers', and others' stories, but also may contribute to new information that have the power to create new stories, reveal multiple courses of action based on different interpretations of stories, including alternative ethical considerations. Such new information might even be an unconsidered personal narrative that requires coherence among not just other narratives, but also among the other elements of WRE. It is this WRE that embraces narrative, as well as other ethical theories and approaches (which are themselves often embedded in narratives), which may untangle some complex ethical issues, arriving at justifiable courses of action through ongoing revision and refinement. Because, we cannot ignore the clinical, social, legal, economical, and ethical elements of VA-ECMO, a framework that recognizes these elements, as well as, patient and caregiver stories, relationships, and values, will best guide shared decision-making and perhaps find a "bridge to somewhere."

4. Finding a bridge to somewhere

To illustrate how the WRE can be a beneficial model for shared decision-making, we present two cases, followed by our ethical analysis.

4.1 Case 1

A critically ill 67-year-old female patient, M.J. presents to the cardiology team with progressive heart disease, profound cardiogenic shock, as a result of a massive acute myocardial infarction secondary to long-standing known coronary artery disease in the setting of previous coronary artery bypass surgery (CABG). As a result of a recently diagnosed, but medically treated breast cancer, she is neither a candidate for a transplant nor is a long-term ventricular assist device a reasonable option. Due to her ability to breathe on her own without ventilator support, she is on VA-ECMO without having to be in a clinically induced coma. Thus, she is alert, at times able to interact with family, but unfortunately has a poor prognosis and would die without ongoing ECMO support. The support is non-beneficial in that it will not be an effective bridge to survival, but simply a means to temporarily sustain a terminal life. M.J. is scared of dying, and feels as though if she gives up now, she will be a disappointment to her loved ones. Because of the patient's insistence to keep living as long as possible, the healthcare team, family, and those closest to the patient are uncomfortable with removing ECHO. The healthcare team sees current benefit in giving the patient time to make end of life plans and spend time with family despite the financial burdens of ECMO. The issue of this case, however, is that M.J. refuses to listen to the healthcare team about her impending prognosis and to consider end of life planning in the event she is no longer able to make decisions.

Although the case of M.J. involves the use of VA-ECMO for a "bridge to nowhere," the healthcare team would like to see this not as a futile endeavor but one that bridge to a peaceful closure to life. For the multitude of patients who do not get to choose their deaths, M.J. has an opportunity to make end of life plans based on her values and needs, and yet the healthcare team is struggling as to why she is not engaged in such planning. When looking at this case through the lens of WRE, the initial moral judgment of the healthcare team may look like "M.J. should remain on ECMO." And, as simply put, there is consensus that removing ECMO from M.J. at this point in time would be unethical given that it is providing benefit by caring for her end of life needs, e.g., seeing family; removing ECMO could lead to moral distress among healthcare professions, emotional and social harm to M.J and her family, potential legal liability, and social distrust. Looking at the benefits versus the risks of financial burden for family, lack of ECMO access for other patients, and amount of teamwork required to sustain M.J.'s life (i.e., "manpower" hours), as well as institutional considerations that may require alternative actions, e.g., transfer of care, before enacting non-beneficial treatment policies for the withdrawal of ECMO.

4.1.1 Initial moral judgment

In the event M.J. becomes incapacitated, we may ask the question, "For how long should M.J. remain on ECMO?" This new scenario and question prompts new moral judgments and ethical, clinical, legal, and social considerations such that "M.J. should not remain on ECMO due to progression of disease and unavoidable harm." This judgment, loaded with clinical and social requirements, leads to concerns about surrogate decision-making and refusal of withdrawal, DNR and ECPR, and OP-ECMO. If M.J.'s family supports her decision for continuing life support even when she no longer has capacity, this will lead to a complex dilemma for the healthcare team and family. The initial moral judgment, then, for the healthcare team will be based on their ability to sustain a quality of life for M.J.

4.1.2 Background beliefs and theories

Before delving into the ethical theories and principles, an analysis of multiple factors, i.e., background beliefs, including existing policies, laws, family beliefs and social theory, clinical information, etc., is essential to work back and forth among the WRE elements. Healthcare professionals are not required to provide futile treatment, and thus, many institutions have non-beneficial treatment or futility policies. Of course, the notion of futility is highly debated and this case, in point, shows how the concept of what is or is not beneficial may depend on the context of the situation (i.e., alert patient, family at the bedside). These conceptual considerations are valuable when working through the WRE, as well as the pragmatic considerations such that medical evidence, laws, and policies are considered. If M.J.'s surrogate or next of kin refuses to withdraw ECMO, the healthcare team may enact a non-beneficial treatment policy with the option to transfer care to another facility that may accept M.J.

Here is where the WRE pushes the healthcare team, ethics committee, or general counsel to find out if transfer of care is even possible, i.e., willingness, accessibility, and availability of other institutions. That is, M.J. may not be mobile, facilities may be at full capacity, they may not take cases like M.J.'s, or they may not have the team to support ECMO. If transfer of care is not possible, legal action is most likely the next course of action. To further complicate the matter, decisions of DNR and whether ECPR should be initiated must also be considered. While ECPR may sustain life, even for a short time, M.J. is still terminal and such interventions will not lead to clinically beneficial results. DNR discussions are essential prior to patients becoming incapacitated; however, given that option is no longer viable, such discussions need to occur with M.J.'s surrogate decision-maker. These policies, standards, and theoretical concepts (e.g., futility), should be considered in light of ethical theories and principles under the WRE model.

4.1.3 Ethical theories and principles

In light of clinical facts, existing policies, and standards, the healthcare team feels that it is best to withdraw support based on ethical considerations. By keeping M.J. "alive" on ECMO (and equally its removal) can violate the ethical principle of non-maleficence ("do no harm"), as would initiating CPR. Quality of life was understood as M.J.'s ability to interact with her family although she understood that ECMO was a non-beneficial treatment. However, due to her current state, and progressive declining health, she no longer has quality of life, and may potentially suffer if she still has brain function with continued ECMO use. Thus, the healthcare team believes it is their ethical obligation to withdraw all support so as to do no harm, despite allowing death to occur, which, to some, is counter to the goals of medical care. In addition, there are justice issues with this scenario; it is unjust utilizing a needed public resource for a patient who is no longer benefitting from that resource, especially when availability and accessibility is limited. Furthermore, the family is accruing a potential financial burden, and may not be fully cognizant of the economic costs of keeping a person alive because they are not wanting to let her go or violate her autonomous wish to be kept alive. The economic burdens, in their mind, may not outweigh their unrelenting desire to keep her alive and abide by her wishes. Besides principle-based considerations, the narrative approach is also valuable in this scenario to better understand the family's interests and values, and whether they are genuinely aware of M.J.s current state.

Furthermore, M.J.'s story may further reveal to the family/surrogate decision-maker and healthcare team that her autonomous wish to be kept alive was only intended to be limited for when she was alert and able to interact with her surroundings. If she and her family's insistence on "doing everything possible" with continued ECMO support and refusal of DNR orders (a concept that, in itself, is somewhat misleading since the patient is, by definition, full cardiopulmonary life-support. As such, the term DNR is the setting of ECMO is often used to place objective limitations on escalation of support—such as initiating or escalating doses of vasoactive medications, new antibiotics, or performing additional invasive procedures) is motivated by cultural, religious, spiritual, or philosophical beliefs, these beliefs would then be brought into the WRE framework and pushing us to move back and forth between these beliefs and ethical theories and principles. Narrative ethics pushes us deeper into the reasoning behind our patients' and surrogates' decisions and beliefs and contextualizing the aforementioned considerations for further reflection and refinement. With deeper understanding, the healthcare team may have to utilize more resources, and justify the use of those resources, e.g., chaplaincy service, while possibly postponing critical decisions and the alleviation of M.J.'s harm and suffering.

4.1.4 Revision, refinement, and reflection

There may be some compromises (not necessarily consensus) among patients, family, and the healthcare team as we move back and forth among these elements of the WRE. For example, the healthcare team may be able to educate the family or surrogate about M.J.'s poor prognosis and the possible suffering she might endure if prolonged on ECMO as supported by their ethical obligation to do no harm. The family or surrogate, possibly feeling guilt, fear, or any number emotions in confronting the death of a loved one, might not want to sacrifice M.J.'s welfare for a previously declared request for continued treatment, and decide to withdraw. Then again, they may compromise and ask to have some more time with MJ, but with the acceptance of a DNR order. They may also be motivated to withdraw or accept a DNR order by recognizing that patients with quality lives can survive if they have access to the ECMO technology that is currently being utilized by M.J. The context of the decisions by which the healthcare will support or reject the family's decision just may depend on the level of harm, whether there is a patient in need of the ECMO unit, or if a transfer of care is possible. Regardless, the WRE should not simply be a tool for just healthcare professionals to come to terms with their initial moral judgments; the WRE should involve the perspectives, stories, and values of all persons who have stake in the decisions to be made. That is, the WRE can be a useful tool for shared decision-making, where considerations are presented by multiple persons and parties.

Moreover, in any of the possible outcomes, the WRE shows us that there does not have to be a single decision, recommendation, or outcome; some outcomes may be ethically preferable than others, however, the best outcome is one that has been carefully vetted through the WRE framework. With new information, the decisions may change, the patient, family and/or surrogates may be understood more fully as stakeholders in a shared decision-making process, and the healthcare team will have recognized that medical decisions, policies, and even laws may be subjected to revision and refinement. More importantly, once more permanent decisions are made such that ECMO is withdrawn, it is important for such decisions to be reflected on, asking "what other considerations might we have failed to consider?"

4.2 Case 2

A 22-year-old, previously healthy, male patient presents with severe cardiac failure due to fulminant myocarditis associated with a viral infection. The patient, T.K. has been experiencing flu-like symptoms for over 3 weeks without seeking appropriate medical attention. After passing out at a fast food restaurant, paramedics arrived on the scene and suspected cardiogenic shock, which was confirmed by his healthcare team. Clinical tests further confirm tachycardia, hypotension, left ventricle dysfunction, severe respiratory failure, and rapidly evolving multi-organ failure. Furthermore, T.K. did not respond to mechanical ventilation. Currently, T.K. is on ECMO as a potential bridge to VAD, however, due to a significant embolic stroke sustained while on ECMO, it is unlikely that he will survive with meaningful quality of life. T.K. has already been resuscitated, and the healthcare team is questioning whether to continue ECMO treatment toward VAD, continue ECMO for a short time ("bridge to nowhere"), withdraw ECMO, or consider OP-ECMO. T.K. currently does not have decision-making capacity; his estranged father is at his bedside and trying to make sense of the situation.

4.2.1 Initial moral judgment

While there are several possible courses of actions, the healthcare team could take their initial moral judgment that is to avoid as much harm to the patient as possible, while establishing a more accurate prognosis regarding T.K.'s quality of life. The team also believes that including T.K.'s father in ongoing discussions about his son's prognosis is ethically appropriate.

4.2.2 Background beliefs and theories

When considering the risks and benefits of the options presented by the healthcare team that are specific to T.K. and his current status, it is clear that without ECMO support, there is no hope of recovery. In regard to their "hope for recovery," the healthcare team reviews all of the clinical facts surrounding T.K.'s situation. For example, it is not uncommon for patients on ECMO to have neurological complications such as ischemic stroke, however, outcomes are limited to few reported cases [6]. The amount of neurological damage due to embolic stroke and quality of life is uncertain until the patient is able to move from critical care to a period of recovery, where further neurological assessment can be done along with rehabilitative interventions. Although, it is initially suspected that T.K. will have a poor quality of life if he survives, uncertainty gives the healthcare team pause. They have seen some patients recover, and others who had to be withdrawn from ECMO with no survivability. T.K.'s young age and prior health status contribute to the team's push to continue ECMO, while being mindful of the inherent and ongoing risks of continued treatment. The team can continue to try to manage the emerging multi-organ distress and provide medication therapy and other interventions to monitor and prevent further neurological damage, while also setting important limits to their efforts. As for using ECMO as a bridge to VAD, the uncertainty of the current health status of the patient prompts a more "wait and see" approach. With that, the team also should realistically consider the higher rates of long-term disability and morbidity and mortality rates with T.K.'s co-morbidities and the surmounting financial burdens to the patient, family, and/or healthcare institution. However, the team's decision should not be isolated from a surrogate decision-maker. Thus, they need to first establish who is the surrogate decision-maker before moving forward in providing continued ECMO support in a "wait and see" approach.

T.K. is unmarried, does not have a significant other in his life, and his only family is a distant cousin who lives three states away and his estranged father. His father left T.K. and his mother, when he was 15 years old. Since the time, T.K.'s mother passed away from metastatic ovarian cancer, and he has been putting himself through college, while working a full-time job as an apprentice carpenter. T.K. talked to his father a few times on the phone over the past 2 years (his father calls every birthday); they met once for coffee about 2 months prior to T.K.'s hospitalization. T.K.'s father wanted to be back in his son's life and has been at his bedside nearly every day since his hospitalization. Given this information, and the legal requirements for next of kin (i.e., parent), the team is comfortable with providing ongoing communication with the father and involving him in shared decision-making regarding his son.

T.K.'s father does not insist that "everything be done" but approaches the situation based on what he feels his son would want. He describes his son as a "fighter," who is resilient, physically and emotionally strong, and would not want to be in a position, where he would have no quality of life or possibility to "fight" for his independence. The father is hopeful for his son's recovery, and willing to put in the work to secure him the resources he needs, however, he has also requested that if nothing more can be done, to simply "let him rest in peace" without "being a guinea pig" for scientific discovery. His reason for leaving his wife was due to her reliance on homeopathic medicine, and for never giving Western medicine a chance. T.K.

resented both of his parents for their actions but was willing to rekindle his relationship with his father, as reported by his father.

4.2.3 Moral principles and theories

In considering the clinical narrative of T.K., his father's narrative, and the healthcare team's initial moral judgment, it would seem as though the initial decisions to continue ECMO and treat the existing co-morbid issues, while engaging T.K.'s father in ongoing conversations about treatments and prognosis aligns with the principles of beneficence and nonmaleficence. T.K.'s father, in considering his son's needs and interests first, recognizes the importance of quality of life, end of life decision-making that is in the best interests of the patient, and the difficult nature of this clinical situation, which could change at any moment. Both the healthcare team and T.K.'s father mutually supports the decision to continue ECMO, treat any underlying problems, monitor the neurological effects from the stroke, and determine next steps. If and when T.K. should continue to decline, and ECMO is no longer beneficial, the team has discussed further options with his father including removal of ECMO. Advance care planning is guided by a care ethics approach, which involves caring for T.K. and his father (e.g., bereavement counseling), as well as the promotion of T.K.'s autonomy through surrogate decision-making, i.e., decisions based on what T.K. would have wanted if he were able to decide for himself.

4.2.4 A need to refine the coherence framework with new information

T.K. continues to decline, including an LV distention and subsequent pulmonary edema, and the neurological effects of the embolic stroke have proven to be severe. T.K.'s father, distraught with the new information, and knowing this is the end for his sons, asks the team to continue ECMO support for purposes of organ procurement, as "my son was a giving person, and I believe he would want to be able to help others." However, with multi-organ failure, a viral infection, prior ischemic stroke, and pulmonary edema, the team suspects there are no viable organs despite recent success cases [28], and thus, the best decision is to remove ECMO and allow T.K. to have dignity at the end of his life. The inconclusive nature of brain death determinations on ECMO, the high probability of non-viable organs that would be otherwise discarded rather than donated, the lack of robust case presentations and evidence-based medicine regarding ECMO patients as organ donors, and the rapid decline of T.K., all contributed to the background belief that ECMO should be withdrawn without pursuing organ procurement. This belief or rather the facts of the case, thus support the initial moral judgment to reduce or avoid unnecessary harm and keep T.K.'s father well-informed. However, the "wait and see" approach needs to be refined given the new clinical information (i.e., T.K.'s new prognosis), and the meaning of "harm" can be elucidated with a deeper examination of the ethical theories and principles as well as the status of the medical interventions (i.e., ECMO is no longer beneficial).

4.2.5 Revision, refinement, and reflection

In considering the new information, the healthcare team discusses removal of ECMO support and the inability to procure viable organs at this time, despite the honorable and altruistic recommendation by T.K.'s father. The team openly discusses the relatively new approaches to organ procurement from patients, who are on ECMO, and some of the ethical and pragmatic concerns with the father. T.K.'s father understands what the team is relaying and is in agreement that more harm than good can arise from organ procurement; however, he does question whether removal of ECMO is necessary, given that T.K. is rapidly declining and has no hope for survival anyways. The team then explains that because ECMO is no longer beneficial, if T.K. were to remain on this technology for any length of time, additional harms, i.e., damage to his body, are likely and the team does not want to contribute to those harms if they can prevent them. Of note, it is difficult for everyone who has cared about T.K. to see him continue without any benefit (moral distress). Even if a non-beneficial treatment policy were to be implemented by the healthcare team, which permits them to forgo treatment that is not a benefit to the patient when family or surrogates insist to continue treatment, having the honest and open conversation prior any discussion surrounding hospital policy is preferable. The team is able to share what they mean by "harm" and have an opportunity to understand the family or surrogate's point of view. Here, T.K.'s father understands that medicine cannot bring back his son, and collectively decides to withdraw ECMO support with the healthcare team. However, ethical considerations should not end simply with this decision; the healthcare team should reflect on the father's experiences: losing his wife who refused Western medicine and losing a son with the limitations of Western medicine. Further care such as grief counseling, support groups, or simply acknowledging this difficult time should be part of the WRE; all persons involved ought to be considered along with those decisions or recommendations that emerge from achieving coherence. That is, the WRE prompts us to see all issues or concerns of a case or situation that involve multiple persons (healthcare team, patients, and family/surrogate).

Part of the ethical framework also prompts the healthcare team, institutions, and others to think critically about future patients, policies, and guidelines that could open up the organ donor pool significantly while giving family and surrogates the opportunity to make such decisions. In the end, while T.K.'s father agrees to the withdraw of ECMO treatment, there is also the possibility of future family members or surrogates who insist on continuing ECMO support in the effort to hold onto hope. In such cases, the WRE can help guide healthcare teams and families to understand the limits of medical technology, the importance of deciding what the patient would have wanted, the harms of continuing non-beneficial treatment, and the resources available for bereavement and support when letting go of a loved one.

The case of T.K. could had a very different outcome; instead of a rapid decline and no benefit of ECMO, to improvement with continued ECMO support, but not without future extensive rehabilitation, and a loss of quality of life (i.e., T.K. no longer able to work, go to school, or have the same capabilities as he did prior to hospitalization). Such decisions, though, should ultimately be left up to the family or surrogate decision-maker as to whether to continue ECMO or to withdraw given the prognosis of a potentially poor quality of life and a lifetime of ongoing care. Advance care planning, then, is essential for patients and families confronted with these ECMO decisions, as is the understanding of "harms" and "quality of life" as every outcome does not lead to a complete recovery without complications. Each patient and family member or surrogate will have different values and interpretations that ultimately ought to be respected by the healthcare team following shared decision-making and a careful consideration of the elements of the WRE, especially as new information requires us to revise, refine, and reflect on previously held judgments and actions.

5. Concluding thoughts

Although our two patients, M.J. and T.K., do not have successful outcomes with ECMO, and are unable to utilize this technology as a bridge to recovery; this does not suggest ECMO for them is simply a "bridge to nowhere." What ECMO became for them was a bridge for careful ethical considerations, meaningful family and surrogate engagement and support, shared decision-making with the healthcare team, and outcomes that preserved the quality of life at the end of life. While ECMO had to be withdrawn, it was not done hastily, and pushes the healthcare community, including clinical ethicists, to critically think about best practices, policies, and ethical guidance, and the future of ECMO for such opportunities as organ donation.

Author details

Julie Aultman[1] and Michael S. Firstenberg[2,3]*

1 Northeast Ohio Medical University, Rootstown, Ohio, United States

2 The Medical Center of Aurora, Aurora, Colorado, United States

3 Adjunct Faculty, College of Graduate Studies, Northeast Ohio Medical University, Rootstown, Ohio, United States

*Address all correspondence to: msfirst@gmail.com

References

[1] Abrams DC, Prager K, Blinderman CD, Burkart KM, Brodie D. Ethical dilemmas encountered with the use of extracorporeal membrane oxygen in adults. Chest. 2014;**145**(4):876-882

[2] Makdisi G, Wang IW. Extra corporeal membrane oxygenation (ECMO) review of a lifesaving technology. Journal of Thoracic Disease. 2015;**7**:E166-E176

[3] Makdisi G, Makdisi PB, Wang IW. New horizons of non-emergent use of extracorporeal membranous oxygenator support. Annals of Translational Medicine. 2016;**4**:76

[4] Makdisi T, Makdisi G. Extra corporeal membrane oxygenation support: Ethical dilemmas. Annals of Translational Medicine. 2017;**5**(5):112

[5] Pavlushkov E, Berman M, Valchanov K. Cannulation techniques for extracorporeal life support. Annals of Translational Medicine. 2017;**5**(4):70. DOI: 10.21037/atm.2016.11.47

[6] Nasr DM, Rabinstein AA. Neurologic complications of extracorporeal membrane oxygenation. Clinical Neurology and Neurosurgery. 2015;**11**(4):383-389

[7] Courtwright AM, Robinson EM, Feins K, et al. Ethics committee consultation and extracorporeal membrane oxygenation. Annals of the American Thoracic Society. 2016;**13**:1553-1558

[8] Bartlett RH, Gattinoni L. Current status of extracorporeal life support (ECMO) for cardiopulmonary failure. Minerva Anestesiologica. 2010;**76**:534-540

[9] Ramanathan K, Cove ME, Caleb MG, Teoh KLK, Maclaren G. Ethical dilemmas of adult ECMO: Emerging conceptual challenges. Journal of Cardiothoracic and Vascular Anesthesia. 2015;**29**(1):229-233

[10] Gamulka BD. Ethical uncertainty: An approach to decisions involving extracorporeal membrane oxygenation. CMAJ. 1994;**150**:565-568

[11] Howe EG. New paradigms in medical ethics. The Journal of Clinical Ethics. 2016;**27**(4):267-280

[12] Shah KB, Levenson JL, Mehra MR. Emergent use of mechanical circulatory support devices: Ethical dilemmas. Current Opinion in Cardiology, Wolters Kluwer Health. 2014;**29**:281-284

[13] Meltzer EC et al. Extracorporeal membrane oxygenation as a bridge to chemotherapy in an orthodox Jewish patient. The Oncologist. 2014;**19**:985-989

[14] Dalle Ave AL, Gardiner D, Shaw DM. The ethics of extracorporeal membrane oxygenation in brain-dead potential organ donors. Transplant International. 2016;**29**:612-618

[15] Nguyen D. Brain death and true patient care. The Linacre Quarterly. 2016;**83**(3):258-282

[16] Morales N. "Dead" man recovering after ATV accident. NBC News. 2008. Available from: http://www.nbcnews.com/id/23768436/ns/dateline_nbc-newsmakers/t/dead-man-recovering-after-atv-accident

[17] Malm S. The girl who wouldn't die: Incredible story of the 19-year-old who woke up as doctors were preparing to harvest her organs. Daily Mail (UK). 2012. Available from: http://www.dailymail.co.uk/ news/article-2219085/Carina-Melchior- The-girl-wouldnt-die-Miracle-Danish-girl-woke-doctors-prepared-organs-donated.html

[18] O'Brien J, Mulder JT. St. Joe's "dead" patient awoke as docs pre- pared to remove organs. Syracuse.com. 2013. Available from: http://www.syracuse.com/news/index.ssf/2013/07/st_joes_fined_over_ dead_patien.html

[19] Joffe AR, Kolski H, Duff J, deCaen AR. A 10-month-old infant with reversible findings of brain death. Pediatric Neurology. 2009;**41**(5):378-382

[20] Webb AC, Samuels OB. Reversible brain death after cardiopulmonary arrest and induced hypothermia. Critical Care Medicine. 2011, 2011;**39**(6):1538-1542

[21] Bein T, Weber-Carstens S, Herridge M. Extracorporeal life support, ethics, and questions at the bedside: How does the end of the pathway look? Intensive Care Medicine. 2015;**41**:1714-1715

[22] Meltzer EC, Ivascu NS, Stark M, Orfanos AV, Acres CA, Christos PJ, et al. A survey of physicians' attitudes toward decision-making authority for initiating and withdrawing VA-ECMO: Results and ethical implications for shared decision making. The Journal of Clinical Ethics. 2016;**27**(4):281-289

[23] Nielsen K. Relativism and wide reflective equilibrium. The Monist. 1993;**76**(3):316-332

[24] Nielsen K. Reflective equilibrium and the transformation of philosophy. Metaphilosophy. 1989;**20**(3/4):235-246

[25] Rawls J. A Theory of Justice. 2nd ed. Cambridge MA: Harvard University Press; 1971

[26] Beauchamp T, Childress J. Principles of Biomedical Ethics. 5th ed. Oxford: Oxford University Press; 2001

[27] McCarthy J. Principlism or narrative ethics: Must we choose between them? Journal Medical Ethics; Medical Humanities. 2003;**29**:65-71

[28] Dewei R, Abu Saleh WK, Al Jabbari O, Ramlawi B, Bruckner BA, Suarez E, et al. Lung procurement from a donor on ECMO support. American Society of Artificial Internal Organs (ASAIO) Journal. 2015;**61**:e40-e41

Chapter 5

Echocardiography Evaluation in ECMO Patients

Luigi Tritapepe, Ernesto Greco and Carlo Gaudio

Abstract

Extracorporeal membrane oxygenation (ECMO) is a special form of organ support for selected cases of cardiovascular and severe respiratory failure. Echocardiography is a diagnostic and monitoring tool widely used in all aspects of ECMO support. The pathophysiology of ECMO, and its distinct effects on cardiorespiratory physiology, requires an echocardiographer with high skills to understand the interaction between the ECMO and the patient. In this chapter, we present the main application of echocardiography in ECMO patients and some general concepts on the ECMO working. ECMO, such as the standard cardiopulmonary bypass employed in cardiac surgery, V-V (veno-venous), can support the insufficient respiratory system by oxygenating and removing carbon dioxide from the blood. VA-ECMO (venous-arterial) can support haemodynamics by providing mechanical circulatory assistance. Today, ECMO can be used as bridge to decision, waiting for the development of the clinical conditions to support with other devices the evolution of cardiorespiratory failure or stop the assistance. Echocardiography (transthoracic (TTE) or transoesophageal (TOE)) can be used primarily to take decisions regarding appropriateness of ECMO support, therefore to control cannula insertion and confirm final position, to modify number and position of the cannulae in case of malfunctioning of these, and, finally, to assess clinical progress and suitability for weaning from ECMO.

Keywords: echocardiography, critical care, ARDS, extracorporeal cardiopulmonary resuscitation, thromboembolism, tamponade, hemodynamic monitoring, VV-ECMO, VA-ECMO

1. Introduction

Cardiac surgeons and/or cardiac anaesthesiologists after cardiac operations prevalently use the ECMO in its VA-ECMO configuration for cardio-circulatory failure [1, 2]. Recently, ECMO in its veno-venous configuration is becoming widely used in ICU by intensivists to treat severe form of respiratory failure (ARDS) [3, 4] after the recent successes obtained with the use of ECMO in the A(H1N1) influenza epidemic [5, 6], linked to the results of CESAR Trial [7].

At the same time, the practice of echocardiographic investigation in intensive care units by the intensivists combined the echocardiographic method to haemodynamic monitoring, favouring the use of echocardiography for the assessment of haemodynamic and respiratory instability [8].

The patient who needs extracorporeal support is thus evaluated by the echocardiographer who establishes the timing of the support, the need for support, and the

PRINCIPAL INDICATIONS FOR THE TWO TYPES OF ECMO	
VA-ECMO	VV-ECMO
Cardiac arrest and cardiogenic shock	Pneumonia
Poisoning and drug overdose	ARDS
Pulmonary embolism	Pulmonary contusion
Hypothermia	Status asthmaticus
Massive pulmonary hemorrhage	Aspiration or inhalation injury
Bridge to transplant, to decision, to recovery, to candidacy	Drowing
Sepsis	

Table 1.
Main indications for the use of ECMO assistance.

contraindications to the support and follows the phases of cannulation and functioning of the extracorporeal support [9].

ECMO is a rescue therapy used to provide cardiac and/or respiratory support for critically ill patients in whom maximal conventional medical management failed [3, 4]. VV-ECMO provides adequate oxygenation and removal of carbon dioxide in isolated refractory respiratory failure, while VA-ECMO is used when support for cardiac and /or respiratory failure is needed [1] (**Table 1**).

1.1 General role of echocardiography

Echocardiography (ECHO) plays a pivotal role in the management of critical patients, particularly those supported with ECMO [9–11]. ECHO can be used to not only evaluate function and diagnose diseases requiring ECMO but also to detect all cardiac complications or vascular diseases that may arise following ECMO [12, 13].

The central role of ECHO is important to identifying various diseases such as cardiac /undiagnosed valve lesions and left ventricular (LV) dysfunction, which could be the cause of severe haemodynamic instability, as well as to exclude them to avoid ECMO support [11].

The detection of aortic dissection represents an absolute contraindication in VA-ECMO, whereas a moderate to severe aortic valve regurgitation (AVR) is a relative contraindication in VA-ECMO, because the LV afterload increase, determining by ECMO itself, leads a worsening in AVR. ECHO provides information on aortic atherosclerosis and then guides the intensivist to decide the suitable cannulation sites (central versus peripheral) or the technique (surgical versus percutaneous) [13]. ECHO also helps to evaluate the right heart morphology for any structural abnormality, which could prevent the positioning of venous cannula for VV-ECMO or VA-ECMO [14].

In addition, as stated above, ECHO has a key role during ECMO cannulation. First, it guides the correct placement of the ECMO cannulae [15]. TTE may not be able to guide ECMO cannulation because of limited spatial resolution, and therefore transoesophageal echocardiography (TOE) represents the examination of choice to guiding the insertion. Echocardiographer and intensivist have to work together in order to correct the final position of the cannulae [15]. In VV-ECMO the position of the tips of the venous cannulae is essential for the correct functioning of the ECMO. Indeed, the drainage cannula must be positioned just before the entrance of the inferior vena cava (IVC) in the right atrium (RA), while the tip of the return cannula must be positioned in the central part of the RA just before the tricuspid valve but far away from the inter-atrial septum [16].

However, the echocardiographic evaluation is also essential for the identification and management of specific complications that may arise during ECMO support and may determine its malfunction. For the problems related to TTE resolution, also involving to the patient's respiratory pathology, the TOE is preferred to make it clear any possible complication [17]. ECHO allows a rapid evaluation not only of the positioning of the cannula but mainly of the cardiac filling, of the cardiac function, and of the cardiac tamponade [16, 17]. Detection of cardiac tamponade and evaluation of the significance of pericardial effusion or collection may be difficult in patients supported with ECMO because the heart is in a partially bypassed state.

In conclusion, ECHO is mandatory during the start of ECMO, cannulae insertion, haemodynamic monitoring, and detection of complications during weaning [16–18].

1.1.1 Ultrasonography for ECMO cannulation

In many cases, cannulation can be performed without ultrasound guidance. However, the use of ultrasound can help to reduce the rate of complications associated with cannulation such as haematoma, retroperitoneal haematoma, vascular damage, cardiac tamponade, and ischemia of the lower leg [19]. In the paediatric patient, the eco-guided cannulation has been shown to reduce complications, especially the need for surgical placement [20, 21].

The ultrasound evaluation of the diameter of the vessels to be cannulated, especially the femoral artery, allows to choose the right size of the cannula, avoiding vascular occlusions distal to the cannulation point, with consequent ischemia, for example, of the lower limb [15, 19]. Cannulation can be carried out echo-guided or echo-assisted, i.e. only by identifying the insertion point. Today the ultrasound shows a greater sensitivity and specificity compared to radiography in identifying the exact point of arrival of the cannulae. The exact position of the femoral arterial cannula allows to optimise the flow, as well as the exact position of the venous cannula in IVC, above the hepatic vein, and contributes to an excellent drainage, clearly optimising hepatic drainage [22] (**Figure 1**). The echocardiography, after the positioning of the cannulae, must be performed to highlight early cardiac tamponade and problems of acute dilatation of the ventricles [14, 16, 23]. The use of colour Doppler also highlights problems of distal perfusion in the lower limb, such as having to provide with dedicated shunts.

Before dilating vein for venous cannulation, it is necessary to make sure that guide wires, percutaneously inserted, are positioned inside the heart or large vessels. Only after ultrasound confirmation, physicians can proceed to advance the cannulae on these wires. However, it is necessary to discriminate the real images from the echocardiographic artefacts generated by these wires and cannulae, before proceeding to the final position of the cannulae. In the peripheral configurations of ECMO, especially in the VA-ECMO, we must assist with ultrasound the placement of the venous cannula in the middle of the right atrium in order to obtain an optimal drainage [13, 14] (**Figure 2**). With TOE, the bi-caval projection is able to orient perfectly on the optimal position of the venous cannula (**Figure 3**). Although the ultrasounds cannot indicate the level of the arterial cannula tip, which reaches the iliac artery from the femoral artery, they can confirm that the guide wire used in percutaneous arterial cannulation is located in the lumen of the aorta, before the femoral artery dilatation, reducing the risk of extra-arterial placement of the cannula.

1.1.2 Cannula position/complications

Therefore, summing up, it is essential to visualise in real time the positioning of the guide wires in the caval districts (IVC and SVC) with the middle oesophageal

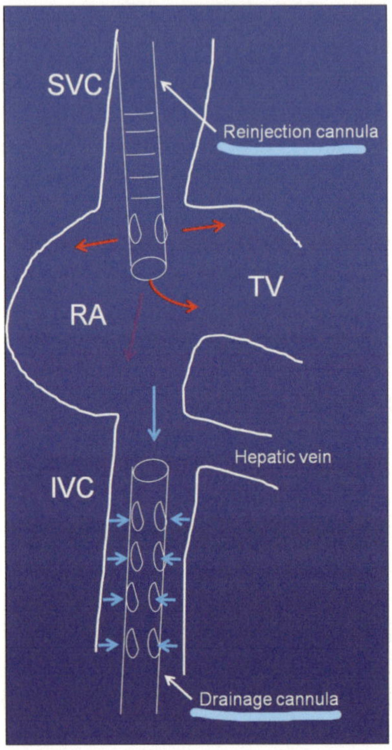

Figure 1.
Cannulation scheme in VV-ECMO. The red arrows indicate the reinfusion of oxygenated blood, the purple arrow indicates the recirculating blood, and the light blue arrows indicate the drainage of the venous blood. SVC, superior vena cava; IVC, inferior vena cava; TV, tricuspid valve; RA, right atrium.

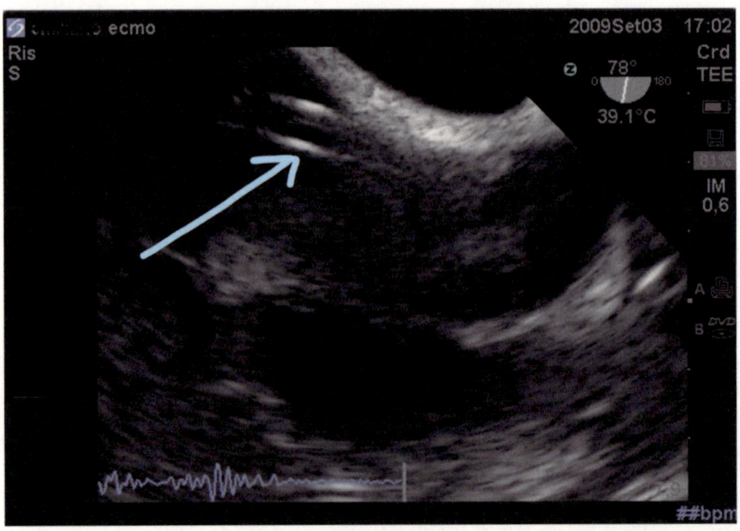

Figure 2.
Bi-caval view of the TOE: the drainage cannula from the IVC is visible in the middle atrium (arrow light blue).

bi-caval projection to the TOE [11] (**Figures 2–4**). This is to avoid incorrect positioning of the cannula in the right ventricle, in the coronary sinus, or, worse, in the left atrium through a patent foramen ovale (PFO) [11, 13, 16]. During the entire positioning manoeuvres of the venous cannulae, particular attention must be paid to the presence of pericardial effusion, from atrial/right ventricular trauma, and to

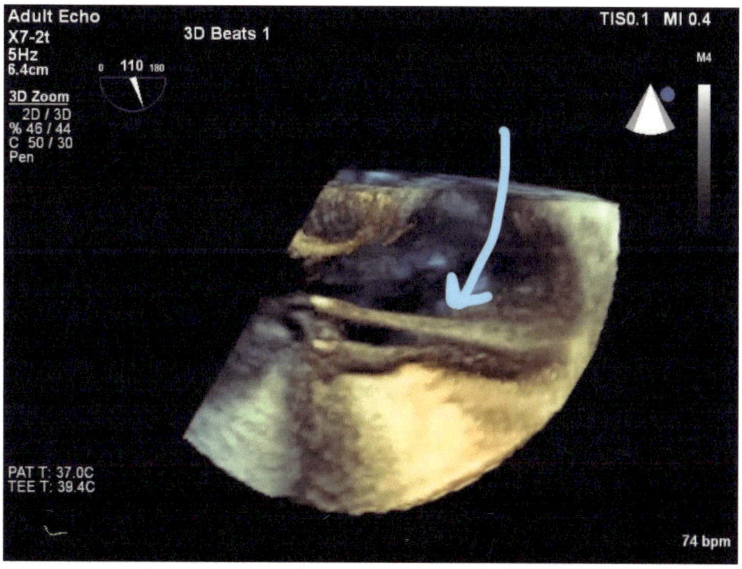

Figure 3.
Bi-caval view to the 3D TOE: the drainage cannula from the IVC can be seen in the middle atrium (arrow light blue).

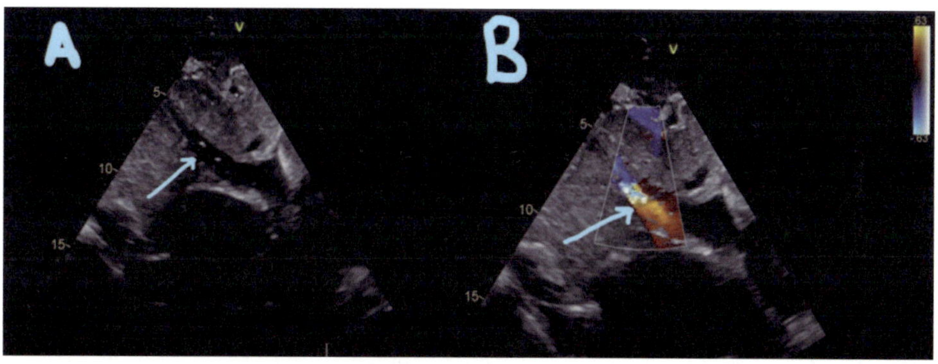

Figure 4.
(A) Drainage cannula in IVC (light blue arrow) and (B) colour Doppler showing the flow in the cannula.

the possible suction of the inter-atrial septum, with the obstruction of the drainage flow, linked to the venous aspiration from an adherent cannula to the septum itself [24, 25]. In the case of loss of oxygen performance of the ECMO, when a recirculation phenomenon is suspected due to a close position of the tips of the drainage and reinfusion cannulae, TOE can guide the correct repositioning of the cannulae [26].

1.1.3 Special cannulation (Avalon® cannula)

Compared to the classic configuration of the VV-ECMO which provides a double cannulation, the development of newer devices, such as the Dual Lumen Bi-Caval catheter (Avalon®, *Maquet Cardiopulmonary GmbH Kehler Str. 31, 76,437 Rastatt, Germany*), allowed VV-ECMO with a single cannula inserted in the right internal jugular vein [27]. This allows greater patient mobility, also reducing the femoral cannula decubitus and the infectious risk that this entails. However, being a stiffer and larger diameter cannula, the placement of the bi-luminal cannula involves greater risks of vessel injury and cardiac tamponade, in addition to the possible malfunction due to migration of the cannula from its original position [28, 29]. It is essential to use the TOE for the correct positioning of the Avalon® catheter. In fact, the tip of the cannula is advanced under the TOE guide until the cannula drainage holes are positioned in the inferior and in the superior venae cave (like a normal two-stage cannula used for cardiopulmonary bypass), and the re-entry is perfectly aligned with the inflow of the tricuspid valve [27]. This alignment is investigated with the colour Doppler which will measure the linear flow in case of correct positioning or a turbulent flow, in case of malposition. It is best to advance and withdraw the cannula under the TOE guide until the flow is laminar and directed through the centre of the tricuspid valve. Particular attention should be paid to visualising the cannula tip in the hepatic vein. A malposition of the cannula will cause recirculation, because the oxygenated blood from the cannula is drained immediately from the suction areas of the cannula to the ECMO circuit before being circulated systematically [28, 30].

1.2 Veno-venous ECMO

In the treatment of severe respiratory failure (severe ARDS), VV-ECMO is a valid option [31]. It can be considered a bridge to the healing of the lung, allowing the therapies to act effectively. Moreover, unlike the VA-ECMO it does not present problems of oxygenation north-south (harlequin syndrome). All this is valid if cardiac function is maintained normal and able to effectively support the systemic circulation. Therefore, before a VV-ECMO is established, a complete evaluation of both the patient's echocardiographic and haemodynamic parameters is essential [11, 16]. Echocardiography, both TTE and TOE, must ensure a correct evaluation of the right ventricular function and evaluate the degree of tricuspid insufficiency and the estimate of pulmonary artery pressure, potentially altered parameters in the course of ARDS, and sepsis [32].

VV-ECMO could improve the performance of the right ventricle and the whole heart. There is an irrelevant modification of the right preload, an increase in the left load due to a reduction in pulmonary pressure with a further increase in SvO_2, and the saturation of the coronary blood. Approximately 20–25% of patients with ARDS develop an acute cor pulmonale (ACP) with right ventricular dilatation, inter-ventricular septum shift, left ventricular hypo-diastolic status, and pulmonary hypertension [32, 33]. This clinical picture is also typical of the right ventricular failure induced by the septic state. Echocardiography helps to choose the right timing for extracorporeal support and allows to follow the evolutionary state (improvement) of the right performance following VV-ECMO support: reduction of pulmonary pressure, increase in right contractility (increased systolic excursion of the tricuspid annular plane (TAPSE)), and improvement of the cardiac output (CO) [11, 16, 34].

TTE echocardiographic evaluation in patients with ARDS may present some resolution problems; therefore, normally the TOE is used, also because of low invasiveness as the patients are already intubated and sedated.

The presence of pulmonary hypertension and sepsis can create the conditions for a rapid deterioration of cardiac function, so that can worsen from initial presence of respiratory failure to cardiorespiratory insufficiency. Through echocardiographic and haemodynamic monitoring, we can anticipate the worsening of the clinical picture and establish a cardiorespiratory support (VA-ECMO).

1.2.1 Echo in VV-ECMO

The right ventricle echocardiographic assessment in the ECMO patients with acute respiratory distress syndrome (ARDS) plays a key role to reduce complications and to improve the outcome [11, 14, 16, 31].

It is simple to understand the role of ECHO in the risk stratification of patients undergoing VV-ECMO. In fact, ARDS requires an initial aggressive ventilatory treatment that brings to haemodynamic instability [33]. Patient presents high CVP associated to fluid accumulation in the pleural and abdominal spaces. ECHO shows a dilatation of the right ventricle with associated pulmonary hypertension. This clinical picture is described as ACP [8, 32, 33]. To minimise the impact of the positive end-expiratory pressure (PEEP) on right ventricular haemodynamic, physicians have choice a right balance between the PEEP value and cardio-circulatory stability. The therapeutic request is the protective ventilation aimed at reducing right ventricular failure related to an increase in the afterload of the right chambers [8, 33]. The aim of the treatment is the reduction of pulmonary arterial hypertension to reduce enlargement of right ventricle and consequent shift of the inter-ventricular septum. Unfortunately, despite implementation of protective lung ventilation, ACP still remains until 25% [32, 33, 34]. VV-ECMO represents a real solution to support both the lung and the right ventricle [35, 36].

The improvement of gas exchange and the reduction of airway pressures both contribute at the reduction of pulmonary vascular resistance with consequent hemodynamic improvement.

The daily evaluation of echocardiography in this case is mandatory.

Because the high acoustic impedance is caused by high PEEP values, TTE cannot be straightforward, and TOE is preferred.

A recently published summary paper on the management of ECMO recommends that physician training in echocardiography be part in the ECMO patient care team [37].

However, the role of echocardiography in ECMO is not widely accepted and is still poorly described in the literature.

The echocardiographic examination of the right ventricle requires a long axis and a short axis view to evaluate the size of the cavity with the relationship of the left ventricle and the kinetics of the septum. The examination can be completed by the Doppler of the right ventricular outflow and tricuspid regurgitation when present, to measure the systolic pressure of the pulmonary artery. The measurement of the TAPSE, simple and useful from prognostic point of view, avoids measuring the fractional area change (FAC) of the right ventricle more complicated. Right ventricle TDI (tissue Doppler imaging) is useful to evaluate diastolic and systolic functions [38].

Moderate to severe right ventricular dilatations, defined as a ratio greater than 0.6 and as a ratio greater than or equal to 1, are associated with paradoxical septum motion at the end systole complicating the left ventricular function [8, 39, 40].

Pulmonary hypertension is usually associated with tricuspid regurgitation, but it also depends on right ventricular systolic function, and its value can be very low when associated with low CO [38, 39]. The right ventricular remodelling in ARDS patients is represented by the thickness of free wall, related to the increase in afterload [40]. Most important is also the detection of a PFO that can complicate the oxygenation of ARDS patients [39] (**Figures 5** and **6**). The displacement of septum due to right ventricular dilatation causes the left ventricular hypo-diastolic status, with a consequent low CO syndrome related to the difficult preload of the left ventricle. This is considered an ECHO evaluation of right ventricular function in pre-ECMO stage.

1.3 VA-ECMO

The purpose of the VA-ECMO is to support cardio-circulatory function in patients with heart failure refractory to medical therapy [1, 36]. Based on the INTERMACS class it belongs to, VA-ECMO can be used in major risk classes, not only as bridge to recovery or bridge to destination therapy (left ventricular assist device (LVAD) or heart transplantation (HTx)) but also as bridge to decision [41] (**Table 2**). In addition, the VA-ECMO can be used in haemodynamic support to

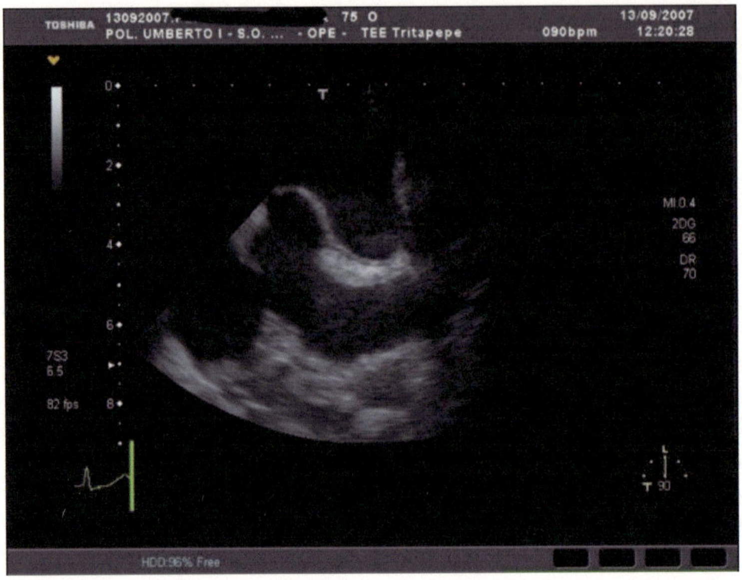

Figure 5.
Bi-caval view in which an aneurysm of the inter-atrial septum is seen.

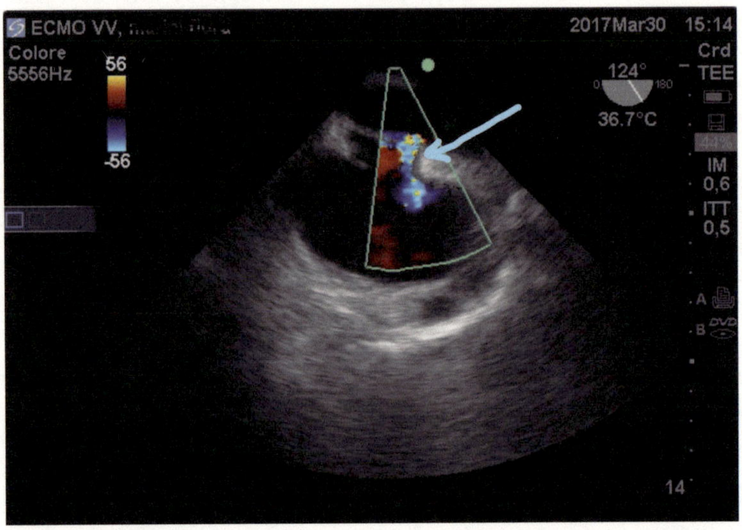

Figure 6.
Colour Doppler bi-caval view in which you see the shunt through the PFO.

refractory cardiac arrest that can result in patient recovery or be used as a procedure for donation of splanchnic organs in non-beating heart [42, 43].

Compared to other mechanical cardiac assistance devices, ECMO has the advantage. of reduced costs and the possibility of being set up easily and quickly on the outside. of the operating room (intensive care unit, cardiac catheterization theatre, or emergency departments) and also during cardiopulmonary resuscitation manoeuvres [43]. However, it is an invasive assistance technique with major problems such as the short duration of assistance, the possible increase of infections, bleeding and thrombosis, and the increase of the afterload of the left ventricle.

The ultrasound evaluation is important before the implantation of the VA-ECMO. However, the conditions of the left ventricle, the degree of aortic

Type	Description
Bridge to decision	Use of VA-ECMO in pts with drug-refractory acute circulatory collapse and at immediate risk of death to sustain life until a full clinical evaluation can be completed and additional therapeutic options can be evaluated
Bridge to recovery	Use of VA-ECMO to keep patient alive until intrinsic cardiac function recovers sufficiently to remove VA-ECMO
Bridge to candidacy	Use of VA-ECMO to improve end-organ function in order to make an ineligible patient eligible for transplantation/LVAD
Brigde to transplantation	Use of VA-ECMO to keep a patient at high risk of death before transplantation alive until a donor organ becomes available

Table 2.
Possible uses of VA-ECMO.

insufficiency, and the presence of mitral and tricuspid valve insufficiencies must be carefully evaluated. The configuration of the VA-ECMO involves peripheral cannulations, already partially described, and central cannulations (right atrium and aorta) that can be performed in the cardiac surgery patient who has problems in weaning from the cardiopulmonary bypass.

1.3.1 Indications to VA-ECMO support: cardiogenic shock

In patients with cardiogenic shock, echocardiographic examination is necessary to determine cause and indication for extracorporeal support [41] (**Table 1**). Even more, the echo exam can identify situations that may contraindicate the placement of circulatory assistance.

The echo examination must be as complete as possible and must highlight the morphology and the systolic and diastolic functions of the ventricles, evaluate the valve continence and the presence of pericardial effusion, and seek, in greater detail, the cause of cardiogenic shock (i.e. regional or global dysfunction of the left ventricle) [39]. In the study of cardiac valvular function, the study of the aortic valve is fundamental since its regurgitation can create unfavourable conditions for the positioning of VA-ECMO, given the increase in the afterload that the VA-ECMO generates. Clearly aortic dissection is an absolute contraindication for VA-ECMO placement. In addition, the morphology and the structure of the right atrium and of the right heart in general must be carefully evaluated. In fact, the presence of leads (pacemaker or ICD), a prominent Chiari network, a PFO, a tricuspid valve prosthesis, they are all elements that can compromise or make atrial cannulation impossible [11].

1.3.2 Monitoring during ECMO performance

The echocardiographic examination must fundamentally focus on the systolic function of the left ventricle. The systolic function is evaluated with conventional parameters such as the size of the left ventricle (LV), ejection fraction (EF), mitral regurgitation dP/dt, and aortic velocity time integral (VTI) [39]. The blood flow of ECMO can be adjusted based on the overall assessment of ventricular systolic function and cardiac preload. Some authors have systematically studied the effect of the flow rate of oxygenation of the extracorporeal membrane on changes in cardiac parameters [44]. A decrease of flow from 4 to 0.7 L/min leads to a 22% increase in the E/E′ ratio (from 5.9 to 7.2; $p < 0.001$), an increase of 17% in EF (from 15 to 17.5%; 0.001), increase of 12 and 45% of VTI (from 8 to 11.6 cm; $p < 0.001$), and increase of 12% of the left ventricular tele-diastolic volume (from 95 to 108 ml, $p < 0.001$) [44, 45].

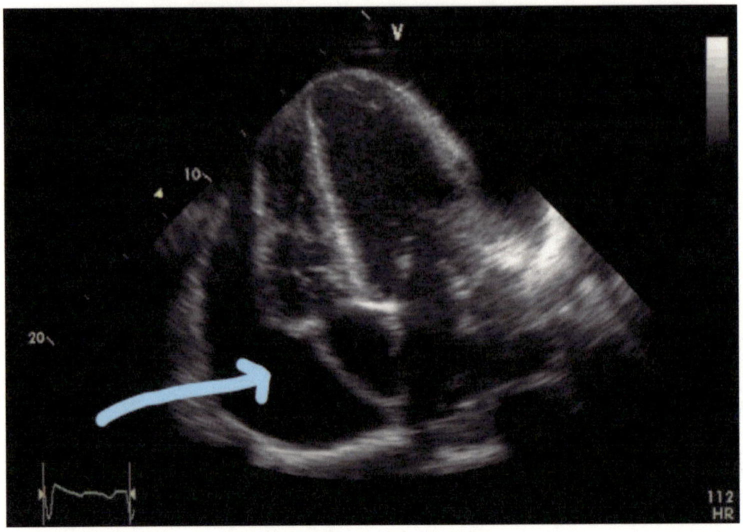

Figure 7.
Presence of abundant pericardial effusion (light blue arrow) at TTE.

A serious problem in the ultrasound evaluation is the detection of an evolving pericardial effusion to the cardiac tamponade (**Figure 7**), due to the passage of wires or cannulae with rupture of the cardiac chambers [11, 14, 16]. Following anticoagulant therapy, necessary in VA-ECMO, the pericardial blood collection can become consistent at many hours from the positioning, and only a series of ultrasound analysis allows the recognition of this clinical situation.

Thrombosis is a major complication during VA-ECMO and can be catastrophic when cerebral embolism occurs [46, 47]. Factors predisposing thrombosis are related to the blood/circuit contact and its activation as well as to the turbulence linked to the lumen of the cannulae [48]. Thrombosis can be more or less evident at ultrasound, and a real pitfall is represented by spontaneous intracavitary echo contrast (smoke) [49]. The evaluation of the opening of the aortic valve guarantees a certain pulsatility to the flow and avoids the stasis linked to the stagnant flow on the closed valve and predictor of thrombosis [46–49]. If the valve does not open, it is necessary to open the valve through changes in the flow of the VA-ECMO, the use of inodilator drugs, or the insertion of the intra-aortic balloon pump (IABP), which also favours the decompression of the left ventricle. Furthermore, in these cases it is necessary to optimise anticoagulation, which can be evaluated with specific point of care (thrombo-elastographic examination (TEG)) [50].

The increase in the afterload generated by the VA-ECMO can promote mitral-aortic valve regurgitation, compromising myocardial oxygenation and favouring the left ventricular distension not good for cardiac functional recovery.

1.3.3 ECHO in VA-ECMO

The difficult management of the patient in VA-ECMO must be accompanied by a continuous echocardiographic evaluation, carried out at least two times a day and whenever there is an unforeseen haemodynamic instability. The study of cardiac function should allow to optimise the flows of the mechanical support and the concomitant therapies. The ECHO evaluation must precede the start of the ECMO, follow the initial support phase, evaluate the evolution of the cardiac function in the stabilisation phase, and evaluate the cardiac functional recovery dictating the weaning time from the extracorporeal support.

1.3.4 ECMO start

At the start of the VA-ECMO, it is necessary to concentrate the attention on the venous drainage to be able to maintain the flow rate. Flow reduction may be due to obstructions (thrombus) or malposition of the cannula or hypovolaemia [11, 48]. A sudden reduction in perfusion pressure and low flow could lead to the search for aortic dissection or severe aortic valve regurgitation resulting in dilation of the left ventricle.

1.3.5 ECMO support

VA-ECMO is usually a medium-short duration assay, allowing the recovery of cardiac function or the bridge to other solutions (LVAD or HTx). At this time, echocardiographic monitoring is essential to monitor cardiac function recovery or lack of it.

One of the major problems, especially in the peripheral configuration of the VA-ECMO, is the distension of the left ventricle, such as to increase the tele-diastolic pressure and compromise the functional recovery of the heart [51, 52]. During peripheral VA-ECMO, LV preload usually decreases, but the LV afterload increases, resulting in a distension of the left ventricle associated with failure to open the aortic valve. The flow thus becomes continuous and non-pulsatile with consequent stasis, tendency to thrombosis, and embolization. This situation compromises the recovery of the heart.

The therapeutic strategy consists in venting the left ventricle [52] (**Figure 8**). The opening of the aortic valve can be done simply by trying to reduce the ECMO flow, but almost always you have to proceed with the IABP or better with the use of Impella® (ABIOMED, Inc., 22 Cherry Hill Drive, Danvers, MA 01923, USA) [53]. The most effective system is the cannulation of the left ventricular apex through a mini-thoracotomy, a procedure that can be performed under ultrasound guidance [52]. Echocardiographic monitoring has a key role in monitoring the distension of the left ventricle which leads to an increase in capillary pressure, interstitial pulmonary oedema, and bi-ventricular insufficiency. An alternative but less effective venting system is represented by an EndoVent in the pulmonary artery that, rather than detecting the left ventricle as it would take, reduces its preload [54]. Another solution for left ventricular decompression, in patients receiving extracorporeal

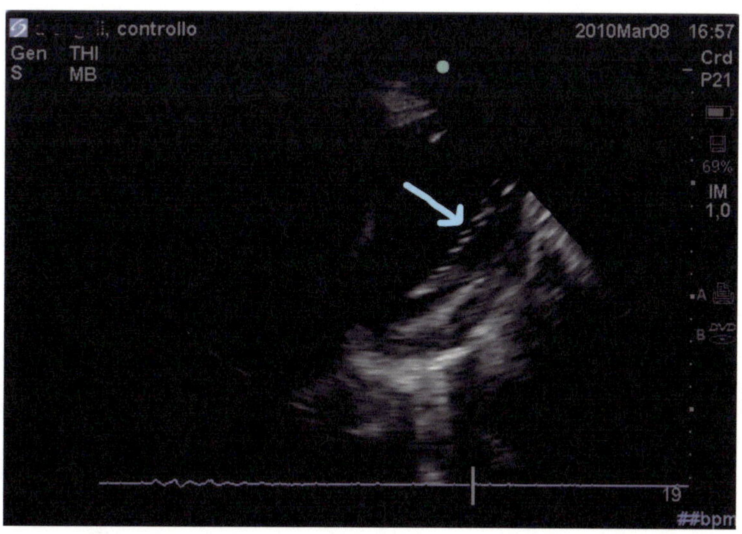

Figure 8.
The light blue indicates the presence of intraventricular vent for the unloading of the left ventricle.

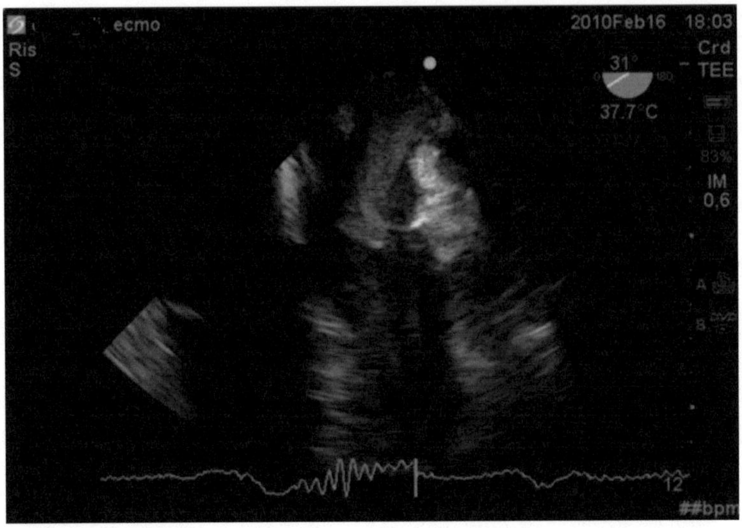

Figure 9.
TOE (4Ch view) of patient in VA-ECMO in which there is an extensive thrombotic formation of the left ventricle and of the left atrium.

membrane oxygenation for myocardial failure, is represented by balloon atrial septostomy, used especially in paediatric patients [55, 56].

Echocardiography, through the evaluation of trans-aortic flow, is a precious instrument to measure CO during ECMO support as all CO monitoring methods are affected by errors.

The evaluation of distal perfusion is mandatory, and in most cases the distal hypoperfusion must be resolved by a retrograde perfusion cannula.

1.3.6 Weaning from ECMO

The echocardiographic evaluation reaches its peak in determining the timing and the possibility of weaning from ECMO [57]. Clearly weaning is possible only if the recovery of cardiac function is associated, as is evident, with the resolution of the pathological conditions determining the use of the VA-ECMO. An indirect sign of recovery of cardiac function is the increase in systolic-diastolic blood pressure. The echocardiographic parameters, which may suggest a safe weaning from the VA-ECMO, are the aortic VTI > 10 cm, the absence of cardiac tamponade, the partial recovery of the EF%, but above all an increase of the Sa wave at the TDI (>6 cm/s) [57, 58].

During the weaning of the VA-ECMO, the flow of ECMO is reduced, and clinical, haemodynamic, and echocardiographic parameters are evaluated. ECMO flows are usually not reduced below 1–2 L/min, due to the increased risk of thrombosis (**Figure 9**) of the low-flow circuit [59, 60]. If the patient remains with stable haemodynamic at low flow, they can be ready to be disconnected from the support. Weaning and de-cannulation are delicate phases, and careful haemodynamic and echocardiographic evaluation is needed to identify and promptly deal with contingent problems.

The ultrasonography evaluation also allows the vascular evaluation after de-cannulation.

1.4 Conclusions

Ultrasounds play a fundamental role in managing patients supported with ECMO, during all the different stages of assistance [10, 11, 14–16, 58], from indication to cannulation, monitoring, and weaning. Either during circulatory or respiratory assistance, ultrasounds are fundamental to evaluate the cardiac function of the patients, providing information that determines appropriate patient selection. They are also needed to choose the best vascular access sites, guide the insertion of cannulas, monitor progress, detect complications, and help in determining recovery and weaning of support [10, 14–16, 34].

Author details

Luigi Tritapepe[1,2,5]*, Ernesto Greco[2,3,5] and Carlo Gaudio[2,4,5]

1 Anaesthesia and Intensive Care, Sapienza University of Rome, Italy

2 Department of Cardiovascular, Respiratory, Nephrology, Anaesthesiology and Geriatric Sciences, Rome, Italy

3 Cardiac Surgery, Sapienza University of Rome, Italy

4 Applied Medical Technical Sciences, Sapienza University of Rome, Italy

5 Policlinico Umberto I Hospital, Rome, Italy

*Address all correspondence to: luigi.tritapepe@uniroma1.it

References

[1] Pellegrino V. Extracorporeal membrane oxygenation. In: Bersten AD, Soni N, editors. Oh's Intensive Care Manual. 7th ed. China: Butterworth Heinemann Elsevier; 2014

[2] Marasco SF, Lukas G, McDonald M, McMillan J, Ihle B. Review of ECMO (extracorporeal membrane oxygenation) support in critically ill adult patients. Heart, Lung & Circulation. 2008;**17**(Suppl):S41-S47

[3] Allen S, Holena D, McCunn M, Kohl B, Sarani B. A review of the fundamental principles and evidence base in the use of extracorporeal membrane oxygenation (ECMO) in critically ill adult patients. Journal of Intensive Care Medicine. 2011;**26**:13-26

[4] Gattinoni L, Carlesso E, Langer T. Clinical review: Extracorporeal membrane oxygenation. Critical Care. 2011;**15**:243

[5] Davies A, Jones D, Bailey M, Beca J, Bellomo R, Blackwell N, et al. Extracorporeal membrane oxygenation for 2009 influenza A(H1N1) acute respiratory distress syndrome. JAMA. 2009;**302**:1888-1895

[6] Firstenberg MS, Blais D, Louis LB, Stevenson KB, Sun B, Mangino JE. Extracorporeal membrane oxygenation for pandemic (H1N1). Emerging Infectious Diseases. 2009;**15**:2059-2060

[7] Peek GJ, Mugford M, Tiruvoipati R, Wilson A, Allen E, Thalanany MM, et al. Efficacy and economic assessment of conventional ventilatory support versus extracorporeal membrane oxygenation for severe adult respiratory failure (CESAR): A multicentre randomised controlled trial. Lancet. 2009;**374**:1351-1363

[8] Caille V, Vieillard-Baron A. The right ventricle during the acute respiratory distress syndrome revisited by echocardiography. The Open Nuclear Medicine Journal. 2010;**2**:119-124

[9] Sedgwick JF, Burstow DJ, Platts DG. The role of echocardiography in the management of patients supported by extracorporeal membranous oxygenation (ECMO). International Journal of Cardiology. 2010;**147**(Suppl):S16

[10] Firstenberg MS, Orsinelli DA. ECMO and echo: The evolving role of quantitative echo in the management of patients requiring extracorporeal membrane oxygenation. Journal of the American Society of Echocardiography. 2012;**25**:641-643

[11] Platts DG, Sedgwick JF, Burstow DJ, Mullany DV, Fraser JF. The role of echo in the management of patients supported by extracorporeal membrane oxygenation. Journal of the American Society of Echocardiography. 2012;**25**:131-141

[12] Douflé G, Roscoe A, Billia F, Fan E. Echocardiography for adult patients supported with extracorporeal membrane oxygenation. Critical Care. 2015;**19**:326-336

[13] Donker DW, Meuwese CL, Braithwaite SA, Broomé M, van der Heijden JJ, Hermens JA, et al. Echocardiography in extracorporeal life support: A key player in procedural guidance, tailoring and monitoring. Perfusion. 2018;**33**(1S):31-41

[14] Guinot PG, Soulignac C, Zogheib E, Guilbart M, Abou-Arab O, Longrois D, et al. Interactions between veno-venous extracorporeal membrane oxygenation and cardiac function: An echocardiographic study upon weaning. British Journal of Anaesthesia. 2016;**117**(6):821-835

[15] Giraud R, Banfi C, Bendjelid K. Echocardiography should be mandatory in ECMO venous cannula placement.

European Heart Journal - Cardiovascular Imaging. 1 Dec 2018;**19**(12):1429-1430. DOI: 10.1093/ehjci/jey142

[16] Tritapepe L. ECMO management guided by echo: Is it feasible? Minerva Anestesiologica. 2016;**82**(10):1023-1025

[17] Zhang Z. Echocardiography for patients undergoing extracorporeal cardiopulmonary resuscitation: A primer for intensive care physicians. Journal of Intensive Care. 2017;**5**:15

[18] Auzinger G, Loveridge R, Willars C, Best T, Kakar V, Hurst T, et al. Transoesophageal echocardiography and extracorporeal membrane oxygenation: Fancy for enthusiasts or indispensable tool? Critical Care. 2014;**18**(Suppl 1):P134

[19] Katz WE, Jafar MZ, Mankad S, Keenan RJ, Martich GD. Transesophageal echocardiographic identification of a malpositioned extracorporeal membrane oxygenation cannula. Journal of Heart and Lung Transplantation. 1995;**14**:790-792

[20] Kuenzler KA, Arthur LG, Burchard AE, Lawless ST, Wolfson PJ, Murphy SG. Intraoperative ultrasound reduces ECMO catheter malposition requiring surgical correction. Journal of Pediatric Surgery. 2002;**37**:691-694

[21] Zreik H, Bengur AR, Meliones JN, Hansell D, Li JS. Superior vena cava obstruction after extracorporeal membrane oxygenation. Journal of Pediatrics. 1995;**127**:314-316

[22] Victor K, Barrett N, Glover G, Kapetanakis S, Langrish C. Acute Budd-Chiari syndrome during veno-venous extracorporeal membrane oxygenation diagnosed using transthoracic echocardiography. British Journal of Anaesthesia. 2012;**108**:1043-1044

[23] Scherer M, Sirat AS, Moritz A, Martens S. Extracorporeal membrane oxygenation as perioperative right ventricular support in patients with biventricular failure undergoing left ventricular assist device implantation. European Journal of Cardio-Thoracic Surgery. 2011;**39**:939-944

[24] Hirose H, Yamane K, Marhefka G, Cavarocchi N. Right ventricular rupture and tamponade caused by malposition of the Avalon cannula for venovenous extracorporeal membrane oxygenation. Journal of Cardiothoracic Surgery. 2012;**7**:36

[25] Yastrebov K, Manganas C, Kapalli T, Peeceeyen S. Right ventricular loop indicating malposition of J-wire introducer for double lumen bicaval venovenous extracorporeal membrane oxygenation (VV ECMO) cannula. Heart Lung Circulation. 2014;**23**:e4-e7

[26] Abrams D, Bacchetta M, Brodie D. Recirculation in venovenous extracorporeal membrane oxygenation. ASAIO Journal. 2015;**61**:115-121

[27] Avalon Laboratories. Avalon Elite_ bi-caval dual lumen catheter. Available from: http://www.avalonlabs.com/html/pulmonary_support.html [Accessed: 25 Nov 2011]

[28] Javidfar J, Wang D, Zwischenberger J, Costa J, Mongero L, Sonett J, et al. Insertion of bicaval dual lumen extracorporeal membrane oxygenation catheter with image guidance. ASAIO Journal. 2011;**57**:203-205

[29] Dolch ME, Frey L, Buerkle MA, Weig T, Wassilowsky D, Irlbeck M. Transesophageal echocardiography-guided technique for extracorporeal membrane oxygenation dual-lumen catheter placement. ASAIO Journal. 2011;**57**:341-343

[30] Chacon MM, Shillcutt SK. Intraoperative transesophageal echocardiography–guided placement of bicaval dual-lumen extracorporeal

membrane oxygenation cannula. CASE (Phila). 2017;**1**(3):116-118

[31] Brodie D, Bacchetta M. Extracorporeal membrane oxygenation for ARDS in adults. The New England Journal of Medicine. 2011;**365**:1905-1914

[32] Bouferrache K, Vieillard-Baron A. Acute respiratory distress syndrome, mechanical ventilation, and right ventricular function. Current Opinion in Critical Care. 2011;**17**:30-35

[33] Tritapepe L. ARDS treatment strategies: After half a century do we still need guidelines? Journal of Emergency and Critical Care Medicine. 2017;**1**:24

[34] Sidebotham D, Allen SJ, McGeorge A, Ibbott N, Willcox T. Venovenous extracorporeal membrane oxygenation in adults: Practical aspects of circuits, cannulae, and procedures. Journal of Cardiothoracic and Vascular Anesthesia. 2012;**26**:893-909

[35] Miranda DR, van Thiel R, Brodie D, Bakker J. Right ventricular unloading after initiation of VV ECMO. American Journal of Respiratory and Critical Care Medicine. 2015;**191**:346-347

[36] Abrams D, Combes A, Brodie D. Extracorporeal membrane oxygenation in cardiopulmonary disease in adults. Journal of the American College of Cardiology. 2014;**63**:2769-2778

[37] Combes A, Brodie D, Bartlett R, Brochard L, Brower R, Conrad S, et al. Position paper for the organization of extracorporeal membrane oxygenation programs for acute respiratory failure in adult patients. American Journal of Respiratory and Critical Care Medicine. 2014;**190**:488-496

[38] Tritapepe L, De Santis V, Pacilli M. The right ventricle and pulmonary artery. In: Sarti A, Lorini FL, editors. Echocardiography for Intensivists. Milan: Springer-Verlag; 2012. pp. 91-97

[39] Hahn RT, Abraham T, Adams MS, Bruce CJ, Glas KE, Lang RM, et al. Guidelines for performing a comprehensive transesophageal echocardiographic examination: Recommendations from the American Society of Echocardiography and the Society of Cardiovascular Anesthesiologists. Journal of the American Society of Echocardiography. 2013;**26**:921-964

[40] Boissier F, Katsahian S, Razazi K, Thille AW, Roche-Campo F, Leon R, et al. Prevalence and prognosis of cor pulmonale during protective ventilation for acute respiratory distress syndrome. Intensive Care Medicine. 2013;**39**:1725-1733

[41] Meuwese CL, Ramjankhan FZ, Braithwaite SA, et al. Extracorporeal life support in cardiogenic shock: Indications and management in current practice. Netherlands Heart Journal. 2018;**26**:58-66

[42] Chen Y-S, Lin J-W, Yu H-Y, Jerng J-S, Ko W-J, Chang W-T, et al. Cardiopulmonary resuscitation with assisted extracorporeal life-support versus conventional cardiopulmonary resuscitation in adults with in-hospital cardiac arrest: An observational study and propensity analysis. Lancet. 2008;**372**:554-561

[43] Cardarelli MG, Young AJ, Griffith B. Use of extracorporeal membrane oxygenation for adults in cardiac arrest (E-CPR): A meta-analysis of observational studies. ASAIO Journal. 2009;**55**:581-586

[44] Aissaoui N, Luyt CE, Leprince P, Trouillet JL, Leger P, Pavie A, et al. Predictors of successful extracorporeal membrane oxygenation (ECMO) weaning after assistance for refractory

cardiogenic shock. Intensive Care Medicine. 2010;**37**:1738-1745

[45] Aissaoui N, Guerot E, Combes A, Delouche A, Chastre J, Leprince P, et al. Two dimensional strain rate and Doppler tissue myocardial velocities: Analysis by echocardiography of hemodynamic and functional changes of the failed left ventricle during different degrees of extracorporeal life support. Journal of the American Society of Echocardiography. 2012;**25**:632-640

[46] Ramjee V, Shreenivas S, Rame JE, Kirkpatrick JN, Jagasia D. Complete spontaneous left heart and aortic thromboses on extracorporeal membrane oxygenation support. Echocardiography. 2013;**30**:E342-E343

[47] Madershahian N, Weber C, Scherner M, Langebartels G, Slottosch I, Wahlers T. Thrombosis of the aortic root and ascending aorta during extracorporeal membrane oxygenation. Intensive Care Medicine. 2014;**40**:432-433

[48] Hajj-Chahine J, Tomasi J, Lanquetot H, Corbi P. Ascending aortic thrombosis in a patient on extra-corporeal membrane oxygenation. European Journal of Cardio-Thoracic Surgery. 2010;**37**:953

[49] Unai S, Nguyen M-L, Tanaka D, Gorbachuk N, Marhefka GD, Hirose H, et al. Clinical significance of spontaneous echo contrast on extracorporeal membrane oxygenation. The Annals of Thoracic Surgery. 2017;**103**:773-849

[50] Mulder MMG, Fawzy I, Lancé MD. ECMO and anticoagulation: A comprehensive review. Netherlands Journal of Critical Care. 2018;**26**(1):6-13

[51] Rupprecht L, Florchinger B, Schopka S, Schmid C, Philipp A, Lunz D, et al. Cardiac decompression on extracorporeal life support: A review and discussion of the literature. ASAIO Journal. 2013;**59**:547-553

[52] Weymann A, Schmack B, Sabashnikov A, Bowles CT, Raake P, Arif R, et al. Central extracorporeal life support with left ventricular decompression for the treatment of refractory cardiogenic shock and lung failure. Journal of Cardiothoracic Surgery. 2014;**9**:60

[53] Koeckert MS, Jorde UP, Naka Y, Moses JW, Takayama H. Impella LP 2.5 for left ventricular unloading during venoarterial extracorporeal membrane oxygenation support. Journal of Cardiac Surgery. 2011;**26**:666-668

[54] Avalli L, Maggioni E, Sangalli F, Favini G, Formica F, Fumagalli R. Extracorporeal membrane oxygenation: An alternative to surgical and transeptal venting in adult patients. ASAIO Journal. 2011;**57**:38-40

[55] Koenig PR, Ralston MA, Kimball TR, Meyer RA, Daniels SR, Schwartz DC. Balloon atrial septostomy for left ventricular decompression in patients receiving extracorporeal membrane oxygenation for myocardial failure. The Journal of Pediatrics. 1993;**122**:S95-S99

[56] O'Connor TA, Downing GJ, Ewing LL, Gowdamarajan R. Echocardiographically guided balloon atrial septostomy during extracorporeal membrane oxygenation (ECMO). Pediatric Cardiology. 1999;**14**:167-168

[57] Aissaoui N, El-Banayosy A, Combes A. How to wean a patient from veno-arterial extracorporeal membrane oxygenation. Intensive Care Medicine. 2015;**41**:902-905

[58] Cavarocchi NC, Pitcher HT, Yang Q, Karbowski P, Miessau J, Hastings HM, et al. Weaning of extracorporeal membrane oxygenation using continuous hemodynamic transesophageal echocardiography.

Journal of Thoracic and Cardiovascular Surgery. 2013;**146**:1474-1479

[59] Konishi H, Misawa Y, Nakagawa Y, Fuse K. Doppler aortic flow pattern in the recovery heart treated by cardiac ECMO. Artificial Organs. 1999;**23**:367-369

[60] Pappalardo F, Pieri M, Arnaez Corada B, Ajello S, Melisurgo G, De Bonis M, et al. Timing and strategy for weaning from venoarterial ECMO are complex issues. Journal of Cardiothoracic and Vascular Anesthesia. 2014;**29**:906-911

Section 3

Special Applications

Chapter 6

Extracorporeal Carbon Dioxide Removal for the Exacerbation of Chronic Hypercapnic Respiratory Diseases

Luis Morales-Quinteros and Antonio Artigas

Abstract

In the past, treatment of acute exacerbations of obstructive disease refractory to medical treatment was invasive mechanical ventilation. As a result of technical improvements, extracorporeal techniques for carbon dioxide removal have aroused as an attractive option to avoid worsening respiratory failure and respiratory acidosis and potentially prevent, shorten the duration of invasive mechanical ventilation (IMV), and serve as rescue therapy in patients with exacerbation of COPD and asthma. In this review, we will present a comprehensive summary of the pathophysiological rationale and evidence of $ECCO_2R$ in patients with severe exacerbations of these pathologies.

Keywords: COPD, asthma, $ECCO_2R$, invasive mechanical ventilation, noninvasive mechanical ventilation

1. Introduction

Patients with obstructive lung diseases, such as asthma and chronic obstructive pulmonary disease (COPD), may experience acute exacerbations with severe hypercapnic respiratory failure. Hypercapnia results from acute worsening of expiratory flow limitation caused by the increased small airway resistance with consequent development of dynamic alveolar hyperinflation and intrinsic PEEP. In the most severe cases, these may be refractory to conventional therapies and mechanical ventilation, becoming life-threatening.

Extracorporeal carbon dioxide removal ($ECCO_2R$) represents an attractive approach in this setting.

The last decade has seen an increasing interest in the provision of extracorporeal support for respiratory failure, as demonstrated by the progressively increasing number of scientific publications on this topic. In particular, remarkable interest has been focused on $ECCO_2R$, due to the relative ease and efficiency in blood CO_2 clearance granted by extracorporeal gas exchangers as compared to oxygen delivery (**Table 1**).

In recent years, new-generation $ECCO_2R$ devices have been developed. More efficient veno-venous (VV-$ECCO_2R$) devices have become available and have replaced the arteriovenous approach, having the advantage of not requiring arterial puncture.

They offer lower resistance to blood flow, have small priming volumes, and have a much more efficient gas exchange [1] with relatively low extracorporeal blood flows

	ECMO	$ECCO_2R$
Cannulas	Large cannulas	Double lumen catheter
Blood flow	High extracorporeal flow (2000–>5000 ml/min)	Low flow, respiratory dialysis (250–1000 ml/min)
Membrane oxygenator	Large membrane oxygenator	Medium size oxygenator
Oxygenation	Full blood oxygenation	No blood oxygenation
CO_2 removal	Full blood decarboxylation	Partial blood decarboxylation
Heparin requirements	High	Higher than ECMO
Setting	High technicity, ECMO center	Regular ICU

Table 1.
ECMO and $ECCO_2R$ differences.

(0.4–1 L/min). With $ECCO_2R$ the patient's $PaCO_2$ is principally determined by the rate of fresh gas flow through the membrane lung [2]. These devices are now comparable to renal dialysis equipment, which is routinely used safely as standard care in ICU.

This approach has been the subject of many animal experiments and human case series demonstrating improved arterial CO_2 and work of breathing [3–6].

2. Pathophysiological rationale for $ECCO_2R$

Both in asthma and COPD exacerbations, diffuse narrowing of the airways results in profound physiologic consequences. Airway narrowing prevents the lungs from completely emptying ("air trapping") due to resistance to expiratory flow and bronchial closure at higher than average lung volumes. Air trapping results in dynamic hyperinflation (DHI) [7] which is the excessive increase in end-expiratory lung volume above the relaxation volume of the respiratory system, generating intrinsic positive end-expiratory pressure (auto-PEEP) [8]. As a result, the patient breathes at higher total lung volumes, depending on increased residual volume [9] which reduces tidal ventilation. The net effect is that the work of breathing increases significantly. The diaphragm, intercostal muscles, and even the abdominal muscles are overloaded causing respiratory muscle fatigue and dyspnea.

Pharmacotherapy with bronchodilators and systemic corticosteroids are the cornerstones of medical therapy, designed to reduce this pathophysiological airflow obstruction and improve symptoms.

Patients suffering from a combination of persistent or worsening hypercapnia, respiratory muscle fatigue, and a decline in mental status require mechanical ventilation (MV) along with lung-protective ventilator strategies (e.g., low-tidal-volume ventilation, relatively short inspiratory time and longer expiratory times) [10, 11].

The goal of mechanical ventilation is to provide adequate gas exchange while waiting for airflow obstruction to respond to bronchodilator therapy. However, mechanical ventilation may aggravate alveolar hyperinflation by worsening DHI, which may lead to worsened hypercapnia, barotrauma, and alveolar rupture leading to pneumothorax and further hemodynamic deterioration [12].

Furthermore, during mechanical ventilation, these patients receive sedatives or neuromuscular blockade to facilitate ventilatory support [13]. Sedation and paralysis preclude mobilization, promoting muscular deconditioning and potentially contributing to the long-term cognitive sequelae of critical illness [14].

When conventional therapeutic options are not successful, novel therapies such as extracorporeal membrane oxygenation are entertained as a possible salvage therapeutic modality.

During exacerbation relieving the native lung from at least part of the CO_2 elimination with $ECCO_2R$ could potentially improve the acid–base balance, reduce patient's work of breathing with a consequent reduction in respiratory rate and ventilatory drive, and lower alveolar ventilation. The application of $ECCO_2R$ may allow lower tidal volumes and respiratory rate, resulting in the extension of the expiratory time, suiting better the high expiratory time constant of the respiratory system with expiratory flow limitation. By these physiological mechanisms, $ECCO_2R$ can counteract the vicious circle of dynamic hyperinflation and its detrimental respiratory and cardiovascular consequences. The derived beneficial effects on respiratory mechanics, ventilatory muscle efficiency, work of breathing, and cardiovascular function may improve gas exchanges and relieve dyspnea, thus potentially preventing NIV failure or facilitate weaning from IMV, and, also by rapidly decreasing and weaning off sedation, reduce the rates of delirium, reduce feeding problems, and allow social contacts with friends and family, as well as allow sufficient physiotherapy to reduce myopathy and critical care illness [14].

3. $ECCO_2R$ technical aspects and principle

$ECCO_2R$ is designed to remove carbon dioxide (CO_2) and, unlike extracorporeal membrane oxygen (ECMO), does not provide significant oxygenation.

The device consists of a drainage cannula placed in a large central vein or artery, a membrane lung, and a return cannula into the venous system (**Figure 1**). Blood is pumped through the membrane lung, and CO_2 is removed by diffusion. A flowing gas known as "sweep gas" containing little or no CO_2 runs along the other side of the membrane, ensuring a diffusion gradient from blood to another side, allowing CO_2 removal.

In contrast to ECMO, where the need for oxygenation requires high blood flow rates, $ECCO_2R$ allows much lower blood flow rates, a result of significant differences in CO_2 and oxygen (O_2) kinetics. Almost all the O_2 in blood is carried by hemoglobin, which displays sigmoidal saturation kinetics. Assuming normal hemoglobin and venous O_2, each liter of venous blood can only carry an extra 40–60 ml of O_2 before the hemoglobin is fully saturated. Blood flows of 5–7 L/min are therefore required to supply enough O_2 for an average adult. Conversely, most CO_2 is transported as dissolved bicarbonate, displaying linear kinetics without saturation. Considering that 1 L of blood is transported around 500 mL of CO_2, a perfectly efficient system flow of 0.5 L/min would be enough to remove all of the CO_2 produced [1, 15, 16]. Also, CO_2 diffuses more readily than O_2 across extracorporeal membranes because of higher solubility. However, in practice, $ECCO_2R$ is usually able to remove up to 25% of carbon dioxide production given the limitations of blood flow, blood CO_2 content, hemoglobin, and membrane efficiency [17].

3.1 VV-$ECCO_2R$

In the veno-venous configuration, blood is drawn from a central vein by a draining cannula, using a centrifugal or roller pump to generate flow across the membrane. CO_2 diffuses into the "sweep gas" and is returned into the venous circulation (**Figure 1A**). Single site cannulation is possible using a double lumen cannula. This approach allows low flow through the use of smaller cannulas (15–19F), commonly introduced via the right internal jugular vein. The setup is very similar to renal

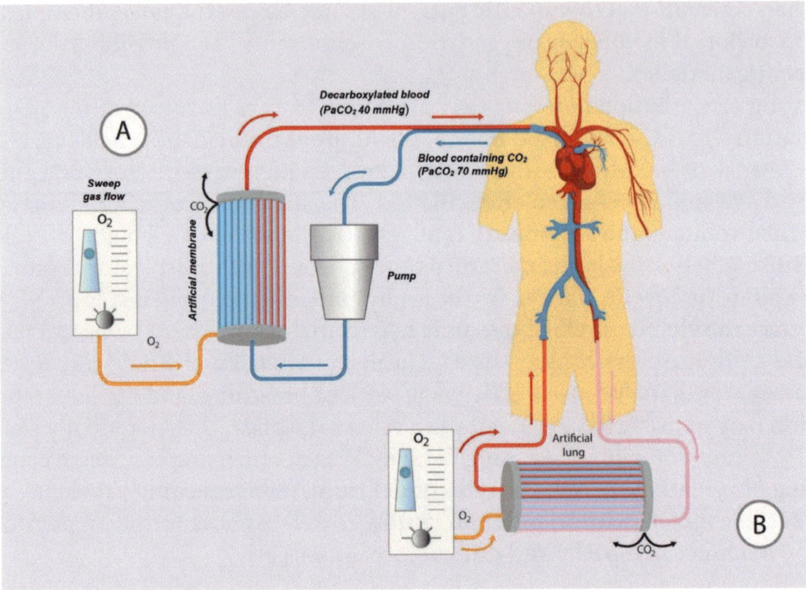

Figure 1.
$ECCO_2R$ common configurations. (A) Minimally invasive veno-venous $ECCO_2R$ system with a single venous vascular access through a double lumen cannula that can be inserted in the internal jugular or femoral vein (B) Pumpless arteriovenous $ECCO_2R$ system with the placement of the membrane in the circuit connecting the femoral artery with the contralateral vein.

replacement therapy, and in fact, some systems are trying to combine the two in one [18, 19] (NCT02590575). One of the advantages of VV-$ECCO_2R$ compared to the AV approach is the less invasiveness by the omission of the arterial cannulation and facilitates early mobilization of patients. It is also possible to set up an $ECCO_2R$ system through cannulation of two central veins, one for drainage and the other for reinfusion (femoral-femoral configuration).

3.2 AV-$ECCO_2R$

One $ECCO_2R$ configuration is through percutaneous cannulation of the femoral artery to the contralateral femoral vein and creating an arteriovenous (AV) bypass, equipped with an artificial gas exchanger membrane across the AV shunt which acts as a "sweep gas" to remove CO_2 that has diffused out of the patient's blood (**Figure 1B**). In this configuration, pumpless systems require an arteriovenous pressure gradient ≥60 mmHg and a cardiac index >3 L/min/m^2, which is unsuitable for hemodynamically unstable patients [16, 20]. Further, cannulation of a major artery can result in distal ischemia [21], although measuring the artery diameter with ultrasound and selecting a cannula that occupies no more than 70% of the lumen reduce this risk [22].

4. Indications and evidence

4.1 Chronic obstructive pulmonary disease

Chronic obstructive pulmonary disease (COPD) is a significant worldwide health burden. Currently, it is the fourth leading cause of death worldwide, is the only leading cause of death that is rising, and will likely become the third cause of death by 2020 [23, 24]. COPD is characterized by progressive destruction in the elastic tissue within the lung, causing respiratory failure.

Acute exacerbations of COPD (aeCOPD) constitute a significant cause of morbidity and mortality among these patients. Patients with moderate to severe acute exacerbations develop alveolar hyperinflation that may lead to increased work of breathing, muscle fatigue, and hypercapnia, creating a vicious loop refractory to medical treatment [25–27]. The standard respiratory support in this setting in order to break this cycle is noninvasive ventilation (NIV). However, despite the significantly decreased mortality with the emergence of NIV, up to 30% of patients with aeCOPD will "fail" and require intubation and invasive mechanical ventilation (IMV) [28–30]. For patients requiring respiratory support with IMV, in-hospital mortality in recent meta-analysis and observational studies has been reported to be as high as 25–39% [31–34].

Patients with COPD requiring IMV develop a considerable reduction in respiratory muscle strength, having a higher risk of prolonged weaning and failure to wean compared to other causes of acute hypercapnic respiratory failure. Up to 60% of the ventilatory time is devoted to these patients to the process of weaning [35], and they are very likely to require a tracheotomy. Having a prolonged time spent under IMV is not surprising an increase in the incidence of ventilator-associated pneumonia and complications associated with the use of invasive mechanical ventilation such ventilator-induced lung injury (VILI), ventilator-associated pneumonia (VAP), ventilator-associated diaphragmatic dysfunction (VIDD), and a range of neurological disorders associated with prolonged sedation and immobilization.

4.1.1 Evidence and clinical trials of ECCO$_2$R in aeCOPD to date

One of the first reports on the application of ECCO$_2$R to support respiratory function of a COPD patient was published in 1990 by Pesenti et al. [36]. However, the technique was abandoned due to technical complications.

As the medical community regained interest in ECCO$_2$R, investigators began applying the technique to prevent intubation or to assist weaning from the ventilator in patients with hypercapnic aeCOPD. Several studies in both VV and AV configurations were published, including a meta-analysis (**Table 2**).

4.1.2 ECCO$_2$R to avoid IMV

Brederlau et al. [37] described their experience in three patients that failed NIV for severe aeCOPD. They applied a pumpless AV ECCO$_2$R device with the goal of avoiding endotracheal intubation. Shortly after beginning ECCO$_2$R, $PaCO_2$ fell significantly (from 91, 109, and 142 mmHg to 52, 59, and 83 mmHg, respectively), while pH rose (from 7.2, 7.19, and 7.06 to 7.41, 7.43, and 7.34, respectively). Simultaneously, the respiratory rate dropped from 38, 45, and 37 breaths/min to 15, 25, and 18 breaths/min, respectively. The ECCO$_2$R flow ranged between 1.1 and 1.6 L/min, with the sweep gas flow varying from 3 to 10 L/min.

Kluge et al. [5] in the same year evaluated the safety and efficacy of using AV pumpless extracorporeal lung assist (PECLA) in 21 COPD patients who did not respond to NIV compared to 21 matched controls. The use of PECLA was associated with a decrease in $PaCO_2$ levels and improved pH after 24 h and obviated the need for intubation and IMV in 90% of the experimental arm. Although the experimental group demonstrated a shorter length of stay, a retrospective analysis with the control group showed no significant difference in mortality at 28 days (19% with ECCO$_2$R vs. 24% without ECCO$_2$R) or 6 months (both groups 33%).

Study	No of patients	ECCO$_2$R characteristics				Time on ECCO$_2$R	Major results
		Configuration	Blood flow (mL/min)	Sweep flow (L/min)	Membrane (material); surface in m^2		
ECCO$_2$R to avoid mechanical ventilation							
Kluge et al. [5]	21	Femoral AV with 13- to 15-Fr arterial cannula and 13- to 17-Fr venous cannula	1100	Not reported	PMP*; 1.3 (iLA®)	9 days	19 (90%) PECLA patients did not require intubation Two major and seven minor bleeding complications during PECLA No significant difference in 28-day (24 vs. 19%, p = 0.85), 6-month mortality (33 vs. 33%), or hospital length of stay (23 vs. 42 days, p = 0.06) Significantly fewer tracheostomies in PECLA group (10 vs. 67%, p = 0.004)
Del Sorbo et al. [4]	25	Modified continuous VV hemofiltration system with membrane lung via 14-Fr single dual-lumen cannula (femoral)	255	8	PLP**; 1.35 (Hemodec DecapSmart®)	1–2 days	Significantly higher risk of intubation in NIV-only group (HR 0.27; 95% CI 0.07–0.98) 13 patients experienced adverse events: 3 had bleeding, 1 had vein perforation, and 9 had device malfunction
Braune et al. [39]	25	VV configuration via a 22 or 24-Fr single dual-lumen cannula (femoral or jugular)	1300	Not reported	PMP; 1.3 (Novalung iLA Activve)	8.5 days	Intubation was avoided in 14 out of all 25 ECCO$_2$R patients (56%) Seven ECCO$_2$R patients were intubated because of progressive hypoxemia and four due to ventilatory failure despite ECCO$_2$R and NIV Nine ECCO$_2$R patients (36%) suffered from major bleeding complications 90-day mortality rates were 28 vs. 28%

Study	No of patients	$ECCO_2R$ characteristics				Time on $ECCO_2R$	Major results
		Configuration	Blood flow (mL/min)	Sweep flow (L/min)	Membrane (material); surface in m^2		
$ECCO_2R$ to wean from mechanical ventilation							
Abrams et al. [3]	5	VV configuration via a 20- to 24-Fr single dual-lumen jugular catheter using lower flow on ECMO system	1700	1–7	PMP; 0.98 (Maquet PALP CardioHelp)	8 days	Mean (SD) time to ambulation after $ECCO_2R$ initiation was 29.4 ± 12.6 h Four patients were discharged home, and one underwent planned lung transplantation Only two minor bleeding complications
Cardenas et al. [42]	1	VV configuration with pediatric dual-lumen jugular cannula	800	10	PMP; 1.8 (Quadrox-d, Maquet)	3.6 days	Patient extubated 48 h after decannulation. No complications reported
Roncon et al. [43]							
$ECCO_2R$ with mixed indications							
Burki [38]	20	VV configuration via a 15.5-Fr single dual-lumen catheter (femoral or jugular)	430	Not reported	PLP with a base of siloxane layer; 0.59 (ALung Hemolung RAS)	2–192 h	20 hypercapnic COPD patients received $ECCO_2R$ in three distinct groups: group 1 ($n = 7$) NIV patients with high risk of IMV; group 2 ($n = 2$) could not be weaned from NIV; and group 3 ($n = 11$) on IMV and failed to wean IMV avoided in all patient in group 1 Both patients in group 2 weaned from NIV In group 3, three patients weaned, and IMV was reduced in two patients One patient died due to a retroperitoneal hemorrhage (during cannulation)

PMP: poly-4-methyl-1-pentene.
***PLP: polypropylene.*

Table 2.
Relevant clinical studies of $ECCO_2R$ in COPD.

In the study by Burki et al. [38], 20 hypercapnic patients with COPD were treated with $ECCO_2R$ using a 15.5-Fr dual-lumen cannula allowing a mean blood flow of 430 mL/min. Of the 20 patients recruited into the trial, 7 were at risk of MV despite NIV, 2 were difficult to wean from NIV, and 11 had failed liberation from MV. None of the patients failing NIV required endotracheal intubation, and both patients with difficult weaning from NIV were weaned. However, only 3 of the 11 IMV patients were liberated successfully. Moreover, significant complications arose in a number of patients: bleeding requiring blood transfusion was reported in three patients, deep vein thrombosis was diagnosed in one patient after removal of the $ECCO_2R$ catheter, one patient experienced pneumothorax due to catheter insertion, and one died from hemorrhage when the iliac vein was perforated during $ECCO_2R$ catheter placement.

Del Sorbo et al. [4] examined 25 patients with NIV + $ECCO_2R$ versus NIV alone (historical controls n = 21) for prevention of intubation in aeCOPD. They reported that $ECCO_2R$ with a 14-Fr dual-lumen catheter and blood flow rates of 177–333 mL/min not only improved respiratory acidosis but also reduced the need for intubation by 75% (12 vs. 33%; p = 0.047) and significantly reduced the in-hospital mortality (8 vs. 35%; p = 0.035). However, this came with a cost of 52% prevalence of $ECCO_2R$-related side effects and led the authors to suggest the end point of future studies should be long-term mortality.

In the ECLAIR study, Braune et al. [39] showed that IMV was avoided in 56% of cases treated with $ECCO_2R$ but was associated with a higher incidence of complications. However, several significant differences must be taken into account. In the latter study, there was an inclusion of patients with relative contraindications to NIV, and there was an unexpectedly high incidence of hypoxemic patients [40].

Finally, Morelli et al. [41] and colleagues confirmed the efficacy of $ECCO_2R$ (with a flow rate of 250–450 mL/min through a 13-Fr dual-lumen cannula) in reducing the $PaCO_2$ in a series of 30 patients with acute hypercapnic respiratory failure due to aeCOPD, who refused endotracheal intubation after failing NIV. The duration of $ECCO_2R$ was 2–16 days, and it was possible to prevent endotracheal intubation in 27 patients.

4.1.3 $ECCO_2R$ to facilitate weaning from IMV

Cardenas et al. [42] made the first attempt to use modern ECLS components for VV $ECCO_2R$ in a patient with aeCOPD. They demonstrated a successful reduction in $PaCO_2$, minute ventilation, and ventilator pressures.

Burki et al. [38] showed that in a subgroup of 11 patients receiving IMV, $ECCO_2R$ allowed the weaning from mechanical ventilator in only 3 patients.

Abrams and colleagues [3] reported five older patients (age 73 ± 8.7 years) with aeCOPD who failed NIV, requiring IMV. After an average of 16.5 ± 5.9 h of IMV, $ECCO_2R$ was initiated. By using a dual-lumen cannula (20–23 Fr) with blood flow rates of 1–1.7 L/min and with a sweep gas flow from 1 to 7 L/min, they were able to extubate all five patients within 24 h of treatment (median duration of MV post $ECCO_2R$ = 4 h, range 1.5–21.5 h). Once extubated, patients were rehabilitated while on $ECCO_2R$, with a mean time to ambulation of 29.4 ± 12.6 h after $ECCO_2R$. Moreover, all patients survived to hospital discharge.

Using a pediatric VV ECMO system (with blood flow rates of 0.9 L/min through a 19 Fr dual-lumen cannula placed in the right jugular vein) in two patients with aeCOPD, Roncon-Albuquerque Jr. et al. reported early extubation after 72 h and patient mobilization out of bed at day 6 [43].

4.1.4 Reviews of ECCO$_2$R in COPD

Sklar et al. [44] reviewed 10 studies of ECCO$_2$R for aeCOPD and a total of 87 patients, to examine cumulative safety and efficacy. They reported that ECCO$_2$R was able to prevent intubation in 65 (93%) of 70 patients and assist in successful extubation of 9 (53%) of 17 patients. There were a total of 11 major complications and 30 minor complications. Half of all patients experienced complications related to ECCO$_2$R, and half of those complications were related to bleeding (21/41). No study showed any evidence of increased mortality or increased length of intensive care unit (ICU) or hospital stay with ECCO$_2$R.

In a recent publication, Taccone et al. [45] performed a systematic review of ECCO$_2$R in adult critically ill patients. Three of the six studies included in the review evaluated patients with COPD that developed hypercapnic respiratory failure [4, 5, 39]. In all the three studies, the reduction of PaCO$_2$ was reported within a few hours following the initiation of ECCO$_2$R. Median values decreased from 73 to 88 mmHg to 34–66 mmHg. Regarding the duration of mechanical ventilation, only one described no significant difference between ECCO$_2$R and the controlled group [4]. The need for endotracheal intubation was significantly reduced from 53/67 (79%) to 16/71 (22% $p < 0.001$). However, neither ICU nor hospital length of stay was statistically significantly reduced.

Based on the existing data, we believe that the ideal trial for ECCO$_2$R should be a randomized controlled trial designed such ECCO$_2$R should be implemented within 12 h of intubation after failing to show improvement (i.e., pH < 7.25 for persistent acidosis) with conventional therapy. Given the risks associated with the technique, it should be instituted once patients fail conventional treatment and require IMV. Patients should be randomized to ECCO$_2$R plus IMV or standard IMV. Given the high rate of mortality associated with invasive mechanical ventilation, the study should be powered to demonstrate a mortality benefit, and secondary endpoints include ventilator-free days, transfusion requirements, and rates of ventilator-associated events.

More data will be forthcoming on the application of ECCO$_2$R in the management of patients with COPD exacerbations from a number of ongoing or planned clinical trials (**Table 3**).

4.2 Severe acute asthma

Asthma is an inflammatory disorder of the airways characterized by airway hyperactivity with bronchospasm, mucosal swelling, and mucus production.

The standard treatment of severe acute asthma consists of measures to reverse airflow obstruction. β_2 agonists and steroids are the mainstays of treatment causing bronchodilation and anti-inflammatory effects, respectively [10]. Other available adjunct therapies including anticholinergics, magnesium sulfate, methylxanthines, ketamine, and heliox have been utilized with varying results [46].

Despite advances in asthma therapy, asthma mortality has remained stable in recent years. One reason is status asthmaticus, which can be unresponsive to initial treatment and may lead to hypercapnic respiratory failure despite maximal therapy.

Status asthmaticus, also known as severe acute asthma or near-fatal asthma, is a condition of progressively worsening bronchospasm and respiratory dysfunction due to asthma, which is unresponsive to standard conventional therapy and may progress to respiratory failure and the need for mechanical ventilation. The current indication of mechanical ventilation in a patient presenting with status asthmaticus is a clinical one and does not require a blood gas assessment. These include certain specific situations including alteration of consciousness, respiratory fatigue, or impending cardiopulmonary arrest.

ClinicalTrials. gov number	Title	Type of study	Hypothesis/primary outcome	Estimated enrollment	Device
$ECCO_2R$ to avoid mechanical ventilation					
NCT02086084	Extracorporeal CO_2 removal as an adjunct to noninvasive ventilation in acute severe exacerbations of COPD	Randomized, controlled trial	Addition of $ECCO_2R$ to NIV will shorten the duration of NIV and reduce the likelihood of intubation Primary outcome: time to cessation of NIV defined as from NIV commencement to 6 h without NIV	24 patients	Hemolung RAS
NCT03584295	Early extubation by $ECCO_2R$ compared to IMV in patients with severe acute exacerbation of COPD (X-COPD)	Interventional, randomized with parallel assignment	Advantage of VV-$ECCO_2R$ in severe acute exacerbation of COPD requiring invasive mechanical ventilation (IMV) to facilitate early extubation in terms of reducing mortality or severe disability Primary outcome: death or severe disability	202 patients	Not specified
NCT02564406	Extracorporeal CO_2 removal in hypercapnic patients	Interventional single-group trial	Retrospectively assess the efficacy and safety of noninvasive ventilation-plus-extracorporeal CO_2 removal in patients who fail NIV and refuse endotracheal intubation Primary outcome: number of patients who avoided endotracheal intubation	35 patients	ProLUNG [Estor]
NCT03692117	Extracorporeal carbon dioxide removal in severe chronic obstructive pulmonary disease exacerbation	Prospective cohort study	Primary outcome: incidence of avoiding endotracheal intubation	30 patients	Not specified
$ECCO_2R$ to facilitate liberation from mechanical ventilation					
NCT02259335	Weaning from mechanical ventilation using extracorporeal CO_2 removal (WeanPRO)	Interventional single-group trial	Weaning success avoiding reintubation after removal of $ECCO_2R$	12 patients	ProLUNG [Estor]
NCT02107222	The PALP™-COPD trial (low flow CO_2-removal ($ECCO_2$-R) in exacerbated COPD) (PALP-COPD)	Multicenter, randomized, controlled trial	To evaluate the clinical effect of PALP in reducing the time on invasive ventilation in patients with an exacerbation of COPD requiring invasive mechanical ventilation	120 patients	PALP

ClinicalTrials.gov number	Title	Type of study	Hypothesis/primary outcome	Estimated enrollment	Device
$ECCO_2R$ as an alternative or adjunct to invasive mechanical ventilation					
NCT03255057	Extracorporeal CO_2 removal for mechanical ventilation avoidance during acute exacerbation of COPD (VENT-AVOID)	Multicenter randomized controlled trial	$ECCO_2R$ can be safely used to avoid or reduce time on invasive mechanical ventilation compared to COPD patients treated with standard-of-care mechanical ventilation alone Primary outcome: ventilator-free days at day 60 from randomization	500 patients	Hemolung
$ECCO_2R$ physiological studies					
NCT02586948	Physiological study of minimally invasive $ECCO_2R$ in exacerbations of COPD requiring invasive mechanical ventilation (EPHEBE)	Interventional single-group trial	The addition of minimally invasive $ECCO_2R$ is likely to limit dynamic hyperinflation in COPD patients requiring invasive mechanical ventilation for an acute exacerbation while improving gas exchange Primary outcome: PEEPi at baseline and after $ECCO_2R$ by the device and adjustment of ventilator settings, expressed in cmH_20	12 patients	Hemolung
NCT02590575	"Low Flow" CO_2 removal on RRT	Interventional single-group trial	Test the effectiveness of a membrane gas exchange device in the veno-venous circulation of continuous renal replacement therapy for the purpose of CO_2 elimination and pH compensation The primary outcome is the modification of the $PaCO_2$ and/or the ventilator settings (tidal volume VT and plateau pressure Pplat)	20 patients	Prismalung

Table 3.
Ongoing clinical studies of $ECCO_2R$ in COPD.

Approximately, 4% of all patients hospitalized for acute asthma require mechanical ventilation, which is associated with increased in-hospital mortality compared with patients who do not require mechanical ventilation (7 vs. 0.2%) [47].

Furthermore, mechanical ventilation may aggravate alveolar hyperinflation as it was described above. To prevent the potential side effects caused by mechanical ventilation, $ECCO_2R$ has been applied as rescue therapy.

Extracorporeal carbon dioxide removal as an adjunct to the ventilator for refractory asthma was first reported in 1981 [48]. Subsequently, there have been several case reports (**Table 4**). In the international Extracorporeal Life Support Organization (ELSO) registry, ECMO was used for asthma in 24 out of 1257 adult patients between 1986 and 2006. Before ECMO was started, the average pH was

7.17 ± 0.16, $PaCO_2$ 119.7 ± 58 mmHg, and PaO_2/FiO_2 244 ± 180 despite mechanical ventilation. Complications were described in 19 of 24 patients (79.2%) with a remarkable number of hemodynamic, hemorrhagic, and mechanical complications [49]. These data show that in patients treated with ECMO for status asthmaticus, hypercapnia, rather than hypoxemia, was the central exchange derangement, suggesting that a less invasive technique like $ECCO_2R$ will be suitable, with fewer complications. Although most of the clinical applications of $ECCO_2R$ for the treatment of obstructive lung diseases have been reported in patients with COPD, several cases describe $ECCO_2R$ in patients with near-fatal asthma [50–54] (**Table 4**).

The first cases reported were by using a pumpless extracorporeal life assist (pECLA) device. Although no complications were described in these case series, a possible major complication may arise as a consequence of the arterial cannulation, such as lower limb ischemia [53]. Brenner et al. reported two cases using a venous double lumen catheter with successful survival results.

Study	$ECCO_2R$ technique	Major findings
Sakai et al. [53]	Extracorporeal lung assist (ECLA); 22-Fr drainage and 18-Fr return femoro-femoral cannula with a median blood flow rate of 1.7–2 L/min	23-year old Gas exchange with IMV before $ECCO_2R$: pH 7.02, $paCO_2$ 100 mmHg, PaO_2 50 mmHg (FiO_2 100%) Weaning achieved after 20 h of ECLA was commenced Extubation 2 days after ECLA No complications reported
Elliot et al. [52]	Femoral AV pumpless extracorporeal lung assist (PECLA) 15-Fr arterial cannula and 17-Fr venous cannula with a mean extracorporeal blood flow of 1.5 L/min	Case 1: 74-year old. Gas exchange with IMV before $ECCO_2R$: pH 6.87, $paCO_2$ 147 mmHg. Extubation after 48 h of ECLA. Complications: Coagulation of membrane that needed changing. Bleeding through femoral artery Case 2: 52-year old. Gas exchange with IMV before $ECCO_2R$: pH 7.2, $paCO_2$ 130 mmHg. $ECCO_2R$ duration: 5 days Extubated on intensive care day 11. No complications reported
Jung et al. [54]	Femoral AV pumpless extracorporeal lung assist (PECLA) 15-Fr arterial cannula and 17-Fr venous cannula with a mean extracorporeal blood flow of >1.5 L/min	42-year old No gas exchange before IMV reported. Patient successfully extubated and transferred from the ICU on day 14 of admission No complications reported
Brenner et al. [50]	Dual-lumen catheter 20–23 Fr bicaval, inserted into the right internal jugular vein with blood flow of 1.3–1.8 L/min	Case 1: 48-year old. Gas exchange with IMV before $ECCO_2R$: pH 6.94, $paCO_2$ 147 mmHg, PaO_2 416 mmHg (FiO_2 100%). Successfully extubated while on $ECCO_2R$ and discharged from ICU. No complications reported Case 2: 59-year old. Gas exchange with IMV before $ECCO_2R$: pH 7.12, $paCO_2$ 78 mmHg, PaO_2 112 mmHg (FiO_2 100%). $ECCO_2R$ duration: 9 days. Ventilator support discontinued on day 28 due to critical illness neuromyopathy
Schneider et al. [51]	Awake dual-lumen catheter 22 Fr bicaval, inserted into the right internal jugular vein with blood flow of 0.6–1.5 L/min	67-year old Gas exchange before $ECCO_2R$ (on NIV): pH 7.24, $paCO_2$ 61 mmHg, PaO_2 289 mmHg (FiO_2 100%) Thirty-four hours after initiating $ECCO_2R$, the patient was weaned entirely from NIV, and the cannula could be removed without any complication. On day 4, the patient was discharged from the ICU without the need for supplemental oxygen and 6 days later, discharged from hospital without any impairment

IMV, invasive mechanical ventilation; NIV, noninvasive mechanical ventilation.

Table 4.
Case series of $ECCO_2R$ for near-fatal asthma.

Taking into account the deleterious effects of mechanical ventilation and sedation, and the advantages of keeping the patient awake, recently, an awake approach using a double lumen cannula has been described [51]. NIV was used as ventilatory support. Thirty-four hours after starting the $ECCO_2R$ system, the patient was weaned entirely from NIV, and the cannula was removed without complications. The patient was discharged from the ICU on day 4 without supplemental oxygen and left the hospital on day 10. Although this is a tempting approach, several issues should be taken into account. Unexpected cannula displacement may be provoked by an interactive patient, resulting in significant hemorrhage and lethal shock, as a time to react is short. Patient discomfort, pain, and anxiety in the "awake" approach might be in such extent that starting deep sedation and mechanical ventilation is inevitable, losing all the advantages described before.

5. Complications

Although $ECCO_2R$ seems to be effective in improving or mitigating hypercapnic acidosis and possibly in reducing the rate of endotracheal intubation, its use is associated with a range of vascular, hematological, and other complications.

Arterial cannulation is associated with higher risk than venous catheterization, with specific complications including distal limb ischemia, compartment syndrome of the lower limb requiring fasciotomy, or limb amputation as devastating consequences [16].

The occurrence of bleeding events is the most frequent complications of $ECCO_2R$. The low flow renders systemic anticoagulation mandatory, increasing the risk of significant bleeding including cerebral, gastrointestinal, and nasopharyngeal bleeds. In the studies of $ECCO_2R$ to date, the rate of clinically significant hemorrhagic complications ranges between 2 and 50% [44].

Thrombocytopenia and heparin-induced thrombocytopenia are also commonly observed.

Conversely, thrombus formation is higher at lower blood flow rates because of increased exposure time to the membrane lung and circuit. Clots may detach and enter the patient's bloodstream, plugging the membrane or obstructing the cannula if anticoagulation is not achieved.

6. Conclusions

In the past, $ECCO_2R$ was a complex technique requiring intensive monitoring and surgical expertise. Due to a high rate of complications, it was avoided by all but a few high expertise centers. With newer simplified system, devices are placed like temporary dialysis catheters and can be inserted by most intensivists.

In summary, minimally invasive $ECCO_2R$ appears very promising for patients with acute exacerbation of obstructive diseases refractory to conventional treatment, but systemic evaluation is needed to prove its efficacy and determine the actual risks.

Acknowledgements

We want to acknowledge Eduardo Radicy for creating the figure for this manuscript. He was not compensated for this work.

Conflict of interest

The authors declare that they do not have conflicting interests.

Nomenclature

AV-$ECCO_2R$	arteriovenous extracorporeal carbon dioxide removal
COPD	chronic obstructive pulmonary disease
CO_2	carbon dioxide
DHI	dynamic hyperinflation
$ECCO_2R$	extracorporeal carbon dioxide removal
ECMO	extracorporeal membrane oxygenation
IMV	invasive mechanical ventilation
NIV	noninvasive ventilation
PECLA	pumpless extracorporeal lung assist
PEEP	positive end-expiratory pressure
PLP	polypropylene
PMP	poly-4-methyl-1-pentene
VV-$ECCO_2R$	veno-venous extracorporeal carbon dioxide removal

Author details

Luis Morales-Quinteros[1*] and Antonio Artigas[1,2,3]

1 Intensive Care Unit, Hospital Universitario Sagrado Corazón, Barcelona, Spain

2 Critical Care Center, Parc Taulí Hospital Universitari, Institut d'Investigació i Innovació Parc Taulí I3PT, Universitat Autònoma de Barcelona, Sabadell, Spain

3 CIBER Enfermedades Respiratorias, Instituto de Salud Carlos III, Madrid, Spain

*Address all correspondence to: luchomq2077@gmail.com

References

[1] MacLaren G, Combes A, Bartlett R. Contemporary extracorporeal membrane oxygenation for adult respiratory failure: Life support in the new era. Intensive Care Medicine. 2012;**38**(2):210-220. DOI: 10.1007/s00134-011-2439-2

[2] Schmidt M, Tachon G, Devilliers C, Muller G, Hekimian G, Bréchot N, et al. Blood oxygenation and decarboxylation determinants during venovenous ECMO for respiratory failure in adults. Intensive Care Medicine. 2013;**39**(5):838-846. DOI: 10.1007/s00134-012-2785-8

[3] Abrams DC, Brenner K, Burkart KM, Agerstrand CL, Thomashow BM, Brodie D. Pilot study of extracorporeal carbon dioxide removal to facilitate extubation and ambulation in exacerbations of chronic obstructive pulmonary disease. Annals of the American Thoracic Society. 2013;**10**:307-314

[4] Del Sorbo L, Pisani L, Filippini C, Fanelli V, Fasano L, Terragni P, et al. Extracorporeal CO_2 removal in hypercapnic patients at risk of noninvasive ventilation failure: A matched cohort study with historical control. Critical Care Medicine. 2015;**43**:120-127. DOI: 10.1097/CCM.0000000000000607

[5] Kluge S, Braune SA, Engel M, Nierhaus A, Frings D, Ebelt H, et al. Avoiding invasive mechanical ventilation by extracorporeal carbon dioxide removal in patients failing noninvasive ventilation. Intensive Care Medicine. 2012:1632-1639. DOI: 10.1007/s00134-012-2649-2

[6] Diehl JL, Piquilloud L, Richard JC, Mancebo J, Mercat A. Effects of extracorporeal carbon dioxide removal on work of breathing in patients with chronic obstructive pulmonary disease. Intensive Care Medicine. 2016;**42**(5):951-952. DOI: 10.1007/s00134-015-4166-6

[7] Pellegrino R, Violante B, Nava S, Rampulla C, Brusasco V, Rodarte J. Expiratory airflow limitation and hyperinflation during methacholine-induced bronchoconstriction. Journal of Applied Physiology. 1993;**75**:1720-1727. DOI: 10.1152/jappl.1993.75.4.1720

[8] Laghi F, Goyal A. Auto-PEEP in respiratory failure. Minerva Anestesiologica. 2012;**78**:201-221

[9] Wagers SS, Jaffe EF, Irving CG. Development structure and physiology in normal and asthmatic lung. In: Middleton's Allergy: Principles and Practice. St Louis: Mosby; 2003

[10] National Heart, Lung and Blood Institute. Expert Panel Report 3: Guidelines for the Diagnosis and Management of Asthma: Full Report 2007. 2017. Available from: http://nhlbi.nih.gov/guidelines/asthma/asthgdln.pdf

[11] Sethi JM, Siegel MD. Mechanical ventilation in chronic obstructive lung disease. Clinics in Chest Medicine. 2000;**21**:799-818. DOI: 10.1016/S0272-5231(05)70185-4

[12] Blanch L, Bernabé F, Lucangello U. Measurement of air trapping, intrinsic positive end-expiratory pressure, and dynamic hyperinflation in mechanically ventilated patients. Respiratory Care. 2005;**50**:110-123

[13] Marhong JD, Telesnicki T, Munshi L, Del Sorbo L, Detsky M, Fan E. Mechanical ventilation during extracorporeal membrane oxygenation. Annals of the American Thoracic Society. 2014;**11**:956-961. DOI: 10.1513/AnnalsATS.201403-100BC

[14] Langer T, Santini A, Bottino N, Crotti S, Batckinsky AI, Pesenti A, et al.

"Awake" extracorporeal membrane oxygenation (ECMO): Pathophysiology, technical considerations, and clinical pioneering. Critical Care. 2016;**20**:150. DOI: 10.1186/s13054-016-1329-y

[15] Gattinoni L, Pesenti A, Kolobow T, Damia G. A new look at therapy of the adult respiratory distress syndrome: Motionless lungs. International Anesthesiology Clinics. 1983;**21**:97-117

[16] Cove ME, MacLaren G, Federspiel WJ, Kellum JA. Bench to bedside review: Extracorporeal carbon dioxide removal, past present and future. Critical Care. 2012;**16**(5):232

[17] Terragni P, Maiolo G, Ranieri VM. Role and potentials of low-flow CO_2 removal system in mechanical ventilation. Current Opinion in Critical Care. 2012;**18**:93-98. DOI: 10.1097/MCC.0b013e32834f17ef

[18] Winiszewski H, Aptel F, Belon F, Belin N, Chaignat C, Patry C, et al. Daily use of extracorporeal CO_2 removal in a critical care unit: Indications and results. Journal of Intensive Care. 2018;**6**:36. DOI: 10.1186/s40560-018-0304-x

[19] May AG, Sen A, Cove ME, Kellum JA, Federspiel WJ. Extracorporeal CO_2 removal by hemodialysis: In vitro model and feasibility. Intensive Care Medicine Experimental. 2017;**5**:20. DOI: 10.1186/s40635-017-0132-7

[20] Flörchinger B, Philipp A, Klose A, Hilker M, Kobuch R, Rupprecht L, et al. Pumpless extracorporeal lung assist: A 10-year institutional experience. The Annals of Thoracic Surgery. 2008;**86**:410-417. DOI: 10.1016/j.athoracsur.2008.04.045

[21] Bein T, Weber F, Philipp A, Prasser C, Pfeifer M, Schmid FX, et al. A new pumpless extracorporeal interventional lung assist in critical hypoxemia/hypercapnia. Critical Care Medicine. 2006;**34**:1372-1377

[22] Zimmermann M, Bein T, Arlt M, Philipp A, Rupprecht L, Mueller T, et al. Pumpless extracorporeal interventional lung assist in patients with acute respiratory distress syndrome: A prospective pilot study. Critical Care. 2009;**13**:R10. DOI: 10.1186/cc7703

[23] Calverley PM, Walker P. Chronic obstructive pulmonary disease. Lancet. 2003;**362**(9389):1053-1061. DOI: 10.1016/S0140-6736(03)14416-9

[24] Chapman KR, Mannino DM, Soriano JB, Vermeire PA, Buist AS, Thun MJ, et al. Epidemiology and costs of chronic obstructive pulmonary disease. The European Respiratory Journal. 2006;**27**(1):188-207. DOI: 10.1183/09031936.06.00024505

[25] Barberà JA, Roca J, Ferrer A, Félez MA, Díaz O, Roger N, et al. Mechanisms of worsening gas exchange during acute exacerbations of chronic obstructive pulmonary disease. The European Respiratory Journal. 1997;**10**(6):1285-1291

[26] Roberts CM, Stone RA, Buckingham RJ, Pursey NA, Lowe D. Acidosis, non-invasive ventilation and mortality in hospitalised COPD exacerbations. Thorax. 2011;**66**(1):43-48. DOI: 10.1136/thx.2010.153114

[27] Oliven A, Kelsen SG, Deal EC, Cherniak NS. Mechanisms underlying CO_2 retention during flow-resistive loading in patients with chronic obstructive pulmonary disease. The Journal of Clinical Investigation. 1983;**71**(5):1442-1449. DOI: 10.1172/JCI110897

[28] Phua J, Kong K, Lee KH, Shen L, Lim TK. Noninvasive ventilation in hypercapnic acute respiratory failure due to chronic obstructive pulmonary disease vs. other conditions: Effectiveness and predictors of failure. Intensive Care Medicine. 2005;**31**(4):533-539. DOI: 10.1007/s00134-005-2582-8

[29] Confalonieri M, Garuti G, Cattaruzza MS, Osborn JF, Antonelli M, Conti G, et al. A chart of failure risk for noninvasive ventilation in patients with COPD exacerbation. The European Respiratory Journal. 2005;**25**(2):348-355

[30] Quinnell TG, Pilsworth S, Shneerson JM, Smith IE. Prolonged invasive ventilation following acute ventilatory failure in COPD: Weaning results, survival, and the role of noninvasive ventilation. Chest. 2006;**129**(1):133-139. DOI: 10.1378/chest.129.1.133

[31] Chandra D, Stamm JA, Taylor B, Ramos RM, Satterwhite L, Krishnan JA, et al. Outcomes of noninvasive ventilation for acute exacerbations of chronic obstructive pulmonary disease in the United States, 1998-2008. American Journal of Respiratory and Critical Care Medicine. 2012;**185**(2):152-159. DOI: 10.1164/rccm.201106-1094OC

[32] Tabak YP, Sun X, Johannes RS, Gupta V, Shorr AF. Mortality and need for mechanical ventilation in acute exacerbations of chronic obstructive pulmonary disease: Development and validation of a simple risk score. Archives of Internal Medicine. 2009;**169**(17):1595-1602. DOI: 10.1001/archinternmed.2009.270

[33] Patil SP, Krishnan JA, Lechtzin N, Diette GB. In-hospital mortality following acute exacerbations of chronic obstructive pulmonary disease. Archives of Internal Medicine. 2003;**163**(10):1180-1186. DOI: 10.1001/archinte.163.10.1180

[34] Demoule A, Girou E, Richard JC, Taille S, Brochard L. Benefits and risks of success or failure of noninvasive ventilation. Intensive Care Medicine. 2006;**32**(11):1756-1765. DOI: 10.1007/s00134-006-0324-1

[35] Nava S, Ambrosino N, Clini E, Prato M, Orlando G, Vitacca M, et al. Noninvasive mechanical ventilation in the weaning of patients with respiratory failure due to chronic obstructive pulmonary disease. A randomized, controlled trial. Annals of Internal Medicine. 1998;**128**(9):721-728

[36] Pesenti A, Rossi GP, Pelosi P, Brazzi L, Gattinoni L. Percutaneous extracorporeal CO_2 removal in a patient with bullous emphysema with recurrent bilateral pneumothoraces and respiratory failure. Anesthesiology. 1990;**72**(3):307-314

[37] Brederlau J, Wurmb T, Wilczek S, Will K, Maier S, Kredel M, et al. Extracorporeal lung assist might avoid invasive ventilation in exacerbation of COPD. The European Respiratory Journal. 2012;**40**(3):783-785. DOI: 10.1183/09031936.00006012

[38] Burki NK, Mani RK, Herth FJF, Schmidt W, Teschler H, Bonin F, et al. A novel extracorporeal CO 2 removal results of a pilot study of hypercapnic respiratory failure in patients with COPD. Chest. 2013;**143**(3):678-686. DOI: 10.1378/chest.12-0228

[39] Braune S, Sieweke A, Brettner F, Staudinger T, Joannidis M, Verbrugge S, et al. The feasibility and safety of extracorporeal carbon dioxide removal to avoid intubation in patients with COPD unresponsive to noninvasive ventilation for acute hypercapnic respiratory failure (ECLAIR study): Multicentre case-control study. Intensive Care Medicine. 2016;**42**(9):1437-1444

[40] Del Sorbo L, Fan E, Nava S, Ranieri VM. $ECCO_2R$ in COPD exacerbation only for the right patients and with the right strategy. Intensive Care Medicine. 2016;**42**(11):1830-1831. DOI: 10.1007/s00134-016-4493-2

[41] Morelli A, D'Egidio A, Orecchioni A, Alessandri F, Mascia L, Ranieri VM. Extracorporeal CO_2 removal

in hypercapnic patients who fail noninvasive ventilation and refuse endotracheal intubation: A case series. Intensive Care Medicine Experimental. 2015;**3**(Suppl 1):A824. DOI: 10.1186/2197-425X-3-S1-A824

[42] Cardenas VJ Jr, Lynch JE, Ates R, Miller L, Zwischenberger JB. Venovenous carbon dioxide removal in chronic obstructive pulmonary disease: Experience in one patient. ASAIO Journal. 2009;**55**(4):420-422. DOI: 10.1097/MAT.0b013e3181a7b55d

[43] Roncon-Albuquerque R Jr, Carona G, Neves A, Miranda F, Castelo-Branco S, Oliveira T, et al. Venovenous extracorporeal CO_2 removal for early extubation in COPD exacerbations requiring invasive mechanical ventilation. Intensive Care Medicine. 2014;**40**(12):1969-1970. DOI: 10.1007/s00134-014-3503-5

[44] Sklar MC, Beloncle F, Katsios CM, Brochard L, Friedrich JO. Extracorporeal carbon dioxide removal in patients with chronic obstructive pulmonary disease: A systematic review. Intensive Care Medicine. 2015;**41**:1752-1762. DOI: 10.1007/s00134-015-3921-z

[45] Taccone FS, Malfertheiner MV, Ferrari F, Di Nardo M, Swol J, Broman LM, et al. Minerva Anestesiologica. 2017;**83**(7):762-772

[46] Wong JJ, Lee JH, Turner DA, Rehder KJ. A review of the use of adjunctive therapies in severe acute asthma exacerbation in critically ill children. Expert Review of Respiratory Medicine. 2014;**8**:423-441. DOI: 10.1586/17476348.2014.915752

[47] Krishnan V, Diettte GN, Rand CS, Bilderback AL, Merriman B, Hansel NN, et al. Mortality in patients hospitalized for asthma exacerbations in the United States. American Journal of Respiratory and Critical Care Medicine. 2006;**174**:633-655. DOI: 10.1164/rccm.200601-007OC

[48] MacDonnell KF, Moon HS, Sekar TS, Ahluwalia MP. Extracorporeal membrane oxygenator support in a case of severe status asthmaticus. The Annals of Thoracic Surgery. 1981;**31**:171-175

[49] Mikkelsen ME, Woo YJ, Sager JS, Fuchs BD, Christie JD. Outcomes using extracorporeal life support for adult respiratory failure due to status asthmaticus. ASAIO Journal. 2009;**55**:47-52. DOI: 0.1097/MAT.0b013e3181901ea5

[50] Brenner K, Abrams DC, Agerstrand CL, Brodie D. Extracorporeal carbon dioxide removal for refractory status asthmaticus: Experience in distinct exacerbation phenotypes. Perfusion. 2014;**29**:26-28. DOI: 10.1177/0267659113494964

[51] Schneider TM, Bence T, Brettner F. "Awake" $ECCO_2R$ superseded intubation in a near-fatal asthma attack. Journal of Intensive Care. 2017;**5**:53. DOI: 10.1186/s40560-017-0247-7

[52] Elliot SC, Paramasivam K, Oram J, Bodenham AR, Howell SJ, Mallick A. Pumpless extracorporeal carbon dioxide removal for life-threatening asthma. Critical Care Medicine. 2007;**35**(3):945-948. DOI:10.1097/01.CCM.0000257462.04514.15

[53] Sakai M, Ohteki H, Doi K, Narita Y. Clinical use of extracorporeal lung assist for a patient in status asthmaticus. Annals of Thoracic Surgery. 1996;**62**(3):885-887

[54] Jung C, Lauten A, Pfeifer R, Bahrmann P, Figulla HR, Ferrari M. Pumpless extracorporeal lung assist for the treatment of severe, refractory status asthmaticus. Journal of Asthma. 2011;**48**(1):111-113. DOI: 10.3109/02770903.2010.528500

Chapter 7

Advances in Extracorporeal Membrane Oxygenation in the Setting of Lung Transplantation

Michael Mazzei, Suresh Keshavamurthy and Yoshiya Toyoda

Abstract

Lung transplantation has become an increasingly important modality for the treatment of severe lung disease. From its inception, the procedure has been refined so that it now represents the standard of care for end stage respiratory failure. The widespread adoption of this treatment option, however, has brought into sharp relief the current organ donor shortage. In tandem with the explosion in lung transplant procedures, a number of support modalities have seen an expanded role. Perhaps one of the most versatile tools in the armamentarium of the pulmonary transplant surgeon is extracorporeal membrane oxygenation (ECMO). This powerful tool is being increasingly implemented in all stages of lung transplantation—from supporting the failing native organ as a bridging tool to transplantation, to stabilizing the patient intra-operatively during the transplant procedure, to rescuing the patient with severe primary graft dysfunction immediately post-transplant. A number of advanced techniques for the application of ECMO in order to optimize the pulmonary transplant procedure are gaining traction—and with ECMO's expanded role in lung transplantation, so also has come a new set of technical and ethical challenges that must also be overcome.

Keywords: ECMO, veno-veno, veno-arterial, bridge to transplantation

1. Introduction

Lung transplantation has become an increasingly important modality for the treatment of severe lung disease. From its inception in 1985, the procedure has been refined so that it now represents the standard of care for end stage respiratory failure. As the efficacy of this treatment has been proven, we have seen the frequency of lung transplantation undergo an exponential rise. In 1993, for example, the International Society for Heart and Lung Transplantation (ISHLT) reports that a total of 1055 lung transplant procedures was performed. A decade later in 2003, that number had nearly doubled to 1934 and in 2013, the number of lung transplant procedures per year rose to 3892 [1]. In the same vein, a study in 2018 analyzing national trends of extracorporeal membrane oxygenation use in the National Inpatient Sample identified an over 360% increase in admissions for ECMO support from 2008 to 2014, among which mortality decreased among total admissions from over 60% down to 43% despite a trend toward an increased risk profile [2]. The widespread adoption of this treatment option, however, has brought into sharp relief the current organ donor shortage; there is currently a yearly potential lung transplant recipient mortality of up to 16% while awaiting organs to become available [3].

In tandem with the explosion in lung transplant procedures, a number of support modalities have seen an expanded role. Perhaps one of the most versatile tools in the armamentarium of the pulmonary transplant surgeon is extracorporeal membrane oxygenation (ECMO). This powerful tool is being increasingly implemented in all stages of lung transplantation—from supporting the failing native organ as a bridging tool to transplantation, to stabilizing the patient intraoperatively during the transplant procedure, to rescuing the patient with severe primary graft dysfunction immediately post-transplant. A number of advanced techniques for the application of ECMO in order to optimize the pulmonary transplant procedure are gaining traction—and with ECMO's expanded role in lung transplantation, so to have come a new set of technical and ethical challenges that must also be overcome.

The goal of this chapter is to discuss some of the recent advances in the application of ECMO in the setting of lung transplantation. We discuss the application of ECMO in the preoperative, perioperative, and postoperative period, and focus in particular on advances such as the use of awake ECMO and various cannulation strategies. We also briefly discuss some of the ethical issues surrounding ECMO for lung transplantation, including cost, quality of life, and the application of ECMO to marginal recipients.

2. VV- and VA-ECMO in lung transplantation

In the setting of lung transplantation, ECMO may be utilized in either a veno-venous (VV) or a veno-arterial (VA) configuration. The VV-ECMO modality is used strictly for respiratory support; this review will explore the current frontiers of usage in in the setting of either pre-operative bridge to transplant, as well as for bridging to graft recovery the subset of patients who develop severe post-transplant primary graft dysfunction (PGD). Alternatively, VA-ECMO may be utilized in the subset of patients with either pulmonary arterial hypertension requiring both cardiac and pulmonary support in the preoperative period, recently transplanted patients exhibiting hemodynamic instability, or in the intra-operative period for cardiopulmonary support [4].

Cannulation strategies for VA- and VV-ECMO are listed here. VV-ECMO is typically achieved via outflow and inflow cannulas in the femoral and internal jugular veins, with the tip of the drainage cannula placed to the level of the inferior vena cava-right atria junction and the tip of the return cannula at the right atrium. Alternatively, VV-ECMO may be achieved via a femoral-femoral cannulation strategy, with the tip of the drainage cannula in inferior vena cava and the tip of the outflow cannula is in the right atrium. Alternatively, a one-site cannulation strategy makes use of a dual lumen Avalon cannula (Avalon Elite, Maquet, Rastatt, Germany) percutaneously placed in the either internal jugular vein or in the subclavian vein [5].

VA-ECMO cannulation may be achieved using either a peripheral or central cannulation strategy. In a peripheral cannulation strategy, the femoral vein and artery are cannulated in a percutaneous fashion, with the tip of the arterial cannula placed in the common iliac artery. Alternatively, the arterial inflow cannula can be placed into the right subclavian artery. Because these peripheral strategies may in some cases only transmit arterial blood flow as far as the aortic arch (where blood oxygenated from the patient's native lungs and transmitted by the patient's heart) this may have the effect of poorly perfusing the heart and lungs (known as the Harlequin Syndrome). In this case, central cannulation of VA-ECMO is an option, with the venous cannula placed directly in the right atrium and the arterial cannula placed in the ascending aorta through a median sternotomy incision [4].

A number of hybrid options also exist for selected scenarios; these include Veno-veno-arterial ECMO (VVA-ECMO) where an additional venous cannula is inserted to offload the left ventricle, typically into the right internal jugular vein. This may also describe the conversion of veno-venous (VV) ECMO to additionally supply cardiac support by the insertion of an arterial cannula. Other triple-catheter strategies include the insertion of a distal perfusion cannula to the cannulated lower extremity in peripheral VA-ECMO in order to decrease limb ischemia. This armamentarium provides the surgeon with a number of different techniques for providing either isolated pulmonary or cardiopulmonary support in the transplant patient.

3. ECMO in the preoperative period

3.1 ECMO as a bridge to lung transplantation

The first successful use of ECMO in the preoperative period prior to lung transplant may be traced back to 1975, when ECMO was described as being initiated to correct a profound hypercapnia in a 19-year-old boy prior to transplantation. While the patient was successfully removed from the oxygenator and weaned from mechanical ventilation, he ultimately died on the eighteenth postoperative day due to a bronchial dehiscence [6]. For the next 20 years, this modality was occasionally described in the literature in case studies; however, it was associated with dismal outcomes and as a result did not gain widespread use.

In the past decade, however, there have been a number of advances in both the technology surrounding ECMO, and the management of the patient on ECMO, such that institutions are increasingly turning back to preoperative ECMO as an acceptable or even preferred modality for bridging patients with end stage respiratory disease to lung transplantation. This shift in management was preempted by a number of forces. First, the institution of the lung allocation score in 2005 allowed for more efficacious allocation of donor organs to those patients most emergently in need of a transplants rather than just the length of time on the waiting list. This meant that patients receiving continuous mechanical ventilation were listed with scores. ECMO was found to serve as a useful tool to stabilize ventilator-dependent patients approaching transplantation. Additionally, multicenter trials in the non-transplant population began to demonstrate the effectiveness of ECMO in ameliorating severe adult respiratory distress syndrome [7]. With the significant improvement in ECMO technologies, an increasing number retrospective and prospective studies have been conducted that show promising outcomes related to the use of ECMO as a bridging strategy [5, 8–17].

Some of those studies are reported here. Much of the initial research consisted of single-center retrospective studies. One of the first studies to demonstrate the efficacy of this therapy reported 17 bridged patients with a 78% 1-year survival after transplant, among whom allograft function did not differ between patients who did and did not receive ECMO bridging support [8]. A 2012 institutional study of 11 patients demonstrated shorter durations of mechanical support, and shorter post-transplant ICU and hospital stay in patients bridged with ECMO; a 1-year survival rate of over 85% after ECMO compared to 50% in patients with traditional mechanical ventilation was highlighted [15]. In 2013, a retrospective review of the medical records of 39 French patients bridged to lung transplantation on ECMO highlighted successful bridging to transplant in over 80% of the population, perioperative survival of 75%, and successful discharge from the hospital in 50%. While 2-year survival was largely a function of the underlying disease state, outcomes were largely similar between the ECMO and non-ECMO use groups, supporting the use of ECMO as a bridge to lung in order to preserve a medium-term survival benefit in the critically ill [14].

A large single-institution study retrospectively reviewed 715 consecutive lung transplants performed between the start of LAS implementation in May of 2005 until September 2011, of which 3.4% were performed on patients with attempted pre transplant ECMO. While patients in the pre-transplant ECMO group had significantly higher lung allocation scores, and median hospital stay was nearly double that for the ECMO group compared to the control group there was no difference in survival, with an overall 2-year survival approaching 75% in both cohorts [16]. A 2017 retrospective single-institution study looking particularly at cardiac outcomes in the population bridged to lung transplantation on ECMO identified a successful bridging rate of 60%, with a 1-year survival of over 90%. This study in particular noted right ventricular systolic dysfunction and worsening volume overload to be associated with unsuccessful bridging, but otherwise identified adequate outcomes [18].

In order to overcome some of the weaknesses of small retrospective cohorts, the question of ECMO's efficacy as a bridging strategy to transplant has been additionally queried of large national databases. A 2015 study of the United Network for Organ Sharing (UNOS) database highlighted 119 patients who were bridged to transplantation using extracorporeal membrane oxygenation compared to 12,339 patients who were not. The study period was divided into four 3-year intervals, and this demonstrated both an increasing number of patients bridged per year with ECMO and progressively increasing survival with each period, as did the number of patients bridged using extracorporeal membrane oxygenation. This highlights that short-term survival with the use of extracorporeal membrane oxygenation as a bridge to lung transplantation continues to significantly improve as it is more widely adopted [19].

The use of bridge-to-transplant with ECMO has also been trialed in small cohorts consisting of patient subsets at increased risk due to the presence of comorbidities. For example, this therapy has been demonstrated as effective in patients with cystic fibrosis; the authors of a 2012 case series of this population demonstrate good perioperative outcomes and describe the early initiation of ECMO soon after development of acute respiratory failure requiring mechanical ventilation as an important part of the treatment algorithm for these patients due to their high risk of ventilator-acquired complications [20]. Furthermore, in the subset of patients with advanced interstitial lung disease and secondary pulmonary hypertension, medical management remains complex and mechanical ventilator support are associated with poor outcomes. Small retrospective reviews, however, suggest that this subset had at least a comparable survival when requiring an extracorporeal membrane oxygenation bridge to that of other high acuity patients placed on extracorporeal membrane oxygenation as a bridge to lung transplantation [21]. Taken in sum, these studies suggest that extracorporeal membrane oxygenation is a feasible tool for use as a bridge to lung transplantation.

3.2 Awake and ambulatory ECMO

One benefit of ECMO compared to normal mechanical ventilation is that extracorporeal membrane oxygenation allows for adequate oxygenation to occur in patients who are awake, spontaneously breathing, and liberated from the ventilator. This could potentially represent a novel bridging strategy in that the complications associated with prolonged mechanical ventilation, such as ventilator-acquired pneumonia, are avoided. For example, a 2012 retrospective, single-center analysis of consecutive potential lung transplant patients receiving awake ECMO support compared with a historical control group receiving conventional mechanical ventilation demonstrated a 6-month survival after lung transplantation at 80% in the awake ECMO group versus 50% in the mechanical ventilation group. They also had shorter postoperative recovery periods [10].

In addition to avoiding mechanical ventilation complications, freedom from the vent also allows for novel rehabilitation efforts, such as ambulation and physical therapy while on ECMO, which could potentially help to stave off deconditioning while awaiting transplantation in the unit. Subjects on awake ECMO usually received a combination of passive and active physiotherapy; emerging research in the field affords preliminary evidence supporting the safety of early mobilization and ambulation in patients on awake ECMO support [22]. For example, a retrospective observational study in which ECMO patients were managed with early aggressive physical therapy, ambulation, and spontaneous breathing led to 30-day, 1-year, and 3-year survival outcomes after transplant of 92, 85, and 80%, respectively [11]. A second retrospective study compared five pre-transplant ECMO patients receiving active rehabilitation and ambulation to patients who were bridged with ECMO but did not receive pre-transplant rehabilitation. A third study of 72 patients receiving ECMO as a bridge to lung transplantation of which daily participation in physical therapy was achieved in 50 patients demonstrated favorable survival in patients receiving ECMO as a bridge to lung transplantation, particularly good outcomes in patients receiving physical therapy and maintaining avoidance of mechanical ventilation, and high rates of successful ambulation and therapy in the overall ECMO group [9]. Pre-transplant physical therapy was associated with shorter mean post-transplant mechanical ventilation, intensive care stay, and overall hospital days [23]. In general, preservation of pre-transplant ambulatory status has been found to improve outcomes in patients bridged to lung transplantation with ECMO [24]. These are encouraging findings support the concept that ambulatory ECMO allows for preservation of vitality while critically ill candidates await donor organs, which may improve outcomes.

Efforts to ambulate patients on ECMO bridging to lung transplant have been aided by the implementation of single-site, dual-lumen cannulation via an Avalon catheter. In conventional VV-ECMO, the outflow and inflow cannulas are placed percutaneously using the Seldinger technique, most commonly in the femoral and internal jugular veins. Alternatively, a one-site cannulation strategy makes use of a dual lumen Avalon cannula (Avalon Elite, Maquet, Rastatt, Germany) percutaneously placed in the either internal jugular vein or in the subclavian vein, under direct imaging such as fluoroscopy or transesophageal echocardiogram. This approach avoids use of the femoral site, which aids in mobilization and may limit the risk of recirculation and groin infectious complications [5]. Downsides include the need for precise placement and orientation of the catheter, requiring fluoroscopic guidance; femoral-femoral or femoral-jugular cannulation is much more expeditious, and suited to emergency situations. The Avalon catheter is also significantly more expensive than more conventional cannulation strategies [4]. Ultimately, however, the complication rate of this approach is comparable to traditional two-site ECMO in most studies [25], and many centers are now routinely using single-site ECMO as a first-line cannulation strategy.

Awake ECMO has been shown to be particularly effective for those patients at elevated risk of deconditioning. For example, the subset of patients requiring lung re-transplantation is a particularly challenging transplantation cohort because of the critical illness often associated with graft failure, as well as the higher likelihood of deconditioning after transplant failure. In a 2014 study looking specifically at this group, re-transplant patients bridged on awake, ambulatory ECMO support demonstrated a mortality of 0% compared to 39% in the group requiring mechanical ventilation The study concludes that awake ECMO bridging for re-transplantation provides comparable results to elective re-transplantation [26]. Larger retrospective studies have also made use of clinical databases such as the United Network for Organ Sharing database. In 2016, a study of all adult patients undergoing isolated lung transplantation in the last decade were identified based on their need for preoperative support: no support versus ECMO, invasive mechanical ventilation, or both, while 1-year survival was decreased in all patients requiring any type of support, mid-term survival was comparable between patients on ECMO alone and those not requiring support, but significantly worse with patients requiring mechanical ventilation with or without ECMO. This highlights the fact that those patients supported via ECMO with spontaneous breathing demonstrate improved survival compared with mechanical ventilation [27].

3.3 CO_2 removal in the bridge-to-transplant population

In patients awaiting lung transplantation, adequate gas exchange may not be sufficiently achieved by ventilation alone if acute respiratory decompensation arises. This may result in a life-threatening hypercapnia. ECMO may serve an additional purpose in patients bridging to lung transplantation as an adjunct for CO_2 removal ($ECCO_2$-R). For some patients, increased CO_2 clearance may spare them the need for mechanical ventilation [28]. A 2016 study of 20 patients (15 invasively ventilated and five noninvasively ventilated patients) demonstrated effective correction of hypercapnia and acidosis within the first 12 hours of therapy. Nineteen patients were successfully transplanted, and hospital and 1-year survival was 75 and 72%, respectively. This highlights $ECCO_2$-R as a feasible rescue therapy that can be associated with high transplantation and survival rates [29].

3.4 Prolonged bridging with ECMO

Outcomes in the unique subset of patient requiring the prolonged use of ECMO prior to lung transplantation have in recent years become the subject of study. For example, in a 2016 review of 974 patients who required prolonged (>14 days) ECMO in the Extracorporeal Life Support Organization international multi-institutional registry, 46% of these patients did not sustain native lung recovery; among these, 40 patients (4.1%) underwent lung transplant with a 50% post-operative in-hospital mortality [30]. While 14 days appears to be the consensus after which ECMO is considered to be prolonged, the upper bounds for the length of time for which ECMO can be continued as a bridging method continue to be tested. For example, a recent case report describes a patient remaining on ECMO for as long as 403 days while waiting for a lung transplant. This required changing the membrane oxygenator 23 times and the cannula 10 times; This therapy was ultimately terminated due to a loss of access for cannula insertion. The authors conclude that it is at least technically feasible to maintain patients awaiting lung transplantation on ECMO for extended periods of time, albeit maintaining for than 1-year may be difficult [31]. While case reports have described successful transplantation after many months on ECMO support, ultimately the outcomes remain dismal in this cohort; for example, as late as 2016 there were no recorded cases of pediatric long-term post-transplant survival after more than 52 days on ECMO support [32].

3.5 Selected issues in bridge-to-transplant

3.5.1 Cost-effectiveness

With the increasing utilization of ECMO in the lung transplant population, the question of utility is growing in importance. Recent studies have examined the cost associated with the use of extracorporeal membrane oxygenation in the setting of lung transplantation. A 2017 study using the Nationwide Inpatient Sample evaluated hospital charges of patients undergoing lung transplant who required ECMO during their hospital course; represented 4.2% of the patients undergoing lung transplantation overall. Median charges for lung transplant recipients who required ECMO were $780,391.50 versus $324,279.80 for non-ECMO recipients; the characteristics particularly associated with exorbitant hospital costs included black recipient race, pulmonary hypertension, and Medicare enrollees [33]. Studies have shown a disproportionately high amount of extracorporeal membrane oxygenation use in the Northeast compared to other parts of the country; this is highlighted as a regional disparity [2].

The economic impact of ambulatory versus either non-ambulatory ECMO strategies or mechanical ventilation as a bridge to lung transplantation is also of interest. In a retrospective 2016 study at a single center, subjects who were rehabilitated while supported with ECMO before lung transplantation were compared with those who were not rehabilitated during ECMO. When hospital cost data for the month before transplantation through 12 months after initial post-transplant hospital discharge were compared, subjects supported with ambulatory ECMO had a 22% (greater than $60,000) reduction in total hospital cost, 73% (greater than $100,000) reduction in post-transplant ICU costs, and 11% (greater than $30,000) reduction in total costs compared with non-ambulatory ECMO subjects [34].

3.5.2 Quality of life

With the increasing use of extracorporeal membrane oxygenation as a bridge to lung transplantation, the impact of preoperative ECMO on quality of life and depressive symptoms has been additionally targeted as an area of study. This question stems from the possibility that, due to complications after ECMO coupled with critical illness in the period up to transplantation may have adverse effects of quality of life in patients after transplantation. This does not appear to be the case; a 2018 single-institution prospective cohort study found that lung transplantation provides substantial quality of life improvements following lung transplantation, and these were generally similar among patients on pre-operative ECMO compared to those patients brought in for transplantation from the outpatient setting [35]. A second study in 2017 examining quality of life in ECMO-bridge lung transplant recipients demonstrated that outcomes after successful transplantation after ECMO are comparable with the general population undergoing lung transplantation in terms of quality of life, lung function, performance tests, and mortality [36].

3.5.3 Quality of the data

The increasing need for multi-institutional analysis of ECMO usage has had the effect of highlighting the dramatic differences in the implementation of ECMO at various programs. A survey of all US lung transplant centers in showed that two-thirds of responding centers used of ECMO as a bridge to transplant. Among these, a patient age greater than 65 was a cutoff in nearly half of centers, but otherwise many centers had no official age cutoff. Additionally, there was little consensus on the upper bounds for an acceptable duration of pre-transplant ECMO therapy, and this varied from as little as 10 days to a policy in which ECMO support duration was not bounded. Overall, the institutional criteria for ECMO initiation, age limits, and duration of support are widely disparate across centers [37].

A systematic review in 2014 highlighted the inconsistencies in design between these studies; while 82 potential studies of ECMO bridging were identified at the time, the vast majorities were excluded and the broad heterogeneity among the studies precluded any wider meta-analysis. In this analysis, the preoperative mortality rate of patients on ECMO ranged from 10–50%. It was ultimately concluded that ECMO support as a bridge could potentially provide reasonable perioperative and 1-year survival outcomes, but no broader statement could be made owing to a general paucity of high-quality data and significant heterogeneity among studies [38].

While these largely retrospective studies are compelling, it is acknowledged that retrospective studies are not the ideal candidates for definitively proving the efficacy of ECMO compared to mechanical ventilation, which has in tandem with ECMO evolved in the past decade to include more advanced strategies of protective lung ventilation. While the challenges of randomizing patients to different therapies in end-stage respiratory failure are apparent, at this point significant equipoise now exists to justify the randomized comparison of ECMO with standard ventilator therapy as a bridging strategy [39].

4. ECMO in the peri- and postoperative period

4.1 ECMO versus cardiopulmonary bypass

While partial or full cardiopulmonary support was initially a necessary aspect of lung transplantation, this has become less of a requirement with improvements in ventilation and operative technique. However, for those cases where cardiopulmonary support remains a necessity (such as failure of single lung ventilation, or right heart failure), VA ECMO is playing an increasing role as an alternative to traditional cardiopulmonary bypass. Cardiopulmonary bypass is at least theoretically responsible for the development of pulmonary injury and has been implicated in adult respiratory distress syndrome [40]. Pulmonary injury during cardiopulmonary bypass has been the subject of a significant amount of research over the past 30 years. At this time, it is theorized that lung damage occurs as the result of an inflammatory cascade triggered by a combination of surgical trauma, the interface of blood products with the extracorporeal circuit, and lung reperfusion injury; this triggers the generation of oxygen free radicals that are in turn sequestered within the lung and lead to pulmonary injury [41, 42].

Other issues related to cardiopulmonary bypass include a need for high-dose heparinization, which can lead to intra- and postoperative bleeding complications, and high blood turnover with a high volume of blood necessary to load the circuit. Cardiopulmonary bypass also requires central cannulation that can preclude other interventions in the operative field such as coronary artery bypass grafting. These issues have led providers to seek alternate supportive options. On its face, ECMO has a number of perceived benefits over cardiopulmonary bypass. With this in mind, there have been a number of studies comparing the efficacy of ECMO to cardiopulmonary bypass in the lung transplant setting [43–50].

The first studies of VA ECMO as a replacement therapy were not initially associated with good outcomes. For example, in 2007 a single institute retrospective study, ECMO was found to have a trend toward increased 90-day mortality rate, a higher incidence of severe graft ischemia/reperfusion injury, and a significantly reduced 1-year survival compared to cardiopulmonary bypass [45]. However, with increasing experience in using ECMO, results have been more promising. A 2012 retrospective study of outcomes of patients treated using ECMO versus cardiopulmonary bypass demonstrated a higher transfusion requirement in the cardiopulmonary bypass group, as well as a significantly higher incidence of in-hospital mortality, the need for hemodialysis, and new postoperative ECMO support. In this study transplantation with cardiopulmonary bypass was identified as an independent risk factor for in-hospital mortality [51].

In a 2014 study comparing differences in 47 lung transplant patient outcomes with intraoperative ECMO versus cardiopulmonary bypass, the ECMO group was required fewer transfusions and had less bleeding, fewer reoperations, and less primary graft dysfunction with no 30-day or 1-year survival differences [44]. Similarly, in a 2014 comparison of 271 consecutive patients who underwent lung transplant using either cardiopulmonary bypass or ECMO, there were differences in 30-day or 6-month mortality, and less postoperative complications among the ECMO group [43]. A number of more recent studies similarly comparing VA ECMO to cardiopulmonary bypass have confirmed the finding of a lower perioperative blood product transfusion requirement and lower 90-day mortality among the extracorporeal membrane oxygenation cohorts [48, 49, 52, 53].

Recently, a meta-analysis of the existing evidence to support ECMO versus cardiopulmonary bypass showed beneficial trends of ECMO regarding blood transfusions, duration of ventilator support and intensive care unit length of stay, 3-month and 1-year mortality; these findings, however, were not statistically significant. At this time, while it appears that ECMO is at least non-inferior to cardiopulmonary bypass in the setting of lung transplantation, the superiority of ECMO remains to be determined and will likely require larger multi-center randomized trials [47].

Outcomes compared between patients requiring intraoperative ECMO versus those not requiring any support are less conclusive; in a 2018 study of 53 patients, while patients who underwent ECMO received more intraoperative transfusions, outside of the immediate postoperative period there were no differences in in-hospital and 6-month complications with similar survival between the two groups [50]. In contrast, however, a 2017 single institution study demonstrated 5-year survival to be 52.8% in intraoperative ECMO recipients versus 70.5% in those not requiring ECMO, with multivariate analysis identifying intraoperative ECMO support as significant risk factors for overall survival [46].

4.2 Postoperative ECMO for primary graft dysfunction

Early primary graft dysfunction, defined as lung injury causing decreased oxygenation during the first 3 days after lung transplant, is a devastating albeit fairly uncommon occurrence. ECMO is a useful adjunct for supporting the patient with primary graft dysfunction, either to recovery or as a bridge to redo transplantation.

One-year survival is compromised in patients with severe primary graft dysfunction compared to those without; in addition to the underlying causal factors contributing to dysfunction in the first place, this is often worsened by the high airway pressures and inspired oxygen concentration necessary to adequately oxygenate the patient via mechanical ventilation. ECMO may be desirable for its ability to avoid these risk factors. In a single-institution study of patients with primary graft dysfunction, successful weaning from ECMO was achieved in 96% of patients, with substantially improved long-term outcomes including a 5-year survival of nearly 50%. While allograft function in the ECMO group was worse than in transplant recipients not requiring ECMO, the benefits of ECMO in pulmonary support in the immediate postoperative period is clear [54]. Furthermore, these trends toward better outcomes after primary graft dysfunction appear to be improving due to ECMO support; in a large database study of the highest-risk transplant patients, patients demonstrate improving outcomes, particularly at high-volume centers [55]. In a review of the UNOS database, the use of postoperative ECMO support for primary graft dysfunction was still associated with a 6-month survival of over 60%, and while the subset of ECMO recipients also requiring dialysis had a only a 25% 6-month survival, if dialysis was not needed survival was over 85% [56].

Unfortunately, while early postoperative ECMO in the setting of primary graft dysfunction is associated with reasonable outcomes, the late implementation of ECMO postoperatively (after 7 days) does not appear to have the same good outcomes. In a 2011 study of late ECMO support in lung transplant patients with infection or graft failure, none of the individuals who received late ECMO support survived to hospital discharge, due to the propagation of uncontrolled infection or organ failure that preempted ECMO support. This suggests that while ECMO can provide early support while awaiting graft recovery, it does not represent a means of reversing complications existing prior to initiation of ECMO [57].

4.3 Routine ECMO prolongation

With increasing comfort with ECMO as postoperative support, the indications for extending its use have continued to expand. In some institutions, for example, intraoperative extracorporeal membrane oxygenation has been adopted for all unstable lung transplantations. Protocols have been proposed in which ECMO is prophylactically extended into the postoperative period based on graft quality and the preoperative presence of pulmonary hypertension. A recent single-institution analysis of this prophylactic protocol identified patients receiving ECMO as having improved survival compared to non-ECMO patients despite higher levels of medical complexity. Prophylactic ECMO prolongation is being increasingly recognized as a safe option for the routine postoperative support of patients with either marginal graft function or underlying pulmonary hypertension [12].

In the same vein, research has been conducted to identify those patients at increased risk of ECMO weaning failure after lung transplantation, in order to identify those patients who might benefit from continued extracorporeal support. Identified risk factors including older donors, longer periods of donor mechanical ventilation, donor PaO_2 prior to organ procurement and longer operative time [58]. In these patients, prophylactic ECMO support postoperatively may be recommended.

4.4 Ex-vivo lung perfusion using ECMO

Ex vivo lung perfusion is another exciting breakthrough for the reconditioning of poor quality grafts as high risk of postoperative primary graft dysfunction. In this setup, retrieved donor lungs are perfused in an ex vivo circuit. This provides an opportunity for transplant surgeons to reassess graft function before transplantation, providing a more accurate window into the likelihood of success in transplantation with high-risk donor lungs. The use of an ex vivo circuit allows time for toxic waste products and inflammatory cytokines to be filtered out, for more optimal recruitment of collapsed lung areas, and for the fluid-overloaded lung tissue to be dehydrated by the perfusate high oncotic pressure [59]. In a 2015 study, lung transplant recipients who received lungs reconditioned in an ex vivo manner demonstrated significantly shorter hospital stay and trends toward shorter length of mechanical ventilation [48, 49].

5. Conclusions

Ultimately, recent advances in ECMO have led it to become a critical tool in the armamentarium of the transplant surgeon, in both the preoperative period as a bridging strategy, as a tool for cardiopulmonary support during the operation, and for the rescue of potentially dysfunctional grafts postoperatively. The use of ECMO in lung transplantation has been need-driven in an incredibly complex and medically challenging complication; innovative thinking by basic scientists and transplant surgeons has led to remarkable improvements in patient outcomes. Continued advances in ECMO technologies, deeper experience with the implementation of ECMO in complicated clinical situations, and further high-quality research will help determine the areas where ECMO can help provide a benefit to lung transplant recipients.

Author details

Michael Mazzei[1], Suresh Keshavamurthy[2]* and Yoshiya Toyoda[2]

1 Department of Surgery, Temple University Hospital, Lewis Katz School of Medicine at Temple University, United States of America

2 Department of Surgery, Division of Cardiovascular Surgery, Temple University Hospital, Lewis Katz School of Medicine at Temple University, United States of America

*Address all correspondence to: skeshavamurthy@gmail.com

References

[1] Yusen RD, Edwards LB, Kucheryavaya AY, Benden C, Dipchand AI, Goldfarb SB, et al. The Registry of the International Society for Heart and Lung Transplantation: Thirty-second official adult lung and heart-lung transplantation report—2015; focus theme: Early graft failure. The Journal of Heart and Lung Transplantation. 2015;**34**(10):1264-1277

[2] Sanaiha Y, Bailey K, Downey P, Seo YJ, Aguayo E, Dobaria V, et al. Trends in mortality and resource utilization for extracorporeal membrane oxygenation in the United States: 2008-2014. Surgery. 2018

[3] Zych B, Garcia-Saez D, Simon AR. Lung donor shortage–how to overcome it? Polish Journal of Cardio-Thoracic Surgery. 2016;**13**(3):195

[4] Jayaraman AL, Cormican D, Shah P, Ramakrishna H. Cannulation strategies in adult veno-arterial and veno-venous extracorporeal membrane oxygenation: Techniques, limitations, and special considerations. Annals of Cardiac Anaesthesia. 2017;**20**(Suppl 1):S11

[5] Javidfar J, Brodie D, Wang D, Ibrahimiye AN, Yang J, Zwischenberger JB, et al. Use of bicaval dual-lumen catheter for adult venovenous extracorporeal membrane oxygenation. The Annals of Thoracic Surgery. 2011;**91**(6):1763-1769

[6] Nelems JM, Duffin J, Glynn FX, Brebner J, Scott AA, Cooper JD. Extracorporeal membrane oxygenator support for human lung transplantation. The Journal of Thoracic and Cardiovascular Surgery. 1978;**76**(1):28-32

[7] Peek GJ, Mugford M, Tiruvoipati R, Wilson A, Allen E, Thalanany MM, et al. Efficacy and economic assessment of conventional ventilatory support versus extracorporeal membrane oxygenation for severe adult respiratory failure (CESAR): A multicentre randomised controlled trial. Lancet (London, England). 2009;**374**(9698):1351-1363

[8] Bermudez CA, Rocha RV, Zaldonis D, Bhama JK, Crespo MM, Shigemura N, et al. Extracorporeal membrane oxygenation as a bridge to lung transplant: Midterm outcomes. The Annals of Thoracic Surgery. 2011;**92**(4):1226-1232

[9] Biscotti M, Gannon WD, Agerstrand C, Abrams D, Sonett J, Brodie D, et al. Awake extracorporeal membrane oxygenation as bridge to lung transplantation: A 9-year experience. The Annals of Thoracic Surgery. 2017;**104**(2):412-419

[10] Fuehner T, Kuehn C, Hadem J, Wiesner O, Gottlieb J, Tudorache I, et al. Extracorporeal membrane oxygenation in awake patients as bridge to lung transplantation. American Journal of Respiratory and Critical Care Medicine. 2012;**185**(7):763-768

[11] Hakim AH, Ahmad U, McCurry KR, Johnston DR, Pettersson GB, Budev M, et al. Contemporary outcomes of extracorporeal membrane oxygenation used as bridge to lung transplantation. The Annals of Thoracic Surgery. Jul 1 2018;**106**(1):192-198

[12] Hashimoto K, Hoetzenecker K, Yeung JC, Jeagal L, Donahoe L, Pierre A, et al. Intraoperative extracorporeal support during lung transplantation in patients bridged with venovenous extracorporeal membrane oxygenation. The Journal of Heart and Lung Transplantation. 2018;**37**(12):1418-1424

[13] Ius F, Tudorache I, Warnecke G. Extracorporeal support, during and after lung transplantation: The history of an idea. Journal of Thoracic Disease. 2018;**10**(8):5131

[14] Lafarge M, Mordant P, Thabut G, Brouchet L, Falcoz PE, Haloun A, et al. Experience of extracorporeal membrane oxygenation as a bridge to lung transplantation in France. The Journal of Heart and Lung Transplantation. 2013;**32**(9):905-913

[15] Nosotti M, Rosso L, Tosi D, Palleschi A, Mendogni P, Nataloni IF, et al. Extracorporeal membrane oxygenation with spontaneous breathing as a bridge to lung transplantation. Interactive Cardiovascular and Thoracic Surgery. 2012;**16**(1):55-59

[16] Toyoda Y, Bhama JK, Shigemura N, Zaldonis D, Pilewski J, Crespo M, et al. Efficacy of extracorporeal membrane oxygenation as a bridge to lung transplantation. The Journal of Thoracic and Cardiovascular Surgery. 2013;**145**(4):1065-1071

[17] Javidfar J, Brodie D, Iribarne A, Jurado J, LaVelle M, Brenner K, et al. Extracorporeal membrane oxygenation as a bridge to lung transplantation and recovery. The Journal of Thoracic and Cardiovascular Surgery. 2012;**144**(3):716-721

[18] Banga A, Batchelor E, Mohanka M, Bollineni S, Kaza V, Mullins J, et al. Predictors of outcome among patients on extracorporeal membrane oxygenation as a bridge to lung transplantation. Clinical Transplantation. 2017;**31**(7):e12990

[19] Hayanga AJ, Aboagye J, Esper S, Shigemura N, Bermudez CA, D'cunha J, et al. Extracorporeal membrane oxygenation as a bridge to lung transplantation in the United States: An evolving strategy in the management of rapidly advancing pulmonary disease. The Journal of Thoracic and Cardiovascular Surgery. 2015;**149**(1):291-296

[20] Hayes D Jr, Kukreja J, Tobias JD, Ballard HO, Hoopes CW. Ambulatory venovenous extracorporeal respiratory support as a bridge for cystic fibrosis patients to emergent lung transplantation. Journal of Cystic Fibrosis. 2012;**11**(1):40-45

[21] Hoopes CW, Kukreja J, Golden J, Davenport DL, Diaz-Guzman E, Zwischenberger JB. Extracorporeal membrane oxygenation as a bridge to pulmonary transplantation. The Journal of Thoracic and Cardiovascular Surgery. 2013;**145**(3):862-868

[22] Polastri M, Loforte A, Dell'Amore A, Nava S. Physiotherapy for patients on awake extracorporeal membrane oxygenation: A systematic review. Physiotherapy Research International. 2016;**21**(4):203-209

[23] Rehder KJ, Turner DA, Hartwig MG, Williford WL, Bonadonna D, Walczak RJ, et al. Active rehabilitation during extracorporeal membrane oxygenation as a bridge to lung transplantation. Respiratory Care. 2013;**58**(8):1291-1298

[24] Bailey KL, Iyengar A, Kwon O, Caceras M, Eisenring C, Ross D, et al. Ambulatory status improves outcomes in patients bridged to lung transplantation with ECMO. The Journal of Heart and Lung Transplantation. 2018;**37**(4):S253

[25] Rubino A, Vuylsteke A, Jenkins DP, Fowles JA, Hockings L, Valchanov K. Direct complications of the Avalon bicaval dual-lumen cannula in respiratory extracorporeal membrane oxygenation (ECMO): Single-center experience. The International Journal of Artificial Organs. 2014;**37**(10):741-747

[26] Lang G, Kim D, Aigner C, Matila J, Taghavi S, Jaksch P, et al. Awake extracorporeal membrane oxygenation bridging for pulmonary retransplantation provides comparable results to elective retransplantation. The Journal of Heart and Lung Transplantation. 2014;**33**(12):1264-1272

[27] Schechter MA, Ganapathi AM, Englum BR, Speicher PJ, Daneshmand MA, Davis RD, et al. Spontaneously breathing extracorporeal membrane oxygenation support provides the optimal bridge to lung transplantation. Transplantation. 2016;**100**(12):2699

[28] Bonin F, Sommerwerck U, Lund LW, Teschler H. Avoidance of intubation during acute exacerbation of chronic obstructive pulmonary disease for a lung transplant candidate using extracorporeal carbon dioxide removal with the Hemolung. The Journal of Thoracic and Cardiovascular Surgery. 2013;**145**(5):e43-e44

[29] Schellongowski P, Riss K, Staudinger T, Ullrich R, Krenn CG, Sitzwohl C, et al. Extracorporeal CO_2 removal as bridge to lung transplantation in life-threatening hypercapnia. Transplant International. 2015;**28**(3):297-304

[30] Posluszny J, Rycus PT, Bartlett RH, Engoren M, Haft JW, Lynch WR, et al. Outcome of adult respiratory failure patients receiving prolonged (≥14 days) ECMO. Annals of Surgery. 2016;**263**(3):573-581

[31] Umei N, Ichiba S, Sakamoto A. Idiopathic pulmonary fibrosis patient supported with extracorporeal membrane oxygenation for 403 days while waiting for a lung transplant: A case report. Respiratory Medicine Case Reports. 2018;**24**:86-88

[32] Bates AR, Hanot J, Carroll A, Muhieldin A, Anton N, Lequier L. D51 pediatric cases II: A pediatric case of prolonged extracorporeal support and successful lung transplantation following invasive pulmonary aspergillosis and influenza infection. American Journal of Respiratory and Critical Care Medicine. 2016;**193**:1

[33] Hayanga JA, Shigemura N, Aboagye JK, Ensor C, Dew MA, Hayanga HK, et al. ECMO support in lung transplantation: A contemporary analysis of hospital charges in the United States. The Annals of Thoracic Surgery. 2017;**104**(3):1033-1039

[34] Bain JC, Turner DA, Rehder KJ, Eisenstein EL, Davis RD, Cheifetz IM, et al. Economic outcomes of extracorporeal membrane oxygenation with and without ambulation as a bridge to lung transplantation. Respiratory Care. Jan 2016;**61**(1):1-7

[35] Kolaitis NA, Soong A, Shrestha P, Zhuo H, Neuhaus J, Katz PP, et al. Improvement in patient-reported outcomes after lung transplantation is not impacted by the use of extracorporeal membrane oxygenation as a bridge to transplantation. The Journal of Thoracic and Cardiovascular Surgery. Jul 1 2018;**156**(1):440-448

[36] Lansink-Hartgring AO, van der Bij W, Verschuuren EA, Erasmus ME, de Vries AJ, Vermeulen KM, et al. Extracorporeal life support as a bridge to lung transplantation: A single-center experience with an emphasis on health-related quality of life. Respiratory Care. 2017;**62**(5):588-594

[37] Tsiouris A, Budev MM, Yun JJ. Extracorporeal membrane oxygenation as a bridge to lung transplantation in the United States: A multicenter survey. ASAIO Journal. 2018;**64**(5):689-693

[38] Chiumello D, Coppola S, Froio S, Colombo A, Del Sorbo L. Extracorporeal life support as bridge to lung transplantation: A systematic review. Critical Care. 2015;**19**(1):19

[39] Del Sorbo L, Ranieri VM, Keshavjee S. Extracorporeal membrane oxygenation as "bridge" to lung transplantation: What remains in order to make it standard of care? American Journal of Respiratory and Critical Care Medicine. 2012;**185**(7):699-701

[40] Asimakopoulos G, Smith PL, Ratnatunga CP, Taylor KM. Lung injury and acute respiratory distress syndrome after cardiopulmonary bypass. The Annals of Thoracic Surgery. 1999;**68**(3):1107-1115

[41] Butler J, Rocker GM, Westaby S. Inflammatory response to cardiopulmonary bypass. The Annals of Thoracic Surgery. 1993;**55**(2):552-559

[42] Clark SC. Lung injury after cardiopulmonary bypass. Perfusion. 2006;**21**(4):225-228

[43] Bermudez CA, Shiose A, Esper SA, Shigemura N, D'Cunha J, Bhama JK, et al. Outcomes of intraoperative venoarterial extracorporeal membrane oxygenation versus cardiopulmonary bypass during lung transplantation. The Annals of Thoracic Surgery. 2014;**98**(6):1936-1943

[44] Biscotti M, Yang J, Sonett J, Bacchetta M. Comparison of extracorporeal membrane oxygenation versus cardiopulmonary bypass for lung transplantation. The Journal of Thoracic and Cardiovascular Surgery. 2014;**148**(5):2410-2416

[45] Bittner HB, Binner C, Lehmann S, Kuntze T, Rastan A, Mohr FW. Replacing cardiopulmonary bypass with extracorporeal membrane oxygenation in lung transplantation operations. European Journal of Cardio-Thoracic Surgery. 2007;**31**(3):462-467

[46] Cosgun T, Tomaszek S, Opitz I, Wilhelm M, Schuurmans MM, Weder W, et al. Single-center experience with intraoperative extracorporeal membrane oxygenation use in lung transplantation. The International Journal of Artificial Organs. 2018;**41**(2):89-93

[47] Hoechter DJ, Shen YM, Kammerer T, Günther S, Weig T, Schramm R, et al. Extracorporeal circulation during lung transplantation procedures: A meta-analysis. ASAIO Journal. 2017;**63**(5):551-561

[48] Machuca TN, Collaud S, Mercier O, Cheung M, Cunningham V, Kim SJ, et al. Outcomes of intraoperative extracorporeal membrane oxygenation versus cardiopulmonary bypass for lung transplantation. The Journal of Thoracic and Cardiovascular Surgery. 2015;**149**(4):1152-1157

[49] Machuca TN, Mercier O, Collaud S, Tikkanen J, Krueger T, Yeung JC, et al. Lung transplantation with donation after circulatory determination of death donors and the impact of ex vivo lung perfusion. American Journal of Transplantation. 2015;**15**(4):993-1002

[50] Pettenuzzo T, Faggi G, Di Gregorio G, Schiavon M, Marulli G, Gregori D, et al. Blood products transfusion and mid-term outcomes of lung transplanted patients under extracorporeal membrane oxygenation support. Progress in Transplantation. 2018;**28**(4):314-321

[51] Ius F, Kuehn C, Tudorache I, Sommer W, Avsar M, Boethig D, et al. Lung transplantation on cardiopulmonary support: Venoarterial extracorporeal membrane oxygenation outperformed cardiopulmonary bypass. The Journal of Thoracic and Cardiovascular Surgery. 2012;**144**(6):1510-1516

[52] Song JH, Park JE, Lee JG, Lee CY, Nam KS, Suh JW, et al. Outcomes of perioperative extracorporeal membrane oxygenation use in patients undergoing lung transplantation. Journal of Thoracic Disease. 2017;**9**(12):5075

[53] Yu WS, Paik HC, Haam SJ, Lee CY, Nam KS, Jung HS, et al. Transition to routine use of venoarterial extracorporeal oxygenation during lung transplantation could improve early

outcomes. Journal of Thoracic Disease. 2016;**8**(7):1712

[54] Hartwig MG, Walczak R, Lin SS, Davis RD. Improved survival but marginal allograft function in patients treated with extracorporeal membrane oxygenation after lung transplantation. The Annals of Thoracic Surgery. 2012;**93**(2):366-371

[55] George TJ, Beaty CA, Kilic A, Shah PD, Merlo CA, Shah AS. Outcomes and temporal trends among high-risk patients after lung transplantation in the United States. The Journal of Heart and Lung Transplantation. 2012;**31**(11):1182-1191

[56] Mulvihill MS, Yerokun BA, Davis RP, Ranney DN, Daneshmand MA, Hartwig MG. Extracorporeal membrane oxygenation following lung transplantation: Indications and survival. The Journal of Heart and Lung Transplantation. 2018;**37**(2):259-267

[57] Marasco SF, Vale M, Preovolos A, Pellegrino V, Lee G, Snell G, et al. Institution of extracorporeal membrane oxygenation late after lung transplantation—A futile exercise? Clinical Transplantation. 2012;**26**(1):E71-E77

[58] Narm KS, Lee S, Suh JW, Kim A, Lee JG, Park MS, et al. Risk factor analysis for intraoperative extracorporeal membrane oxygenation weaning failure after lung transplantation. The Annals of Thoracic Surgery. 2018;**105**(1):242-248

[59] Van Raemdonck D, Neyrinck A, Cypel M, Keshavjee S. Ex-vivo lung perfusion. Transplant International. 2015;**28**(6):643-656

Chapter 8

Extracorporeal Cardiopulmonary Resuscitation

Abdelaziz Farhat, Cindy Darnell Bowens, Ravi Thiagarajan and Lakshmi Raman

Abstract

ECMO, or extracorporeal membrane oxygenation, is an advanced life support technique that provides cardiac and pulmonary support similar to cardiopulmonary bypass. ECPR (extracorporeal cardiopulmonary resuscitation) is the rapid deployment of VA-ECMO when conventional cardiopulmonary resuscitation fails to provide return of spontaneous circulation. Evidence in the literature is sparse, but with expanding reported applications, ECPR has shown promise to improve outcomes of cardiac arrest. ECPR is superior to conventional CPR for both survival and neurologic outcomes. ECPR has been successfully used to manage arrests secondary to cardiac and non-cardiac causes. Arrests secondary to primary cardiac causes have the best overall outcome. Other determinants of outcomes of ECPR include duration of low flow state and on-ECMO complications. A narrow list of ECPR contraindications exists, and includes severe neurologic injury and irreversible primary disease process. Various complications can occur with ECPR, and include mechanical, cardiovascular, pulmonary, hematologic, renal, and neurologic complications. Neurologic complications are the most serious, and significantly affect mortality or quality of life. ECPR is a nascent field, and substantial work remains to be done to optimize its application. Given the small number of patients at each institutional level, this is a field ripe for collaborative work and rewarding results.

Keywords: extracorporeal membrane oxygenation, cardiopulmonary resuscitation, ECPR, cardiac arrest

1. Background

ECMO, or extracorporeal membrane oxygenation, is an advanced life support technique that provides cardiac and pulmonary support similar to cardiopulmonary bypass. Venous blood is drained and pumped through a membrane where gas exchange occurs. Oxygenated blood is returned back to the patient either through venous circulation in VV-ECMO (venovenous ECMO) or arterial circulation in VA-ECMO (venoarterial ECMO).

ECPR (extracorporeal cardiopulmonary resuscitation) is the rapid deployment of VA-ECMO during cardiopulmonary resuscitation (CPR) when conventional CPR fails to provide return of spontaneous circulation (ROSC) [1]. The first reported use of ECMO in CPR was in 1976. Since then, the use of ECPR has become well-described in adults and children, with a continuously expanding list of diagnoses.

ECPR literature is limited, more so for pediatrics. Reports are mainly single center experiences, registry retrospective analyses, and a few meta-analyses. Small sample sizes and lack of standardization impede drawing conclusions on utilization and care processes for ECPR. Regardless, utilization of ECPR continues to expand. The Extracorporeal Life Support Organization (ELSO) reports more than a total of 10,000 ECPR patients since 1990, of which more than 5000 are pediatric or neonatal runs [2]. ECPR cases make up approximately 10% of all ECMO runs recorded over this time frame. Most ECPR cases originate in the intensive care unit, but there is growing literature demonstrating widening the use to emergency room arrests and out-of-hospital arrests [3, 4].

With expanding application, ECPR has shown promise to improve outcomes of cardiac arrest. ELSO recognizes that ECMO can be considered for select patients in cardiac arrest. In 2015, the American Heart Association (AHA) cautiously pointed out that while the evidence is still lacking, ECPR may reasonably be considered in potentially reversible situations [5].

This chapter explores the current utility of ECPR, and provides a literature summary of its indications and limitations. The chapter will also describe current use and outcomes in adults and children. Finally, complications of ECPR will be reviewed. A special focus will highlight neurologic complications and their influence on meaningful outcomes after ECPR.

2. ECPR is superior to conventional CPR

ECPR use for victims of cardiac arrest consistently demonstrates a survival benefit over conventional CPR [5–8]. This survival benefit is more pronounced as the duration of CPR increases. In contrast to arrest survivors who only receive conventional CPR, patients rescued with ECPR have higher survival rates at discharge and at 6-12 months post discharge [9]. Arrest victims rescued with ECPR are also more likely to have better neurologic outcome, when compared to patients rescued with conventional CPR [10].

3. Indications

The goal of ECPR is to augment cardiac output during the low flow phase of CPR, restoring oxygenation and perfusion in the setting of cardiac arrest. In some cases ECPR alone may be therapeutic, and in other cases it allows maintenance of perfusion while further treatment is explored.

At this time, no universal criteria exist for the deployment of ECPR. AHA recommendations are limited to heart disease amenable to either recovery or transplantation, in a setting where the arrest occurs in a highly supervised environment [11]. Their only other recommendation is for use in out of hospital cardiac arrest in the setting of severe hypothermia if appropriate expertise, equipment, and protocols are available. ELSO recommends ECPR in arrest victims "with an easily reversible event and have had excellent CPR" [12]. The UK Resuscitation Council considers ECPR as a "rescue therapy for patients in whom initial ALS measures are unsuccessful to facilitate specific interventions" such as coronary interventions or thrombectomies [13].

Centers that offer ECPR use center-specific processes, based on experience and availability of resources. ECPR is most commonly available to in-hospital cardiac arrest. Arrests in the emergency department can also be managed with ECPR. In some settings with appropriate resources, experience, and planning, out-of-hospital cardiac arrest has been managed with out-of-hospital ECPR [4, 14].

4. Contraindications

Contraindications to ECPR vary between institutions, and a unified consensus does not exist. ECMO-related prognostic factors in the current literature are unreliable with regards to ECPR outcomes. On their own, most of these factors do not provide sufficient evidence to support denial of life-saving ECPR to a victim of arrest. The only absolute contraindications to ECPR are the presence of a valid "Do Not Resuscitate" order and the absence of appropriate staff/equipment to initiate ECPR. All contraindications to ECMO use, such as extreme prematurity, also apply.

Otherwise, a range of situations can be proposed as relative contraindications for ECPR:

1. Severe neurological impairment prior to cardiac arrest: Exact definitions of impairment will vary between providers and institutions. In a similar vein, conditions that place a patient at high risk for severe neurologic injury despite good CPR (such as severe primary pulmonary hypertension or patients with cavopulmonary circulation) may be a reason to not offer ECPR. Determinations to preclude a child from ECMO candidacy may involve a discussion with family, and should contain an understanding the perceived and expected quality of the child's life.

2. Known irreversible disease process: When cardiac arrest occurs in the setting of a known irreversible and untreatable disease process, ECPR will only prolong suffering. Providers must work with the appropriate subspecialists to understand primary disease prognosis in order to determine if ECPR is an appropriate choice should the patient arrest.

3. Severe immunosuppressed state: While literature is limited, certain groups of severely immunocompromised patients tend to do worse on ECMO. Patients with immunosuppression in the setting of solid organ transplantation or high-dose steroid regimens may have outcomes comparable to the general population. In contrast, patients with solid tumors, hematological malignancies, or acquired immunodeficiency syndrome (AIDS) do much worse on ECMO. In one study, survival to discharge was 7–20% [15]. This highlights the need to understand primary disease prognosis, and determine ECMO candidacy prior to arrest.

4. Severe coagulopathy: Management of ECMO post-resuscitation requires use of anticoagulation to maintain appropriate circuit function. In cases of severe coagulopathy, the physician must balance the management of the coagulopathy and the circuit anticoagulation. If the coagulopathy is difficult to treat, devastating and fatal hemorrhagic side effects may occur [16].

5. Prolonged total arrest time: There is no consensus on a cut-off time, but as shown in **Figure 1**, prolonged low-flow states are associated with lower survival [17]. Neurologic outcomes are also worse. The impact is magnified if combined with failure to initiate chest compressions in a timely fashion after arrest. While a prolonged resuscitation may be not futile, each institution must consider its capabilities and available resources before establishing a cutoff time. This decision will also likely be patient-dependent.

6. Lack of access for cannulation: Anatomic or other vascular anomalies that preclude successful cannulation render a patient a non-candidate for ECPR.

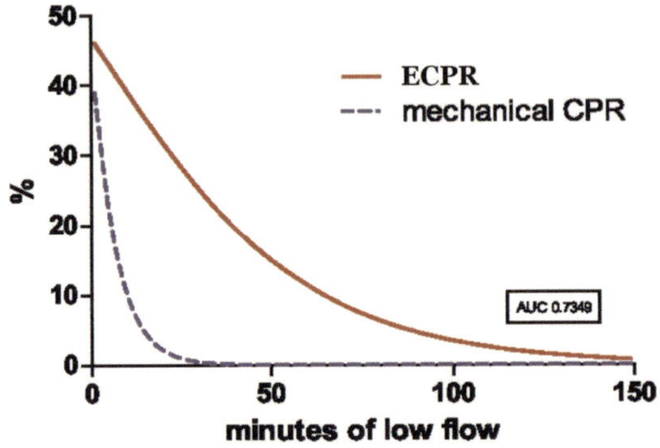

Figure 1.
Estimated survival rates for extracorporeal membrane oxygenation (ECPR) patients after every given low-flow time (red line). Survival with conventional CPR (dashes) is demonstrated as a comparison. Wengenmayer T, et al. Influence of low-flow time on survival after extracorporeal cardiopulmonary resuscitation Crit Care. 2017;21(1):157. Published under terms of the Creative Commons Attribution 4.0 International License.

5. The ECPR experience

According to recent reviews of the ELSO registry, ECPR is currently most commonly used in patients who suffer cardiac arrest secondary to a primary cardiac cause [7]. This is independent from patients who fail to wean off cardiopulmonary bypass. These patients include arrests post cardiac surgery, such as surgery for congenital heart disease (CHD). CHD patients rescued with ECPR include both single and two-ventricle patients. This cardiac cohort also includes patients with structurally normal hearts but develop heart failure in the setting of myocarditis, cardiomyopathy, arrhythmias, pulmonary arterial hypertension, and heart transplant graft failures.

A variety of non-cardiac causes of arrest have also been supported by ECPR. These include arrests in the setting of septic and other forms of non-cardiogenic shock. Arrests that occur in the setting of pneumonia, ARDS, acute airway compromise, toxic ingestions, severe hypothermia, and trauma have also been supported with ECPR.

In some situations where the cause of arrest is unclear, ECPR allows for preserving the patient while the diagnosis can be clarified. For example, ECMO support allows for time to perform head imaging or other diagnostic testing that helps with clarifying treatment or prognostication. If a negative prognosis is uncovered, there is time to involve palliative care, if desired, and allows family another opportunity for closure.

Some institutions have reported ECPR use as a temporary measure for organ perfusion while organ procurement organizations work to facilitate organ placement [18, 19]. This is usually in situations where brain death is quickly identified after placement on ECMO. Viability of the organs is preserved, and the transplanted organs have a high rate of good functional recovery [20].

6. Application of ECPR

6.1 Process

The real-life application of ECPR varies between centers [21]. At a minimum, a core group that consists of a code team, a cannulation team (surgeon or interventionalist to cannulate), and an ECMO specialist must be available. Support staff including additional nursing, pharmacy, and OR staff may be needed. Location of the cannulation procedure will depend on center experience and appropriateness of available space. For example, the procedure can happen in the intensive care unit, in the catheterization lab, or in the operating room. Some centers have reported experience with cannulating in other locations, such as in the emergency department, in the IR suite, or on regular hospital wards. Most reported experiences follow a similar algorithm.

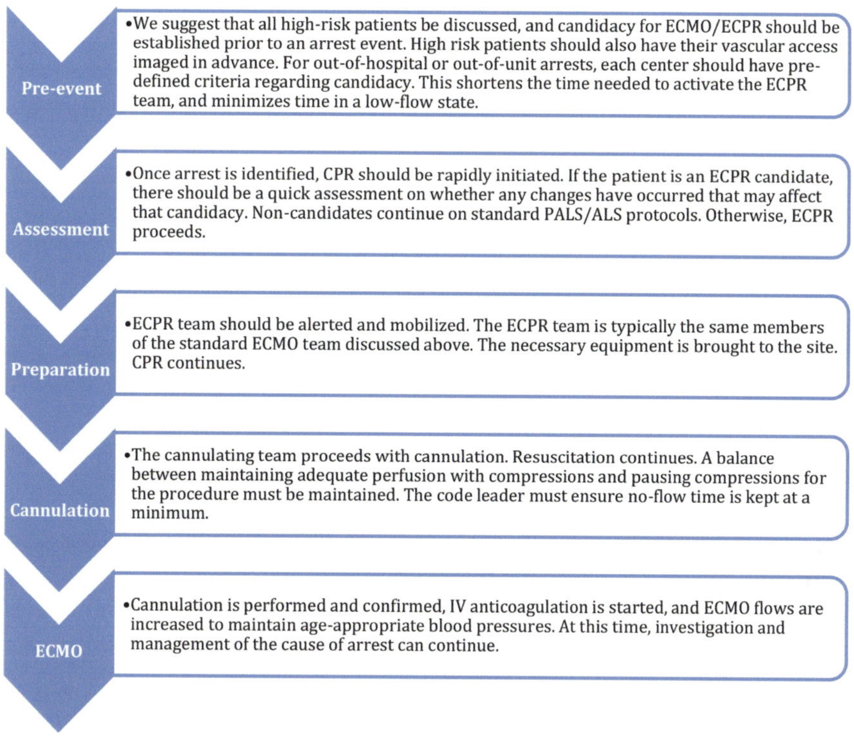

6.2 ECMO cannulation

Cannulation technique for ECPR depends on anatomy, experience and training of the cannulating provider, and circumstances necessitating support [22]. In almost all cases, ECPR patients require VA cannulation. If the patient has an open sternum, central cannulation is the easiest approach. In smaller children, the right carotid artery and internal jugular vein are the most common choice. In adults and adult-sized children, femoral cannulation is technically feasible. Femoral cannulation can limit the no-flow time due to minimal or no interruptions in compressions. Placed cannulas should support at least 120-150 mL/kg/min flow in order to provide an appropriate cardiac index in smaller children. In larger children and adults, the cannulas should support 3.5 to 5 L/min depending on the underlying etiology of cardiac arrest. If cannula sizes are deemed to be insufficient for flow, additional venous drainage can be added.

6.3 Initial management: post arrest care

The goal of post arrest care is to safeguard neurologic function and prevent secondary organ injury, while working towards the diagnosis and management of

Management goal	Reasoning
Maintain normal oxygenation	Elevated PO2 contributes to oxidative stress, and adult studies associate hyperoxia with decreased survival [24]. Hypoxia is associated with worse neurologic and overall outcomes.
Maintain normocarbia	Hypocapnia has been associated with worse outcomes in adults, and hypercapnia has been associated with decreased survival in pediatrics [24].
Maintain normotension	Post-ROSC hypotension is associated with decreased survival to discharge and worse neurologic outcomes [25]. Severe hypertension may adversely affect cardiac output, and has also been associated with neurologic injury [26].
Targeted temperature management	Aggressively avoid hyperthermia, which is associated with poor outcomes [27]. At this time, there is insufficient evidence to recommend hypothermia over goal-directed normothermia.

Table 1.
Post arrest care.

Continuous telemetry	Assists with close monitoring of rhythm status
Exhaled CO_2 monitor	Allows for capturing CO_2 changes early
Continuous pulse oximetry	Assists with maintaining normoxia
Cerebral NIRS (near-infrared spectrometry) monitor	May be useful in identifying periods of increased vulnerability to developing neurologic injury [28]
Electroencephalogram (EEG)	Discontinuous or isoelectric tracings are associated with worse neurologic outcome. EEG data in this setting is limited but may be useful in prognostication in consort with other criteria.
Arterial blood pressure monitor	Assists with close monitoring of hemodynamics thus avoiding hypotension
Central venous pressure monitor	Assists with assessment of volume status
Continuous temperature monitor	Rectal or bladder monitor: may allow for capturing temperature changes early

Table 2.
Monitoring modalities.

the cause of arrest. The AHA recommends adopting a systems-based, protocolized, goal-directed approach to the management of post-arrest patients [23]. This includes ECPR patients.

Table 1 highlights the most important care recommendations from the AHA, and **Table 2** includes monitoring modalities to be considered. These are based on the best available evidence, which may be limited to expert opinion in some cases. All recommendations are continuously reviewed and updated by the AHA as more evidence becomes available.

6.4 Initial management: A systems approach

Critical care management of post-ECPR ECMO patients should involve a multidisciplinary team that includes ECMO nurse/therapist, bedside staff, intensivists, and surgeons. Post arrest management should be implemented per local protocols. Like all ECMO patients, sedation, ventilation, anticoagulation, nutrition, and infection control should be cautiously monitored:

1. Neurological/Sedation: Soon after resuscitation, it is imperative to determine the patient's neurologic status, as this will guide further decision making

and management. Close monitoring of the neurologic exam is imperative. Evaluate for signs of seizures, and EEG should be obtained if there is any suspicion. Near-infrared spectroscopy (NIRS) monitors can be used to follow cerebral oxygenation, possibly serving as an indicator of neurological activity and overall perfusion. In infants, routine bedside head ultrasounds should be considered, since these are simple and inexpensive assessments that can provide important information about development of neurologic injury. For all patients, head imaging such as with computed topography should be considered as indicated by exam and other clinical findings. Analgesia and sedation should be appropriately used to provide comfort; muscle relaxants use should be minimized to cases of safety or medical concerns.

2. Cardiovascular: Continuous cardiac and hemodynamic monitoring is important. Peripheral perfusion should be monitored, especially in patients with femoral cannulation. Volume must be judiciously used to maintain cardiac preload. Systemic vascular resistance should be balanced to the patient's needs, with judicious use of inotropy if cardiac contractility needs augmentation. All patients should be monitored for need for LV decompression as discussed below. In patients with absent pulsatility, the LV must be monitored for clot formation.

3. Pulmonary: Maintain functional residual capacity to facilitate oxygenation of pulmonary blood flow, balancing that with allowing for lung rest. Gentle pulmonary toilet is warranted, balancing secretion clearance with avoiding trauma and bleeding.

4. Gastrointestinal/Renal: Nutrition should be considered as indicated; we promote early enteral feeding if able. Gastric drainage and stool output must be monitored for bleeding. Urine output should be monitored closely, with promotion of diuresis as needed. In case of renal failure, hemofiltration or dialysis must be considered.

5. Infection: Routine indicators of infection are unreliable: vital signs are influenced or controlled by the circuit, and lab parameters can be affected by the circuit. Assessment of the patient must include diligent monitoring of all sites of cannula or line insertion, as well as all wounds. Routine monitoring of CBC with differential is recommended. Surveillance cultures, as well as antibiotic prophylaxis, should be done per institutional protocol.

6.5 Initial management: Anticoagulation

Most ECMO centers have their own institutional protocols for ECMO anticoagulation, usually an amalgam of center experience, ELSO guidelines, and published literature. We suggest utilizing an anticoagulation expert when setting up such a protocol, and recommend reviewing institutional practices regularly with the goal of keeping up-to-date with the literature.

Anticoagulation in this patient population starts with the cannulation procedure. A bolus of unfractionated heparin (typically 50–100 units per kg) is given directly to the patient prior to cannula placement. Afterwards, an unfractionated heparin infusion is started, usually 28–30 units/kg/hr. in neonates and infants, and 20 units/kg/hr. in larger children. Of note, neonates may need higher doses of unfractionated heparin secondary to naturally lower antithrombin III (ATIII) plasma concentrations. Less heparin may be required in patients who have a coagulopathy.

Anticoagulation monitoring differs between centers [29, 30]. Labs can include partial thromboplastin time (PTT), anti-Xa, and thromboelastography (TEG). ATIII levels may be monitored dependent on the clinical situation. Platelets, fibrinogen, and plasma free hemoglobin are adjunct values that can be monitored, and can help with management of a circuit's anticoagulation. The patient's coagulable state must be taken into consideration, and this may alter dosing and target lab values. **Table 3** lists the most common parameters used in monitoring anticoagulation.

Some centers report the use of direct thrombin inhibitors, such as bivalirudin, as an alternative to unfractionated heparin infusions [31]. Direct thrombin inhibitors (DTI) have the advantage of not requiring ATIII for action and can inhibit clot-bound thrombin. However, DTIs do not act on the contact pathway, which may be an issue in low-flow parts of a circuit (such as a bridge or a pigtail for lab draws). DTIs are titrated to a PTT of 1.5–2 times normal, and so it is important to establish a baseline value prior to use.

6.6 Special consideration: left heart decompression

Patients managed with ECMO, more so in the setting of cardiac disease or ECPR, can develop myocardial dysfunction and left heart failure [32]. In ECMO patients who develop poor left heart function, the team must work to offload the heart [33]. This is necessary to prevent complications such as worsening cardiac function or pulmonary edema [34].

Management of ECMO-related LV distension should start with exclusion of poor cannula positioning and eliminating mechanical issues with the ECMO circuit [35]. Pump function should be adjusted to maintain appropriate flows. LV distension can be secondary to volume overload, and so volume status should be addressed accordingly. In case of poor cardiac muscle function, inotropes to improve contractility and vasodilators to decrease LV afterload can be utilized.

If offloading the left heart cannot be achieved medically, and cardiac output remains compromised, the institution of an interventional approach may be required. Several interventional decompression strategies have been described and are listed in **Table 4**. Evidence-based guidelines are lacking with regards of absolute indications, timing of intervention, and management method. The following is a non-comprehensive list of indications from the literature:

1. Elevated LA pressure and LVEDP despite maximal medical management

2. Severe distension of LA or LV (can include LV thrombus in setting of stasis)

3. Poor left outflow tract ejection/closed aortic valve

4. Refractory pulmonary edema or pulmonary hemorrhage

5. Aortic valve regurgitation

6. Elevated LV wall stress

7. LV or RV dysfunction

6.7 ECPR program

Several authors have discussed the essential components of an ECMO program, which are needed before ECPR can be offered as a treatment option [21, 47]. With

Lab parameter	Description	Goals
Activated Clotting Time (ACT)	Assesses whole blood clotting	Normal: 80–160 sec ECMO target: 180–240 seconds
Activated Partial Thromboplastin Time (aPTT)	Assesses the intrinsic pathway	Normal: 30–40 sec ECMO target: 1.5x normal
Anti-Xa level	Assesses clotting activity	ECMO target: 0.35–0.70 units/ml
Thromboelastography (TEG)	Assessment of whole blood clotting, fibrinolysis and platelet activity	

Table 3.
Monitoring anticoagulation.

Strategy	Reference
Intra-aortic balloon pump	Aso et al. [36]
Pulmonary artery vent	Fouilloux et al. [37]
Percutaneous trans-septal LA decompression	Aiyagari et al. [38], O'Byrne et al. [39]
Trans-septal LA decompression with BAS and LA vent insertion	Eastaugh et al. [40]
Transaortic vent	Hong et al. [41]
Static over-the-wire balloon dilation	Baruteau et al. [42], Eastaugh et al. [40]
Blade balloon septostomy	Johnston et al. [43]
Atrial stenting	Haynes et al. [44]
Direct surgical LA or LV venting	Guirgis et al. [45], Sandrio et al. [46]

Table 4.
Interventional decompression strategies for ECMO-related left heart dysfunction.

ECPR, time is of the essence. In order to successfully offer ECPR, a well-established protocol needs to be in-place and needs to be followed each time. There are several reported characteristics of a successful ECPR program, independent of the quality and capability of the ECMO team. An ideal team should be able to respond to situations in a consistent manner while maintaining that quality despite negative situations or hardship.

Consistency is maintained by continued training of all members of the team. Ongoing training must be both theoretical and hands-on. Simulation is a unique, effective way to incorporate the necessary training and dispense it to all members of the team in a way that can model real-life situations [48–52]. Leaders of the team must be able to keep up with the most up-to-date literature in ECMO and ECPR. Continued improvement of team performance is also assisted with maintaining quality improvement projects focused on outcomes-based factors related to each institution. On-the-spot debriefing after each event is a good way to identify concerns that need to be addressed.

7. Complications

ECPR, like all other forms of extracorporeal life support, is associated with a host of mechanical and non-mechanical complications. Frequency and severity for most ECPR-specific complications are not reported in the literature at this time –reports generally include all ECMO patients as a single group. The ELSO website has a comprehensive list of reported ECMO and ECPR complications, including mechanical, neurologic, cardiovascular, infectious, immunologic, hematologic, metabolic, pulmonary, and renal [53].

Here we will highlight some of the better studied complications.

7.1 Neurologic complications

Neurologic complications on ECMO have been extensively documented due to their significant burden and influence on outcomes. In pediatric patients treated with ECMO, there is a 7% prevalence of intracranial hemorrhages and a 6% prevalence of cerebral infarctions. Overall ECMO survival drops by half in patients who develop neurological injury. Survivors have multiple long-term morbidities, including seizures and global developmental delay.

ECPR specific neurologic injuries are more prevalent and more significant than with routine ECMO. The ELSO database reports 12% incidence of seizures, 11.8% incidence of hemorrhage or infarct, and 11% incidence of brain death. Hemorrhages and infarcts were associated with lower survival. Severe acidosis, non-cardiac arrest etiology, and on ECMO CPR were risk factors for the neurologic injuries. Unfortunately, registry datasets are not granular and more specific associations are difficult to identify.

Literature reporting of neurodevelopmental outcomes post ECMO and ECPR is limited, and there is a varied approach to assessment and documentation [54]. However, overall trends appear encouraging. Favorable neurologic outcomes have been shown in up-to 65% of ECPR survivors. Favorable outcomes in these reports are defined as normal function or mild cerebral disability, showing that a good quality of life is attainable for arrest patients treated with ECPR. Further work is needed to uncover determinants of good outcomes.

7.2 Acute kidney injury and renal replacement therapy

Acute kidney injury (AKI) is common in critically ill patients, and patients treated with ECMO are especially prone to developing AKI. ECMO patients with AKI and subsequent fluid overload have a higher risk of longer ECMO runs and greater mortality [7]. Fluid overload management differs between centers, and includes fluid restriction, diuresis, slow continuous ultrafiltration (SCUF). None of these methods are efficient in removing solutes, and so continuous renal replacement therapy may be needed when fluid overload coincides with AKI. It should be noted that aggressive early CRRT may be associated with worse outcome [55], and indicates that judicious fluid management must always be an ongoing balance tailored to each patient.

8. Outcomes

ECPR is superior to conventional CPR. Overall survival to discharge in pediatric patients treated with ECPR in the ELSO registry is approximately 40%; **Table 5** shows a breakdown of this data. Other reports of ECPR survival vary across the literature, and the quoted numbers range between 23%-55%. In contrast, overall reported survival rates for conventional CPR in pediatrics range between 16 to 30%. The large range of variability is due to differences between institutional experience, expertise, and reporting on these patients. Superior survival rates persist with longer term follow-up and have been demonstrated up-to 12 months after discharge.

A major indicator of quality of life in survivors of ECPR is neurologic outcome. While work is limited, there is indication that these outcomes may be positive, and perhaps better than in patients rescued by conventional CPR. Several reviews have shown that survival with minimal neurologic damage was more frequent in patients rescued with ECPR. This trend remained true even after performing propensity score matching for patients across these groups.

8.1 Determining outcomes

Several pre-ECMO factors have been identified as important to determining outcomes of ECPR. Disease process leading to arrest is one such factor. Post-cardiac surgery patients, or patients who arrest in the setting of another primary cardiac process, have consistently demonstrated the best survival when rescued with ECPR versus conventional CPR. Patients who arrest in the setting of neonatal respiratory disease also have favorable outcomes. Patients who arrest in the setting of sepsis have higher mortality rates than patients with a pure cardiac process, but have better survival than if managed with CPR alone [57]. Patients with arrest in the setting of a respiratory illness also do well [58]. Patients with gastrointestinal conditions, who are usually patients with complex multiorgan disorders, tend to have worse outcomes. Patients with oncologic disease and other immunosuppressed processes also do worse [15].

Time to full support is another important predictor of survival of patients rescued with ECPR [17]. Longer time spent in a low flow state is associated with drastic drops on survival to hospital discharge. Post-discharge, patients with longer low flow times have worse neurologic outcomes and higher post-discharge mortality. Duration in a low flow state is a highly modifiable factor, and should be minimized in order to achieve the best outcomes. It is important to establish ECMO candidacy for all high risk patients, so that ECMO can be deployed quickly in the setting of an arrest. In centers that offer ECPR, a rapid response team must be available at all times, in order to minimize the time needed to establish ECMO flow. This team must be highly trained and very adaptable, highlighting the need for an ongoing development program for any center that offers ECPR. In addition to the presence of a rapid response team, ECMO equipment must be readily available for utilization at all times. During the resuscitation, pauses in compressions are needed to allow for cannula insertion. Duration and frequency of such pauses must be limited as much as possible, since any no-flow time dramatically decreases survival as well.

It is important to note that prolonged resuscitation may not be futile if ECPR is utilized, highlighting the importance of choosing the right patients for ECPR therapy [59].

Location of arrest can influence survival. Arrests that occur in the intensive care unit, have the best outcomes post management with ECPR. Outside the intensive care unit, outcomes worsen, perhaps related to the quality of resuscitation provided and the duration it may take to establish access for ECMO. Locations where ECPR can be offered will be dependent on institutional logistics and resource availability. Regardless, there should be advance coordination to ensure the equipment and

	Total runs	Survive ECLS	Survival to discharge
Neonatal ECPR	1718	1140 (66%)	708 (41%)
Pediatric ECPR	3946	2262 (57%)	1675 (42%)
Total	5664	3402 (60%)	2383 (42%)

Table 5.
ECPR runs per the ELSO database, 1990–2018 [56].

personnel needed can be deployed smoothly. Literature has shown that it is possible to successfully offer ECPR in the emergency department with such arrangements.

On-ECMO complications also influence survival, regardless whether it is a planned run or ECPR [57]. Neurologic complications are associated with high mortality post-ECPR. Inability to achieve and maintain adequate perfusion while on ECMO, noted by metabolic and lactic acidosis, has been tied to worse outcomes [60, 61]. Similarly, cardiac arrest during the ECMO run is also associated with poor outcomes. Renal failure and the need for renal replacement therapy have an association with inferior outcomes [58]. Severe coagulopathy and DIC also worsen survival – maintaining anticoagulation for the circuit and avoidance of fatal hemorrhage is a fine balance, and coagulopathy raises the risk of fatal hemorrhages [16, 62].

9. Special mention: out-of-hospital ECPR

Out of hospital cardiac arrests (OHCA) have very high mortality rates and very poor neurologic outcomes for both pediatric and adult patients [63, 64]. As a result, there has been growing interest in applying ECPR to OHCA. Overall survival rates vary for OHCA ECPR. Reported survival rates range from 12 to 30%, but patient numbers are very limited and there is extreme selection bias in this cohort [4]. ELSO reports that about half of all OHCA ECPR were reported in Europe, followed by the Asia-Pacific region, and lastly North America [65]. Almost all published experience is exclusively adult experience [66].

Application of ECPR for OHCA varies across different centers. Some institutions provide a "scoop and run" strategy, with quick transport to the emergency department for cannulation in select patients with OHCA [67]. Other centers have a different approach, with the ability to "stay and treat" by initiating ECPR on the scene of the OHCA [68]. The different styles of application are dependent on availability of resources, feasibility, and local experience.

Provision of ECPR to OHCA presents challenges with cost-effectiveness, optimal candidacy, and timing of deployment. However, if done in settings with the appropriate resources utilizing an aggressive strategy with optimum patient selection, survival can possibly be favorable [14]. However, evidence remains inconclusive and requires further study [66].

10. Conclusion and future directions

ECPR has emerged as an exciting rescue therapy, promising to improve outcomes of cardiac arrest. It has shown superiority over conventional CPR, with better survival to discharge and better longer-term survival. It has also shown better neurologic outcomes. As overall experience grows, we expect to see increased uses and even better outcomes.

Nonetheless, this is an emerging field and there is a lot left to learn. Especially in pediatrics, knowledge gaps include:

1. Ideal ECPR candidacy

    a. Definition of refractory arrest, i.e. how long should conventional CPR continue before ECPR should be considered

    b. Inclusion and exclusion criteria for higher risk populations, including immunosuppressed patients and trauma patients

c. Inclusion and exclusion criteria for out-of-hospital cardiac arrest

d. Assessment of futility in possible ECPR candidates

2. Team preparedness: specific nature of training to maintain ECPR team competency to decrease low flow time

3. Optimal approach to comprehensive post arrest care for ECPR patients

4. Approach to neuroprotection and neuroprognostication post-ECPR

5. Functional and neurodevelopmental post-discharge status of patients rescued with ECPR, and how to improve such outcomes

At this time, most ECMO and ECPR research is observational in nature. Generalization of pediatric data is hindered by the heterogeneity of patient ages and diagnosis, as well as variability of practice between different institutions. Because of the small numbers of patients overall and per institution, the field is ripe with opportunity for collaborative work. International registries and large research collaboratives may be able to provide enough patients to power larger investigations. More data will help empower decisions to treat children with ECPR, refine the caliber of care they receive, and improve their future quality of life.

Author details

Abdelaziz Farhat[1]*, Cindy Darnell Bowens[1], Ravi Thiagarajan[2] and Lakshmi Raman[1]

1 Children's Medical Center and University of Texas Southwestern Medical Center, Dallas, TX, USA

2 Children's Hospital Boston and the Harvard Medical School, Boston, MA, USA

*Address all correspondence to: abdelaziz.farhat@utsouthwestern.edu

References

[1] Conrad SA, Rycus PT. Extracorporeal membrane oxygenation for refractory cardiac arrest. Annals of Cardiac Anaesthesia. 2017;**20**:S4-S10

[2] Barbaro RP et al. Pediatric extracorporeal life support organization registry international report 2016. ASAIO, American Society for Artificial Internal Organs. 2017;**1992**(63):456-463

[3] Singer B, Reynolds JC, Lockey DJ, O'Brien B. Pre-hospital extra-corporeal cardiopulmonary resuscitation. Scandinavian Journal of Trauma, Resuscitation and Emergency Medicine. 2018;**26**(1):26

[4] Hutin A et al. Early ECPR for out-of-hospital cardiac arrest: Best practice in 2018. Resuscitation. 2018;**130**:44-48

[5] Pappalardo F, Montisci A. What is extracorporeal cardiopulmonary resuscitation? Journal of Thoracic Disease. 2017;**9**:1415-1419

[6] Dennis M et al. Extracorporeal cardiopulmonary resuscitation for refractory cardiac arrest: A multicentre experience. International Journal of Cardiology. 2017;**231**:131-136

[7] Thiagarajan RR, Laussen PC, Rycus PT, Bartlett RH, Bratton SL. Extracorporeal membrane oxygenation to aid cardiopulmonary resuscitation in infants and children. Circulation. 2007;**116**:1693-1700

[8] Meaney PA et al. Higher survival rates among younger patients after pediatric intensive care unit cardiac arrests. Pediatrics. 2006;**118**:2424-2433

[9] Kim SJ, Kim HJ, Lee HY, Ahn HS, Lee SW. Comparing extracorporeal cardiopulmonary resuscitation with conventional cardiopulmonary resuscitation: A meta-analysis. Resuscitation. 2016;**103**:106-116

[10] Lasa JJ et al. Extracorporeal-cardiopulmonary resuscitation (E-CPR) during pediatric In-hospital cardiopulmonary arrest is associated with improved survival to discharge: A report from the American Heart Association's get with the guidelines®—Resuscitation registry (GWTG-R). Circulation. 2016;**133**:165-176

[11] Link Mark S et al. Part 7: Adult advanced cardiovascular life support. Circulation. 2015;**132**:S444-S464

[12] ELSO ECPR Supplement to the ELSO General Guidelines Extracorporeal Life Support Organization (ELSO) Guidelines for ECPR Cases. 2013. Available online: https://www.elso.org/Portals/0/IGD/Archive/FileManager/6713186745cusersshyerdocumentselsoguidelinesforecprcases1.3.pdf

[13] Adult Advanced Life Support. Available at: https://www.resus.org.uk/resuscitation-guidelines/adult-advanced-life-support/ [Accessed: 8-12-2018]

[14] Lamhaut L et al. A pre-hospital extracorporeal cardio pulmonary resuscitation (ECPR) strategy for treatment of refractory out hospital cardiac arrest: An observational study and propensity analysis. Resuscitation. 2017;**117**:109-117

[15] Schmidt M et al. Six-month outcome of Immunocompromised patients with severe acute respiratory distress syndrome rescued by extracorporeal membrane oxygenation. An international multicenter retrospective study. American Journal of Respiratory and Critical Care Medicine. 2018;**197**:1297-1307

[16] Werho DK et al. Hemorrhagic complications in pediatric cardiac patients on extracorporeal membrane oxygenation: An analysis of the

extracorporeal life support organization registry. Pediatric Critical Care Medicine: A Journal of the Society of Critical Care Medicine and the World Federation of Pediatric Intensive and Critical Care Societies. 2015;**16**:276-288

[17] Wengenmayer T et al. Influence of low-flow time on survival after extracorporeal cardiopulmonary resuscitation (eCPR). Critical Care. 2017;**21**(1):157

[18] Organ Donation in Cardiac Arrest Patients Treated with Extracorporeal CPR: A Single Centre Observational Study. PubMed—NCBI. Available at: https://www-ncbi-nlm-nih-gov.foyer.swmed.edu/pubmed/28596083 [Accessed: 2-12-2018]

[19] Puślecki M et al. "Extracorporeal membrane oxygenation for greater Poland" program: How to save lives and develop organ donation? Transplantation Proceedings. 2018;**50**:1957-1961

[20] Carter T et al. Outcome of organs procured from donors on extracorporeal membrane oxygenation support: An analysis of kidney and liver allograft data. Clinical Transplantation. 2014;**28**:816-820

[21] Laussen PC, Guerguerian A-M. Establishing and sustaining an ECPR program. Frontiers in Pediatrics. 2018;**6**:152

[22] Harvey C. Cannulation for neonatal and pediatric extracorporeal membrane oxygenation for cardiac support. Frontiers in Pediatrics. 2018;**6**

[23] Callaway CW et al. Part 8: Post-cardiac arrest care: 2015 American Heart Association guidelines update for cardiopulmonary resuscitation and emergency cardiovascular care. Circulation. 2015;**132**(18 suppl 2):465-482

[24] del Castillo J et al. Hyperoxia, hypocapnia and hypercapnia as outcome factors after cardiac arrest in children. Resuscitation. 2012;**83**:1456-1461

[25] Trzeciak S et al. Significance of arterial hypotension after resuscitation from cardiac arrest*. Critical Care Medicine. 2009;**37**:2895-2903

[26] Müllner M et al. Arterial blood pressure after human cardiac arrest and neurological recovery. Stroke. 1996;**27**:59-62

[27] Zeiner A et al. Hyperthermia after cardiac arrest is associated with an unfavorable neurologic outcome. Archives of Internal Medicine. 2001;**161**:2007-2012

[28] Bouglé A et al. Determinants and significance of cerebral oximetry after cardiac arrest: A prospective cohort study. Resuscitation. 2016;**99**:1-6

[29] Mazzeffi MA et al. Bleeding, thrombosis, and transfusion with two heparin anticoagulation protocols in Venoarterial ECMO patients. Journal of Cardiothoracic and Vascular Anesthesia. 2018:S1053-0770(18)30597-4. DOI: 10.1053/j.jvca.2018.07.045

[30] Cho HJ, Kim DW, Kim GS, Jeong IS. Anticoagulation therapy during extracorporeal membrane oxygenator support in pediatric patients. Chonnam Medical Journal. 2017;**53**:110-117

[31] Netley J et al. Bivalirudin anticoagulation dosing protocol for extracorporeal membrane oxygenation: A retrospective review. The Journal of Extra-Corporeal Technology. 2018;**50**:161-166

[32] Martin GR, Short BL, Abbott C, O'Brien AM. Cardiac stun in infants undergoing extracorporeal membrane oxygenation. The Journal of Thoracic and Cardiovascular Surgery. 1991;**101**:607-611

[33] Hacking DF et al. Elective decompression of the left ventricle

in pediatric patients may reduce the duration of Venoarterial extracorporeal membrane oxygenation. Artificial Organs. 2015;**39**:319-326

[34] Becker JA, Short BL, Martin GR. Cardiovascular complications adversely affect survival during extracorporeal membrane oxygenation. Critical Care Medicine. 1998;**26**:1582-1586

[35] Ostadal P et al. Increasing venoarterial extracorporeal membrane oxygenation flow negatively affects left ventricular performance in a porcine model of cardiogenic shock. Journal of Translational Medicine. 2015;**13**(1):266

[36] Aso S, Matsui H, Fushimi K, Yasunaga H. The effect of intraaortic balloon pumping under Venoarterial extracorporeal membrane oxygenation on mortality of cardiogenic patients: An analysis using a Nationwide inpatient database. Critical Care Medicine. 2016;**44**:1974-1979

[37] Fouilloux V, Lebrun L, Macé L, Kreitmann B. Extracorporeal membranous oxygenation and left atrial decompression: A fast and minimally invasive approach. The Annals of Thoracic Surgery. 2011;**91**:1996-1997

[38] Aiyagari RM, Rocchini AP, Remenapp RT, Graziano JN. Decompression of the left atrium during extracorporeal membrane oxygenation using a transseptal cannula incorporated into the circuit. Critical Care Medicine. 2006;**34**:2603-2606

[39] O'Byrne ML et al. Middle-term results of trans-catheter creation of atrial communication in patients receiving mechanical circulatory support. Catheterization and Cardiovascular Interventions. 2015;**85**:1189-1195

[40] Eastaugh LJ et al. Percutaneous left atrial decompression in patients supported with extracorporeal membrane oxygenation for cardiac disease. Pediatric Critical Care Medicine: A Journal of the Society of Critical Care Medicine and the World Federation of Pediatric Intensive and Critical Care Societies. 2015;**16**:59-65

[41] Hong TH et al. Successful left-heart decompression during extracorporeal membrane oxygenation in an adult patient by percutaneous transaortic catheter venting. Korean Journal of Thoracic and Cardiovascular Surgery. 2015;**48**:210-213

[42] Baruteau A-E et al. Percutaneous balloon atrial septostomy on top of venoarterial extracorporeal membrane oxygenation results in safe and effective left heart decompression. European Heart Journal Acute Cardiovascular Care. 2018;**7**:70-79

[43] Johnston TA, Jaggers J, McGovern JJ, O'Laughlin MP. Bedside transseptal balloon dilation atrial septostomy for decompression of the left heart during extracorporeal membrane oxygenation. Catheterization and Cardiovascular Interventions. 1999;**46**:197-199

[44] Haynes S, Kerber RE, Johnson FL, Lynch WR, Divekar A. Left heart decompression by atrial stenting during extracorporeal membrane oxygenation. The International Journal of Artificial Organs. 2009;**32**:240-242

[45] Guirgis M, Kumar K, Menkis AH, Freed DH. Minimally invasive left-heart decompression during venoarterial extracorporeal membrane oxygenation: An alternative to a percutaneous approach. Interactive Cardiovascular and Thoracic Surgery. 2010;**10**:672-674

[46] Sandrio S et al. Extracorporeal life support with an integrated left ventricular vent in children with a low cardiac output. Cardiology in the Young. 2014;**24**:654-660

[47] Moll V et al. Rapid development and implementation of an ECMO program. ASAIO, American Society for Artificial Internal Organs. 1992, 2016;**62**:354-358

[48] Weems MF et al. The role of extracorporeal membrane oxygenation simulation training at extracorporeal life support organization centers in the United States. Simulation in Healthcare: The Journal of the Society for Simulation in Healthcare. 2017;**12**:233-239

[49] Thompson JL et al. Construction of a reusable, high-fidelity model to enhance extracorporeal membrane oxygenation training through simulation. Advances in Neonatal Care. 2014;**14**:103-109

[50] Anderson JM et al. Simulating extracorporeal membrane oxygenation emergencies to improve human performance. Part I: Methodologic and technologic innovations. Simulation in Healthcare: The Journal of the Society for Simulation in Healthcare. 2006;**1**:220-227

[51] Johnston L, Oldenburg G. Simulation for neonatal extracorporeal membrane oxygenation teams. Seminars in Perinatology. 2016;**40**:421-429

[52] Chan S-Y et al. Prospective assessment of novice learners in a simulation-based extracorporeal membrane oxygenation (ECMO) education program. Pediatric Cardiology. 2013;**34**:543-552

[53] Extracorporeal Life Support Organization—ECMO and ECLS > Registry > Support Documents > ECLS Complications Code. Available at: https://www.elso.org/Registry/SupportDocuments/ECLSComplicationsCode.aspx [Accessed: 9-12-2018]

[54] Mehta A, Ibsen LM. Neurologic complications and neurodevelopmental outcome with extracorporeal life support. World Journal of Critical Care Medicine. 2013;**2**:40-47

[55] Wolf MJ, Chanani NK, Heard ML, Kanter KR, Mahle WT. Early renal replacement therapy during pediatric cardiac extracorporeal support increases mortality. The Annals of Thoracic Surgery. 2013;**96**:917-922

[56] Extracorporeal Life Support Organization—ECMO and ECLS > Registry > Statistics > International Summary. Available at: https://www.elso.org/Registry/Statistics/InternationalSummary.aspx [Accessed: 2-12-2018]

[57] Conrad SJ, Bridges BC, Kalra Y, Pietsch JB, Smith AH. Extracorporeal cardiopulmonary resuscitation among patients with structurally Normal hearts. ASAIO, American Society for Artificial Internal Organs. 1992, 2017;**63**:781-786

[58] Huang S-C et al. Eleven years of experience with extracorporeal cardiopulmonary resuscitation for paediatric patients with in-hospital cardiac arrest. Resuscitation. 2012;**83**:710-714

[59] Kelly RB, Porter PA, Meier AH, Myers JL, Thomas NJ. Duration of cardiopulmonary resuscitation before extracorporeal rescue: How long is not long enough? ASAIO, American Society for Artificial Internal Organs. 1992, 2005;**51**:665-667

[60] Kolodziej A, Burchett A, Tribble T, Grigorian AY, Guglin M. Lactic acid is the Most important factor predicting survival on VA ECMO. The Journal of Heart and Lung Transplantation. 2017;**36**:S347

[61] Park SJ et al. Blood lactate level during extracorporeal life support as a surrogate marker for survival. The Journal of Thoracic and Cardiovascular Surgery. 2014;**148**:714-720

[62] Fletcher-Sandersjöö A et al. Incidence, outcome, and predictors of intracranial hemorrhage in adult patients on extracorporeal membrane oxygenation: A systematic and narrative review. Frontiers in Neurology. 2018;**9**:548

[63] Nolan JP et al. European resuscitation council guidelines for resuscitation 2010 section 1. Executive summary. Resuscitation. 2010;**81**:1219-1276

[64] Sakamoto T et al. Extracorporeal cardiopulmonary resuscitation versus conventional cardiopulmonary resuscitation in adults with out-of-hospital cardiac arrest: A prospective observational study. Resuscitation. 2014;**85**:762-768

[65] Haas NL, Coute RA, Hsu CH, Cranford JA, Neumar RW. Descriptive analysis of extracorporeal cardiopulmonary resuscitation following out-of-hospital cardiac arrest-An ELSO registry study. Resuscitation. 2017;**119**:56-62

[66] Holmberg MJ et al. Extracorporeal cardiopulmonary resuscitation for cardiac arrest: A systematic review. Resuscitation. 2018;**131**:91-100

[67] Poppe M et al. The incidence of “load&go” out-of-hospital cardiac arrest candidates for emergency department utilization of emergency extracorporeal life support: A one-year review. Resuscitation. 2015;**91**:131-136

[68] Lamhaut L et al. Extracorporeal cardiopulmonary resuscitation (ECPR) in the prehospital setting: An illustrative case of ECPR performed in the louvre museum. Prehospital Emergency Care. 2017;**21**:386-389

Chapter 9

Extracorporeal Membrane Oxygenation as a Bridge to Cardiac Transplantation

Nandini Nair and Enrique Gongora

Abstract

Extracorporeal membrane oxygenation (ECMO) is a technique used for temporary support of patients with end-stage heart or lung failure. This review will focus on the venoarterial ECMO system and its use as a bridge to other long-term durable devices and/or cardiac transplantation. It can be used as a bridge to decision because it helps to gain time to stabilize the patient for further evaluation for long-term treatment such as durable mechanical circulatory pumps or transplantation. ECMO is evolving as a treatment for patients waiting on the transplant list. Increasing utilization of ECMO in adults has revealed some of the common complications such as bleeding and coagulopathy which impact survival in this patient population. The use of VA ECMO as a technique for rescuing patients from cardiogenic shock is very attractive. However, considering the extensive set of complications and the mortality it brings with it makes it a less attractive option as a direct bridge to cardiac transplant. The literature currently on this subject is very scanty and limited to a few studies of small numbers of patients. Further definitive research is needed for consensus on the role of VA ECMO as a bridge to cardiac transplant.

Keywords: ECMO, bridge to transplantation, extracorporeal life support

1. Introduction

Extracorporeal membrane oxygenation (ECMO) is a technique used for temporary support of patients with end-stage heart or lung failure. It can be used as a bridge to decision because it helps to gain time to stabilize the patient for further evaluation for long-term treatment such as durable mechanical circulatory pumps or transplantation. The use of ECMO as a direct bridge to cardiac transplantation may unmask the complications in these critically ill patients leading to unfavorable posttransplant outcomes in some instances; however, it is now becoming the mainstay of treatments for patients waiting on the transplant list. The history of ECMO starts with the advent of the heart-lung machine invented by Gibbon [1, 2]. Further modifications leading to devices that are sustainable for longer periods of time gave rise to the technique of ECMO used today [3–5].

The use of ECMO in humans was first initiated in the pediatric population [3, 4]. Adult ECMO gained importance and is being used increasingly since the first randomized clinical trial by Peek et al. which showed a positive outcome in adults with respiratory failure [6]. This has been followed by many reports of success in H1N1 influenza patients [7]. Anselmi et al. recently reported the use of ECMO in pregnant patients [8]. Increasing utilization of ECMO in adults has revealed some of the common complications such as bleeding and coagulopathy which impact survival in this patient population. The delicate balance between adequate anticoagulation and bleeding complications presents one of the greatest challenges of ECMO therapy today.

The ELSO (Extracorporeal Life Support Organization) was established in 1989. The ELSO was formed as an offshoot of a study group that began in 1984 discussing cases. The ELSO focuses on collection and sharing of data and has fostered a rich collaboration among the majority of centers performing ECMO. The ELSO has hence remained a good resource for surgeons, neonatologists, nurses, perfusionists, respiratory therapists, biomedical engineers, critical care physicians, and heart failure cardiologists.

A total of 73,000 ECMO procedures were recorded by the ELSO as of early 2016 of which greater than 25% were performed in adult patients [9]. From 2006 to 2011, adult ECMO volumes increased greater than four times in the United States [10]. Adult ECMO has increased in volume due to its usefulness in improving survival in ARDS (acute respiratory distress syndrome) patients [11]. Additionally, with the improvement in technology, highly specialized hospitals have evolved the capabilities to transport critically ill patients from rural areas to their critical care units making it possible for rural populations to be able to receive advanced care [12, 13].

This review will focus on the venoarterial ECMO system and its use as a bridge to other long-term durable devices and/or cardiac transplantation.

2. The ECMO circuit

The ECMO circuit (**Figure 1**) in its most basic form consists of a pump that is capable of pumping blood it receives from the drainage cannula to the membrane oxygenator which then leads to a heat exchanger. The oxygenated temperature-optimized blood is then returned to the patient by the return cannula. ECMO cannulation can be done centrally through the right atrium and ascending aorta or peripherally via the femoral artery and vein. The type of cannulation used whether central or peripheral influences the outcomes as the complications differ. When central cannulation is used, bleeding requiring transfusions is higher. In central cannulation higher rates of reoperation are also noted. Increased complications will decrease survival and increase resource utilization. On the other hand, peripheral cannulation has been noted to produce fewer bleeding complications. It can be

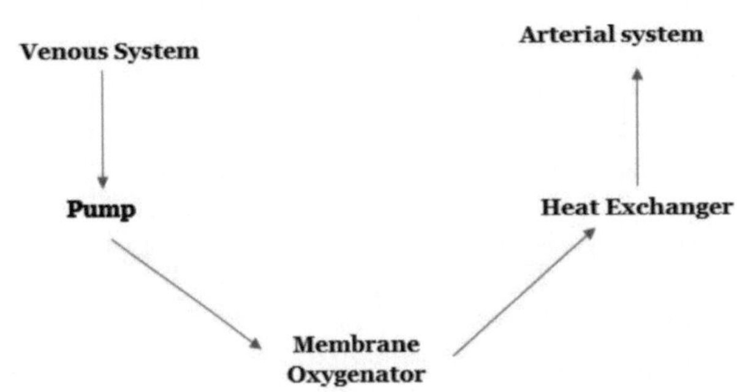

Figure 1.
VA-ECMO circuit.

placed in a shorter time and at the bedside. However, the complication of limb ischemia occurs equally in both types of cannulations.

ECMO circuits are set up depending on the organs that need to be bypassed. When both heart and lungs have to be bypassed, the venoarterial ECMO (VA-ECMO) is used as shown in (**Figure 1**). The VA-ECMO circuit provides both gas exchange and hemodynamic support as blood is pumped from the venous to the arterial systems. On the other hand, if only the lungs need to be bypassed, the veno-venous circuit (VV-ECMO) facilitates only gas exchange with no hemodynamic support. In VV-ECMO blood is removed taken out of the venous system and oxygenated and pumped back into it.

VA-ECMO is designed to provide cardiac and pulmonary support. Deoxygenated blood is drained from the venous system, and oxygenated blood is returned into the arterial circulation, in a similar fashion to standard cardiopulmonary bypass. In the VA-ECMO system, central cannulation is achieved by draining blood directly from the right atrium and returning oxygenated blood to the proximal ascending aorta. Peripheral cannulation uses blood drained from the proximal femoral vein/jugular vein which is oxygenated and then returned to the carotid/axillary/femoral artery. The Seldinger technique is used typically to achieve the cannulations.

Two types of pumps are currently available for use in ECMO circuits. They are centrifugal pumps and roller pumps. Centrifugal pumps are smaller and pump blood by providing a pressure differential across a pump head that contains a magnetically driven impeller revolving at speeds up to 3000 revolutions per min. On the other hand, roller pumps push blood across the circuit by progressively compressing segments of tubing along a curved pathway. Centrifugal pumps have been associated with a lesser degree of hemolysis compared with roller pumps and decreased requirement of anticoagulation. Therefore, centrifugal pumps are being increasingly used in in adult patients.

3. Indications and contraindications for VA-ECMO

The major indication for VA-ECMO is cardiogenic shock as defined in the ELSO guidelines [14]. This includes inadequate tissue perfusion due to hypotension and low cardiac output despite volume repletion, inotropes, vasopressors, and intra-aortic balloon counterpulsation use. Common causes for cardiogenic shock are acute myocardial infarction (AMI), myocarditis, peripartum cardiomyopathy, acute decompensation of chronic heart failure, and postcardiotomy shock.

Septic shock is an indication in some centers. The guidelines on prognostication of survival without ECMO are based on the IABP score in postcardiotomy patients [15] and the Samuels score also in postcardiotomy patients [16]. In a retrospective analysis, Samuels et al. [16] showed that early insertion of mechanical support reduces multi-organ failure in these patients. In hospital mortality, correlates with increasing inotropic support needed to get patients off cardiopulmonary bypass following cardiac surgery. The combination of pharmacological criteria together with hemodynamic presentation should be used for mechanical support initiation in cardiogenic shock. Earlier institution of mechanical support devices tends to lower incidence of postoperative multi-organ failure and improve discharge rates [16].

The advantage of VA-ECMO is that it provides quick biventricular support and can be achieved at the bedside for poor oxygenation, biventricular failure, refractory malignant arrhythmias, and heart failure with severe pulmonary failure. VA-ECMO can be used as a bridge to recovery, AMI after revascularization, myocarditis, postcardiotomy shock, chronic heart failure, and non-revascularizable AMI.

ECMO can be used as a bridge to cardiac transplant as well as durable mechanical circulatory support: ventricular assist device (VAD) and the total artificial heart (TAH).

The absolute contraindications for VA-ECMO would be unrecoverable heart and the patient not being a candidate for cardiac transplant or VAD. Chronic organ dysfunctions such as emphysema, cirrhosis, and end-stage renal failure are all considered absolute contraindications. Compliance in terms of financial and medical strategies and cognitive, psychiatric, or social limitations are considered contraindications. Prolonged CPR without adequate tissue perfusion is also an absolute contraindication.

The relative contraindications for ECMO would be inability to tolerate anticoagulation, advanced age, and obesity. Advanced age is a gray area as there are no defined cutoffs due to lack of existing data in older patients.

4. Complications during VA-ECMO support

Complications encountered during ECMO support include lack of a fine balance between anticoagulation and bleeding, limb ischemia, disseminated intravascular coagulation (DIC), heparin-induced thrombocytopenia (HIT), bleeding from a preexisting surgical site requiring reexploration, and progression of preexisting renal failure.

4.1 Anticoagulation and bleeding

Interaction of blood with non-endothelial surfaces leads to inflammation and prothrombosis. ECMO therefore leads to consumptive coagulopathy as well as a dilution of coagulation factors resulting in decreased fibrinogen levels. The inflammatory response secondary to ECMO gives rise to a hypercoagulable state, requiring anticoagulation to prevent thrombosis of the circuit. The delicate balance between adequate anticoagulation and bleeding complications presents one of the greatest challenges of ECMO therapy today. Different anticoagulation protocols are used across the centers. Uniformity in these protocols is lacking [17].

ECMO has historically been the mainstay of resuscitation in pediatric care. Adult ECMO protocols have hence evolved from the pediatric practice of anticoagulation in ECMO. Higher flow and larger cannula sizes in adult ECMO contribute less to turbulence, stasis, and thrombogenicity. Simple circuits with minimum number of connectors create less turbulence, while larger cannulas especially on the venous side reduce stasis and thrombogenicity, therefore requiring lower levels of anticoagulation. This suggests that anticoagulation protocols used in the pediatric population may not be optimal in adults.

Survival on ECMO appears to be more favorable in the younger population, and bleeding and coagulopathy appear to be the most common complications which raise the question if the coagulation system changes in its character and dimensions with advancing age. Interestingly, aging is accompanied by increases in plasma concentrations of factors VII and VIII and fibrinogen progressively [18, 19]. Coagulation cascade upregulation with age may increase thrombosis in pathological states demanding special attention when designing anticoagulation therapy for adult and especially older patients on ECMO.

Genetic polymorphisms and ethnic variations further complicate and influence drug metabolism and efficacy which need to be accounted for while developing anticoagulation protocols and selecting anticoagulants [20]. Clinical significance and predictive value of hypercoagulability markers need to be defined in different age groups in prospective studies in order to be able to define optimal anticoagulation regimens. Research is needed in areas of optimizing anticoagulation protocols in adults with respect to age, gender, race, ethnicity, and technical aspects. If tailored appropriately adult ECMO therapy could probably achieve better success with far less aggressive anticoagulation than that used in the pediatric population.

4.2 Roller versus centrifugal pumps

Though centrifugal pumps are increasingly used, they are not without disadvantages. Centrifugal pumps are continuous flow pumps (CF pumps) and produce shear stress leading to acquired von Willebrand factor deficiency and bleeding complications. A recent retrospective analysis demonstrated an increased risk for nonsurgical bleeding (gastrointestinal, pulmonary, and neurological) with centrifugal pumps despite lower levels of heparin anticoagulation [21]. This study used patients supported on ECMO for 5 days for comparison of bleeding complications using centrifugal and roller pumps. The underlying etiology can be multifactorial but needs further research for specific delineation of inciting factors.

4.3 Limb ischemia

Femoral arterial cannulation carries an increased risk of profound distal limb ischemia. Some of the causes that lead to lower limb ischemia during ECMO support are acute embolism, dissection/perforation or rupture of the common femoral artery (CFA) or the iliac artery, thrombosis, pseudoaneurysm, hyperperfusion, and ischemia after decannulation usually due to distal embolization [22]. This problem has been solved to a large extent by prophylactically placing an ipsilateral perfusion catheter [22]. In a small study using 43 patients who underwent femoral artery cannulation, placement of a prophylactic superficial femoral artery [SFA] catheter in ten patients produced no limb ischemia. Of the rest of the patients (n = 33) who did not receive prophylactic SFA cannulation, seven patients had limb ischemia. Four of these patients underwent fasciotomy and decannulation leading to amputation in one patient. The three patients who received SFA cannulation for limb ischemia did not need amputation [23]. Foley et al. also showed that age was a predictor for limb ischemia [23]. Patients who developed limb ischemia were significantly younger than those patients without limb ischemia. This has been attributed to the size of the arterial cannula with respect to the femoral artery size in younger patients. CFA diameter was noted to increase with age. It was considered to be related to BSA and gender with increasing diameters found in males and those who have a larger BSA [24]. However, the data presented by Foley et al. found no correlation between the rate of limb ischemia and BSA, BMI, or size of the cannula as compared to the earlier literature [23, 24].

Accurate insertion of the arterial cannula in the CFA is of paramount importance to minimize risk of ipsilateral limb ischemia. One of the important aspects is to avoid improper retrograde SFA cannulation leading to significant flow limitation and in extreme cases to complete occlusion. Additionally, measurement of pressure in the SFA after placing the patient on ECMO support will identify the patients who actually need a catheter for antegrade perfusion [25]. Such an approach may reduce the extra effort and insertion of an additional catheter in all patients prophylactically.

Considering the limited data in the current literature, the use of prophylactic SFA cannulation in younger individuals may be a reasonable approach with or without direct SFA pressure measurements especially if it can be done at the bedside. Duplex ultrasonography or direct SFA pressure measurements done at the time of ECMO placement may be an alternative to an early decision on which patients need the SFA cannulation. The existing literature does not seem to report a direct correlation with mortality in these patients which is another area of investigation that needs future attention.

4.4 Heparin-induced thrombocytopenia

Thrombocytopenia is a devastating complication in patients on VA-ECMO support. The etiology of platelet reduction in ECMO is still ambiguous. HIT has been considered one of the causative mechanisms. Current literature has very little to offer in this area. The incidence and mortality secondary to HIT in VA-ECMO patients is very poorly represented. In a recent retrospective study on VA-ECMO patients hospitalized for >3 days with high clinical suspicion of HIT and positive anti-PF4/heparin antibodies, the prevalence of HIT in patients on VA-ECMO support was estimated as 0.36%. Mortality rate was noted as 33.3%, which was not statistically different from the mortality observed in patients on VA-ECMO support without HIT [26]. HIT is a complication that appears to have a low prevalence; its effects are devastating if untreated. Bivalirudin and argatroban have been used to successfully treat this condition in VA-ECMO patients in small studies [27–29]. Further investigations in larger populations are required in this patient population for standardized regimens to be incorporated into the guidelines.

4.5 Disseminated intravascular coagulation

Extracorporeal cardiopulmonary resuscitation (eCPR) with VA-ECMO has become a reality in today's medicine to rescue patients in refractory cardiac arrest. DIC therefore becomes an important issue in this subset of patients who experience serious abnormalities in coagulation and thrombosis. Survival of adults supported by eCPR in adults is lower than that noted in patients supported on VA-ECMO [30]. In a retrospective analysis of eCPR patients it was noted they had consistently higher DIC scores and the mean DIC scores was significantly different between survivors and non-survivors [31]. It may be reasonable to use DIC scores in prognostication in these patients. Further studies are warranted in this area. Such prognostication remains very important as it can curtail excessive use of blood products.

5. ECMO as a bridge to transplantation

Cardiac transplant still remains the gold standard in treatment of end-stage heart failure. The scarcity of donors has led to the generation of a whole field of mechanical circulatory support devices which has brought in a new era in the treatment of advanced heart failure. The use of continuous flow LVADs as a bridge to transplantation (BTT) has become more popular and the mainstay of patients waiting on the transplant list [32]. More recently, VA-ECMO is being increasingly used as a rescue therapy [33, 34] However, this trend has now led to the use of ECMO as a direct bridge to transplantation in adults. This seems to be an attractive pathway for critically ill advanced heart failure patients waiting on the transplant wait list to get a heart very quickly it raises many questions about the feasibility of such an approach in the population. Though there is a very small portion of the patients on the wait list who would be bridged directly on VA-ECMO to cardiac transplant, the lack of extensive literature and evidence for posttransplant survival of patients supported on ECMO makes this proposition questionable. Due to the large number of candidates waiting on the transplant list and too many high priority status 1A candidates in the wait list, the most recent organ allocation system has placed VA-ECMO bridge as the highest priority for cardiac transplant on the wait list [35]. This has a major disadvantage because of poor early and midterm posttransplant survival as compared to patients supported on CF-VADs [36]. It is therefore probably too early to use VA-ECMO as the highest priority for transplant organ availability/allocation.

BTT in the adult population has remained controversial despite small studies reporting varied survival rates posttransplantation in this population. The decision to use CF-LVADS as a BTT was based on various studies which showed improvements in functional status and quality of life in this population [37]. Such data is lacking in adults supported on VA-ECMO as BTT.

Therefore, the new system of allocation may reduce the transplant wait list mortality but may on the other hand increase the posttransplant mortality leading to a waste of organs in the setting of donor organ shortage. The most recent large retrospective analysis of the UNOS database showed a deceased survival in the early/mid posttransplant period [36]. Other studies from different countries have a wide variety of data which are limited.

The literature on use of VA-ECMO as a direct bridge to heart transplantation in adults is scanty. The use of VA-ECMO in posttransplant primary graft failure showed poor outcomes [38–40]. Since patients supported on ECMO are critically ill and the time to finding an organ is short, the extensive social and psychological evaluation required for transplant evaluation is not possible which could lead to suboptimal candidate selection.

Studies from France reported varying survival rates ranging from 51 to 70.4% at 1-year posttransplant in patients bridged on VA-ECMO [38, 41, 42]. Some of the caveats of these reports are the wait list mortality was not reported in the study by Jasseron et al. [38], while the duration of pretransplant ECMO support was not reported in the study by Rousse et al. [41] In the study Barth et al. [42], the survival was 100% at 1-year posttransplant though there were several adverse events and the study had a n = 8 with a mean age of 41 years. In a case series reported from Taiwan, 73% survived to hospital discharge in a cohort of 15 patients [43]. Mishra et al. [44] have reported a 1-year survival of 70%. A small study from Spain on posttransplant outcomes of patients bridged on ECMO showed no increase in mortality [45]. In France the special urgency wait list did improve the wait list mortality but also showed a significant increase in the posttransplant mortality [46].

6. Conclusions

The use of VA-ECMO as a technique for rescuing patients from cardiogenic shock is very attractive. However, considering the extensive set of complications and the mortality it brings with it makes it a less attractive option as a direct bridge to cardiac transplant. The literature currently on this subject is very scanty and limited to a few studies of small numbers of patients. The existing literature from France suggests a higher rate of posttransplant deaths even though the wait list mortality was reduced which does not seem to be an optimal way for organ allocation. In the light of present findings, further definitive research is needed for a consensus on the role of VA-ECMO as a bridge to cardiac transplant.

Acknowledgements

This work was funded from an internal faculty fund to Dr. Nandini Nair, TTUHSC, Lubbock TX.

Conflict of interest

Drs. Nandini Nair and Enrique Gongora have no conflict of interests to declare with relevance to this work.

Author details

Nandini Nair[1*] and Enrique Gongora[2]

1 Division of Cardiology, Department of Internal Medicine, Texas Tech Health Sciences Center, Lubbock, TX, United States

2 Department of Cardiothoracic Surgery, Memorial Cardiac and Vascular Institute, Hollywood, FL, United States

*Address all correspondence to: nandini.nair@gmail.com

References

[1] Milller BJ, Gibbon JH Jr, Greco VF, Smith BA, Cohn CH, Allbritten FF Jr. The production and repair of interatrial septal defects under direct vision with the assistance of an extracorporeal pump-oxygenator circuit. The Journal of Thoracic Surgery. 1953;**26**:598-616

[2] Miller BJ, Gibbon JH, Fineberg C. An improved mechanical heart and lung apparatus; its use during open cardiotomy in experimental animals. The Medical Clinics of North America. 1953;**1**:1603-1624

[3] Bartlett RH, Gazzaniga AB, Jefferies MR, Huxtable RF, Haiduc NJ, Fong SW. Extracorporeal membrane oxygenation (ECMO) cardiopulmonary support in infancy. Transactions—American Society for Artificial Internal Organs. 1976;**22**:80-93

[4] Bartlett RH, Roloff DW, Cornell RG, Andrews AF, Dillon PW, Zwischenberger JB. Extracorporeal circulation in neonatal respiratory failure: A prospective randomized study. Pediatrics. 1985;**76**:479-487

[5] Bartlett RH, Gattinoni L. Current status of extracorporeal life support (ECMO) for cardiopulmonary failure. Minerva Anestesiologica. 2010;**76**:534-540

[6] Peek GJ, Mugford M, Tiruvoipati R, Wilson A, Allen E, Thalanany MM, et al. CESAR trial collaboration efficacy and economic assessment of conventional ventilatory support versus extracorporeal membrane oxygenation for severe adult respiratory failure (CESAR): A multicentre randomised controlled trial. Lancet. 2009;**374**:1351-1363

[7] Paden ML, Conrad SA, Rycus PT, Thiagarajan RR. ELSO registry extracorporeal life support organization registry report 2012. ASAIO Journal. 2013;**59**:202-210

[8] Anselmi A, Ruggieri VG, Letheulle J, Robert AL, Tomasi J, Le Tulzo Y, et al. Extracorporeal membrane oxygenation in pregnancy. Journal of Cardiac Surgery. 2015;**30**:781-786

[9] Extracorporeal Life Support Registry report (international summary). Extracorporeal Life Support Organization. Ann Arbor; 2015

[10] Maxwell BG, Powers AJ, Sheikh AY, Lee PH, Lobato RL, Wong JK. Resource use trends in extracorporeal membrane oxygenation in adults: An analysis of the Nationwide Inpatient Sample 1998-2009. The Journal of Thoracic and Cardiovascular Surgery. 2014;**148**:416-421

[11] The Australia and New Zealand Extracorporeal Membrane Oxygenation (ANZ ECMO) Influenza Investigators, Davies A, Jones D, Bailey M, Beca J, Bellomo R, et al. Extracorporeal membrane oxygenation for 2009 influenza A (H1N1) acute respiratory distress syndrome. Journal of the American Medical Association. 2009;**302**:1888-1895

[12] Bermudez CA, Rocha RV, Sappington PL, Toyoda Y, Murray HN, Boujoukos AJ. Initial experience with single cannulation for venovenous extracorporeal oxygenation in adults. The Annals of Thoracic Surgery. 2010;**90**:991-995

[13] Staley LL, Dobberpuhl J, Pierce CN, Scott RL, Jaroszewski DE, Arabia FA. Bridge to decision: SWAT team approach used by Mayo Clinic Arizona's cardiac transport team. Progress in Transplantation. 2010;**20**:118-124

[14] ELSO Adult Cardiac Failure Supplement to the ELSO General

Guidelines. 2013. Available from: https://www.elso.org/Resources/Guidelines.aspx

[15] Hausmann H, Potapov EV, Koster A, Krabatsch T, Stein J, Yeter R, et al. Prognosis after the implantation of an intra-aortic balloon pump in cardiac surgery calculated with a new score. Circulation. 2002;**106**(12 Suppl 1): I203-I206

[16] Samuels LE, Kaufman MS, Thomas MP, Holmes EC, Brockman SK, Wechsler AS. Pharmacological criteria for ventricular assist device insertion following postcardiotomy shock: Experience with the Abiomed BVS system. Journal of Cardiac Surgery. 1999;**14**:288-293

[17] Bembea MM, Annich G, Rycus P, Oldenburg G, Berkowitz I, Pronovost P. Variability in anticoagulation management of patients on extracorporeal membrane oxygenation: An international survey. Pediatric Critical Care Medicine. 2013;**14**(2):e77-e78

[18] Bauer KA, Wiess LM, Sparrow D, Vokonas PS, Rosenberg RD. Aging-associated changes in indices of thrombin generation and protein C activation in humans. Normative aging study. The Journal of Clinical Investigation. 1987;**80**:1527

[19] Mari D, Mannucci PM, Coppola R, Bottasso B, Bauer KA, Rosenberg RD. Hypercoagulability in centenarians: The paradox of successful aging. Blood. 1995;**85**:3144

[20] Yasuda SU, Zhang L, Huang S-M. The role of ethnicity in variability in response to drugs: Focus on clinical pharmacology studies. Clinical Pharmacology & Therapeutics. 2008;**84**:417

[21] Halaweish I, Cole A, Cooley E, Lynch WR, Haft JW. Roller and centrifugal pumps: A retrospective comparison of bleeding complications in extracorporeal membrane oxygenation. ASAIO Journal. 2015;**61**:496-501

[22] Makdisi G, Makdisi T, Wang IW. Use of distal perfusion in peripheral extracorporeal membrane oxygenation. The Annals of Translational Medicine. 2017;**5**:103

[23] PJ1 F, Morris RJ, Woo EY, Acker MA, Wang GJ, Fairman RM, et al. Limb ischemia during femoral cannulation for cardiopulmonary support. Journal of Vascular Surgery. 2010;**52**:850-853

[24] Sandgren T, Sonesson B, Ahlgren A, Länne T. The diameter of the common femoral artery in healthy human: Influence of sex, age, and body size. Journal of Vascular Surgery. 1999;**29**:503-510

[25] Huang SC, Yu HY, Ko WJ, Chen YS. Pressure criterion for placement of distal perfusion catheter to prevent limb ischemia during adult extracorporeal life support. The Journal of Thoracic and Cardiovascular Surgery. 2004;**128**:776-777

[26] Kimmoun A, Oulehri W, Sonneville R, Grisot PH, Zogheib E, Amour J, et al. Prevalence and outcome of heparin-induced thrombocytopenia diagnosed under veno-arterial extracorporeal membrane oxygenation: A retrospective nationwide study. Intensive Care Medicine. 2018;**44**:1460-1469

[27] Ljajikj E, Zittermann A, Morshuis M, Börgermann J, Ruiz-Cano M, Schoenbrodt M, et al. Bivalirudin anticoagulation for left ventricular assist device implantation on an extracorporeal life support system in patients with heparin-induced thrombocytopenia antibodies. Interactive Cardiovascular and Thoracic Surgery. 2017;**25**(6):898-904

[28] Fernandes P, O'Neil M, Del Valle S, Cave A, Nagpal D. A 24-hour perioperative case study on argatroban use for left ventricle assist device insertion during cardiopulmonary bypass and veno-arterial extracorporeal membrane oxygenation. Perfusion. 2018;**25**:267659118813043

[29] Rougé A, Pelen F, Durand M, Schwebel C. Argatroban for an alternative anticoagulant in HIT during ECMO. Journal of Intensive Care. 2017;**5**:39

[30] Squiers JJ, Lima B, DiMaio JM. Contemporary extracorporeal membrane oxygenation therapy in adults: Fundamental principles and systematic review of the evidence. The Journal of Thoracic and Cardiovascular Surgery. 2016l;**152**:20-32

[31] Ruggeri L, Franco A, Alba AC, Lembo R, Frassoni S, Scandroglio AM, et al. Coagulation derangements in patients with refractory cardiac arrest treated with extracorporeal cardiopulmonary resuscitation. Journal of Cardiothoracic and Vascular Anesthesia. 2018

[32] Fukuhara S, Takeda K, Polanco AR, Takayama H, Naka Y. Prolonged continuous-flow left ventricular assist device support and post-transplant outcomes: A new challenge. The Journal of Thoracic and Cardiovascular Surgery. 2016;**151**:872-880.e1-5

[33] McCarthy FH, McDermott KM, Kini V, Gutsche JT, Wald JW, Xie D, et al. Trends in U.S. extracorporeal membrane oxygenation use and outcomes: 2002-2012. Seminars in Thoracic and Cardiovascular Surgery. 2015;**27**:81-88

[34] Thiagarajan RR, Barbaro RP, Rycus PT, Mcmullan DM, Conrad SA, Fortenberry JD, et al. Extracorporeal life support organization registry international report 2016. ASAIO Journal. 2017;**63**:60-67

[35] Adult heart allocation—Organ Procurement and Transplantation Network. 2018. Available from: https://optn.transplant.hrsa.gov/learn/professional-education/adult-heart-allocation/

[36] Fukuhara S, Takeda K, Kurlansky PA, Naka Y, Takayama H. Extracorporeal membrane oxygenation as a direct bridge to heart transplantation in adults. The Journal of Thoracic and Cardiovascular Surgery. 2018;**155**:1607-1618

[37] Baskin-Bey ES, Kremers W, Stegall MD, Nyberg SL. United network for organ sharing's expanded criteria donors: Is stratification useful? Clinical Transplantation. 2005;**19**:406-412

[38] Jasseron C, Lebreton G, Cantrelle C, Legeai C, Leprince P, Flecher E, et al. Impact of heart transplantation on survival in patients on venoarterial extracorporeal membrane oxygenation listing in France. Transplantation. 2016;**100**:1979-1987

[39] Pennington DG, McBride LR, Kanter KR, Miller LW, Ruzevich SA, Naunheim K, et al. Bridging to heart transplantation with circulatory support devices. The Journal of Heart Transplantation. 1989;**8**:116-123

[40] Kolla S, Lee WA, Hirschl RB, Bartlett RH. Extracorporeal life support for cardiovascular support in adults. ASAIO Journal. 1996;**42**:M809-M819

[41] Rousse N, Juthier F, Pinçon C, Hysi I, Banfi C, Robin E, et al. ECMO as a bridge to decision: Recovery, VAD, or heart transplantation? International Journal of Cardiology. 2015;**187**:620-627

[42] Barth E, Durand M, Heylbroeck C, Rossi-Blancher M, Boignard A, Vanzetto G, et al. Extracorporeal life support as a bridge to high-urgency heart transplantation. Clinical Transplantation. 2012;**26**:484-488

[43] Chung JC, Tsai PR, Chou NK, Chi NH, Wang SS, Ko WJ. Extracorporeal membrane oxygenation bridge to adult heart transplantation. Clinical Transplantation. 2010;**24**:375-380

[44] Mishra V, Fiane AE, Winsnes BA, Geiran O, Sørensen G, Hagen TP, et al. Cardiac replacement therapies: Outcomes and costs for heart transplantation versus circulatory assist. Scandinavian Cardiovascular Journal. 2017;**51**:1-7

[45] Barge-Caballero E, Almenar-Bonet L, Villa-Arranz A, Pérez-Villa F, Segovia-Cubero J, Delgado-Jiménez J, et al. Impact of short-term mechanical circulatory support with extracorporeal devices on postoperative outcomes after emergency heart transplantation: Data from a multi-institutional Spanish cohort. International Journal of Cardiology. 2014;**176**:86-93

[46] Dorent R, Epailly E, Sebbag L. The effect of graft allocation system on outcomes in heart transplantation in France: Has the time come to take calculated survival benefit into account? The Journal of Heart and Lung Transplantation. 2011;**30**:1299-1300

Chapter 10

ECMO Weaning Strategies to Optimize Outcomes

Jorge Silva Enciso and Kimberly N. Hong

Abstract

Survival to discharge in patients presenting with cardiogenic shock who are managed using extracorporeal membrane oxygenation (ECMO) remains low at ~50%. This speaks to the acuity and severity of individuals being placed on ECMO, as well as the time dependent risk for complications associated with this therapy. Although some patients are able to be weaned from ECMO to either recovery, left ventricular assist device or heart transplantation, other individuals do not survive after device removal, suggesting that current protocols may not be identifying individuals with enough intrinsic cardiac recovery to maintain adequate end-organ perfusion. The decision to wean an individual from ECMO is complex and entails several factors that are dynamic and evolving daily while on full circulatory support. Objective clinical, hemodynamic and biological markers are needed to be controlled prior to trialing device weans but many times the decision relies on clinical experience and intuition. The purpose of this chapter will be to: (1) outline the survival and risks associated with ECMO which encourages early weaning trials and (2) identify patient factors related to either successful weaning or early referral for durable mechanical support or transplant.

Keywords: venoarterial ECMO, weaning, cardiac recovery, echocardiography, hemodynamics

1. Introduction

Cardiogenic shock to date remains associated with a significant mortality (50–80%) even after revascularization [1]. For these patients and in those with other forms of refractory cardiogenic shock or cardiac arrest, circulatory support with the use of venoarterial extracorporeal membrane oxygenation (VA-ECMO) has been utilized to stabilize and improve their survival. Its rapidly expanding use across many centers has favorably altered outcomes in severely critically ill patients and in many instances it serves as a bridge to decision or recovery [2]. However, weaning of VA-ECMO represents a significant challenge depending on the initial indication for its use. Moreover, there is a paucity of data on factors that predict weaning success from VA-ECMO and no clear guidelines to determine which patients will survive after device removal.

With the rapid evolving technology of short term mechanical circulatory support and the increasing number of ECMO use across many centers, there needs to be a clear understanding of the indications, hemodynamic impact, limitations and risks associated with its application to determine who will be a good candidate for device wean and removal.

IntechOpen

In this chapter we will review the basic principles of VA-ECMO function, predictors of survival, conditions conducive towards successful weaning and lastly, weaning strategies.

2. Venoarterial extracorporeal membrane oxygenation function

VA-ECMO support is a well-established technology that allows for full cardiopulmonary support with the goal to recover organ injury. Patients who may require this therapy include: refractory cardiogenic shock (CS), cardiac arrest (CA), refractory ventricular arrhythmia, acute or decompensated biventricular failure (AHF), pulmonary hypertension associated with right ventricular failure, fulminant myocarditis, and postcardiotomy cardiogenic shock (PCCS) [3].

The primary goal of VA-ECMO is restoration of tissue perfusion and avoidance of permanent end organ dysfunction. It has a unique hemodynamic effect due to its dual circulatory support circuit. The venous drainage cannula reduces flow through the lung vasculature, decreasing stress on the right heart while the arterial outflow cannula increases flow to the systemic arterial vasculature and the afterload to the left ventricle proportionate to the pump speed/flow. With incremental changes in speed and flow, the increased afterload reduces aortic valve opening and, in cases of severe left ventricular dysfunction, severe right ventricular dysfunction or asystole, the aortic valve may not open at all. The implications of the latter include increased LV end diastolic pressure and the development of pulmonary edema.

3. Venoarterial extracorporeal membrane oxygenation outcomes

VA-ECMO has been shown to increase survival to hospital discharge in patients with advanced heart disease with some cases having favorable long-term survival [4]. However, outcomes differ depending on the underlying etiology of cardiopulmonary collapse at the time of VA-ECMO cannulation. In a large national inpatient database from Japan with 5263 patients receiving ECMO, the in-hospital mortality was 37.9%, with 64.4% weaned off the device. Cardiac arrest at the time of hospital presentation was recognized as the primary factor for poor survival compared to cardiogenic shock alone. Moreover, higher age and smaller BMI were associated with in hospital mortality. The majority of patients presenting with cardiogenic shock had underlying ischemic heart disease, followed by heart failure, valvular heart disease and myocarditis. Notably, the preponderance of patients discharged from the hospital after weaning from ECMO were those with heart failure (31.1%) and myocarditis (41.9%) compared to those with ischemic heart disease (20.3%). In-hospital mortality after weaning however remained elevated with about half of the patients who were weaned dying in the hospital. This high mortality suggests non-modifiable risk factors with persistence of critical illness even after weaning VA-ECMO, as well as differences in survival depending on the underlying etiology of shock, with those having ischemic heart disease at the time of presentation experiencing a 79.1% in-hospital mortality [5].

In patients presenting with PCCS, VA-ECMO is a viable salvage strategy associated with increased survival to hospital discharge. In a meta-analysis of 21 studies with 1866 patients, survival to hospital discharge was achieved in 20.8–65.4% of patients placed on VA-ECMO [6]. Even more, PCCS patients undergoing VA-ECMO have an acceptable 5-year survival of 55.8% compared to other types of cardiogenic shock [7].

These findings drastically differ to those presenting with acute myocardial infarction associated CS (AMI-CS) where their survival to hospital discharge remains low (33–59%) [8]. This could potentially be mitigated by early intervention at the time of AMI-CS presentation and VA-ECMO support, specifically in those undergoing simultaneous revascularization. In a study of 334 patients with ST elevation AMI, the group that underwent early VA-ECMO support at the time of percutaneous intervention had a lower 30-day mortality compared to those without the support (30.1 vs. 41.7%) with a strong benefit in those with profound shock—defined as systolic blood pressure <75 mmHg despite intravenous inotropic agent administration and intra-aortic balloon pump (IABP) support associated with altered mental status and respiratory failure—compared to those without (72 vs. 39.1% for 30-day death) [9]. Among notable predictors for 30 days mortality were the presence of advanced heart failure (defined as NYHA ≥ III), post intervention TIMI flow grade ≤2 and profound cardiogenic shock.

Lastly in those with AHF, outcomes on VA-ECMO are less promising depending on the original insult. For those with acute presentations, outcomes on VA-ECMO are more favorable compared to those with a chronic cardiomyopathy [10–12]. Specifically, those with fulminant myocarditis and CS or CA survival to discharge ranged from 60 to 88% [10], compared to only 56% in those with chronic cardiomyopathy [11, 12]. In those with long standing heart failure though the decision to bridge to another salvage strategy is of paramount importance as their cardiac reserve is limited (characterized by low cardiac index and cardiac power) with 77–79% requiring more advanced MCS support including durable VAD to allow for both short-term and long-term survival [11, 12]. Nevertheless, the high mortality rates in patients who receive VA-ECMO heighten the importance of limiting patient selection to those who can be weaned from device support.

When patients present with CS, inserting a VA-ECMO as a bridge to decision device allows for assessment of neurological and end-organ recovery, making short-term prognostication possible. In many instances, commencing support prior to hemodynamic deterioration and multiorgan failure or cardiac arrest can allow for transition to viable long-term therapies including VAD or heart transplantation. Studies have shown that in patients presenting with refractory cardiogenic shock requiring mechanical circulatory support, 56% survive with 26% of patients transitioning to an implantable VAD, 11% undergoing heart transplantation and 18% showing cardiac recovery [12, 13].

4. Venoarterial extracorporeal membrane oxygenation complications

Although ECMO can improve survival to hospital discharge, several studies show significant morbidity with rates increasing with prolonged duration on support. A meta-analysis of 20 studies including 1866 patients demonstrated bleeding as one of the most common complications (40.8%), followed by requirement of dialysis (46%), significant infection (30.4%), limb ischemia (16.9%), and stroke (5.9%). Vascular complications, bleeding and blood transfusions were associated with significant in-hospital mortality [6]. Many of the complications relate to the vascular access site, with femoral cannulation requiring surgical intervention in 20% of the cases [14]. A negative downstream effect of cannulation is distal ischemia which can lead to arterial thrombosis and gangrene. This complication can be mitigated by preemptively placing a small antegrade perfusion cannula to bypass the area of obstruction from the ECMO arterial cannula [15]. Moreover, vascular complications can lead to unsuccessful weaning trials as serious bleeding events increase the need for blood product transfusions and the incidence of thrombotic events. Specifically, thrombotic events were noted to occur in 17% of patients, mostly as lower extremity arterial thromboses, and can impact the duration on support, increase morbidity and affect overall outcomes [16, 17].

LV distention in VA-ECMO. When contemplating weaning trials to assess for LV recovery, consideration should be taken on the loading effect that VA-ECMO has on the left ventricle. Proper unloading of the LV can avoid complications from LV distention including pulmonary edema, worsening oxygenation, increased left ventricular wall stress, reduced myocardial blood flow and ventricular arrhythmias. In fact, acute pulmonary edema in the setting of peripheral VA-ECMO has been associated with mortality, with many patients dying within hours after implant or requiring conversion to central VA-ECMO [18]. In a study of 121 patients on ECMO with LV distention, 16% required decompression with an Impella device and cardiac recovery was inversely related to the degree of LV distention. Furthermore, those presenting with LV distention requiring decompression had lower survival in the first 30 days following VA-ECMO compared to those not requiring decompression. More so, the study noted that those presenting with acute decompensated heart failure had a delayed LV decompression strategy which was associated lower survival [19]. This may suggest that more aggressive unloading is required upfront when clinical signs of LV distention are present. In one study, adding an Impella device improved 30-day survival in those presenting with AMI compared to other groups. Additionally, in those with cardiogenic shock due to acute decompensated systolic heart failure, unloading can help to stabilize and bridge them to the next strategy. In a series of 52 patients with ADHF, 71% required an LV venting device with the vast majority transitioned to a durable device support [12].

5. Factors associated with successful weaning from VA-ECMO

Determining successful weaning from VA-ECMO relies on multiple variables which can be partitioned into pre-implant and during support factors.

5.1 Pre-ECMO factors

Patient selection. Many risk scores have identified several variables that rely on clinical and biochemical markers. The SAVE score is a tool that discriminates between survivors and non-survivors of refractory cardiogenic shock on VA-ECMO. While younger patients, acute myocarditis, post-heart transplant, refractory arrhythmias and high diastolic blood pressure are protective factors, those with chronic renal disease, prolonged intubation, pre-ECMO organ failure, lower pulse pressure and lower bicarbonate are associated with poor survival. (http://www.save-score.com/) [20]. Similarly to SAVE, the ENCOURAGE survival score utilizes predictors for those presenting with CS due to AMI, however unlike SAVE it places more weight placed on gender, body mass index, Glasgow coma score and level of serum lactate. Survival was also directly proportional to the patient's risk score (probabilities of survival were 80%, 58, 25, 20, and 7% for classes 0–12, 13–18, 19–22, 23–27, and ≥28, respectively [21].

5.2 During ECMO factors

Once VA-ECMO support is initiated, there is a very narrow window to assess end organ function recovery and decide on need for advanced therapies. In a cohort of 124 consecutive patients receiving VA-ECMO for CS, about two thirds of the deaths occurred during the first 4 days due to multiorgan failure, however those who were supported for more than 6 days had a reduced in-hospital mortality, with 50%, achieving successful device wean. In addition, prolonged support provided an opportunity for improved patient selection with 60% reaching cardiac recovery, 26% undergoing heart transplantation and 14% ventricular assist device (VAD) implant. After a median follow up of 2.4 years, survival at 1 year was 78% for those who achieved cardiac recovery, 51% for those who underwent heart transplant and 75% with VAD implant [18].

LV unloading. Ventricular decompression with an IABP during implant can allow for weaning and survival, bridge to LVAD or transplantation, while its non-use has been associated with increased risk for death during support or after VA-ECMO is withdrawn [22]. A recent meta-analysis of 17 observational studies comprising 3997 patients with 42% receiving an LV unloading device (IABP 92%, percutaneous VAD 5.5%, trans-septal left atrial cannulation 3%) showed a reduction in mortality when utilizing LV unloading devices compared to those without LV unloading (54 vs. 65%, RR 0.79, CI 95% 0.72–0.87). Secondary outcomes for limb ischemia, bleeding, need for renal replacement therapy, multiorgan failure, stroke or transient ischemic attack were not different among all cohorts [23].

Echocardiography. Several echocardiographic indicators exist when considering a weaning trial. Improvement in underlying LV function with an ejection fraction ≥35%, LV outflow tract velocity-time integral >10 cm, tissue Doppler peak systolic velocity of the mitral annulus ≥6 m/s, absence of LV dilatation, and no cardiac tamponade while on minimal support have been shown as good predictors of successful weaning [24, 25]. Similarly, significant improvement in right ventricular function during weaning identifies greater opportunity for survival. In a study of 46 patients on VA-ECMO, RV ejection fraction (RVEF) was assessed by 3D echocardiography. RV free wall strain, RV fractional area change, and central venous pressure were found to be independently associated with RVEF. A cutoff RVEF of >24.6% was found to be a predictor for weaning success after first cannulation with lower values associated with increased all-cause mortality at 30 days (HR 15.86; 95% CI, 3.56–70.73; $p < 0.001$) [26].

Hemodynamics parameters. Multiple hemodynamic variables have been found to be predictive of successful weaning. Presence of a pulse pressure greater than 50 mmHg, elevated systolic pressure greater than 100 mmHg has been associated with good prognosis and survival [25]. Maintaining a perfusion mean arterial pressure (MAP) >60 mmHg with minimal inotropic support is critical [27]. Right heart catheterization data shows that a pulmonary capillary wedge pressure <24, PVR < 1.1 WU, mean pulmonary arterial pressure <25, transpulmonary gradient <10 are recommended parameters to achieve prior to a weaning trial and that inotropic agents as well as pulmonary vasodilators can be of assistance during weaning efforts [26].

Biomarkers. Serological markers of poor perfusion have been associated with worse prognosis. Lactate has been recognized as a biomarker for macrovascular tissue perfusion and early clearance at 24 hours after VA-ECMO initiation has been correlated with weaning and survival [28]. Loforte et al., analyzed 228 patients supported on VA-ECMO primarily post-cardiotomy CS. The authors found that blood lactate level (>3 mmol/L) and a CK-MB index of 10% 72 hours after ECMO initiation, was predictive of a 50% probability of 30-day mortality [29]. An elevated creatinine on the day of withdrawal or weaning trial has been associated with poor outcome with a four-fold risk of death when the level is above 1.4 mg/dL [18].

Tissue perfusion. Derangements in the microvasculature have been noted in both severe sepsis as well as cardiogenic shock, with measures of microcirculation emerging as new markers for tissue perfusion [30]. In those supported by VA-ECMO, there is observational data suggesting that preserved microcirculation at time of VA-ECMO cannulation may be more specific than hemodynamic measures for identifying successful VA-ECMO weaning and survival. This discordance between the micro and macro-circulation has been described previously as a loss of hemodynamic coherence in part due to heterogeneous flow the organs receive during support, alterations in capillary density and presence of tissue edema [31]. Specifically, one study which assessed microcirculation serially, found that even in the presence of preserved lactate, tissue perfusion as estimated by parameters of microcirculation did not improve on VA-ECMO and those with compromised microcirculation—measured as perfused capillary density and proportion of perfused vessels—could not be weaned from VA-ECMO [32]. A separate study looking specifically at 28-day survival in cardiogenic shock patients placed on VA-ECMO, found that while MAP, pressor requirement and lactate did not differ, microcirculation was better preserved in survivors compared to non-survivors within 12 hours of VA-ECMO support [33]. However, further research is needed to determine if microcirculatory assessment can help guide timing of VA-ECMO weaning.

5.3 Post VA-ECMO wean

Survival post VA-ECMO is predicated on correcting the underlying cause for shock or cardiac arrest, ultimately allowing device removal. However, weaning does not always signify that individuals will survive. Individual factors have to be considered to predict long term survival such as age, comorbidities, complications arising during circulatory support, underlying ventricular function and end organ function. On the latter, renal failure (signified by elevated creatinine level) or hepatic failure (marked by elevated total bilirubin and elevated INR) at the time of wean can impact short-term and long-term survival with multiorgan failure being the predominant mode of death after weaning [22]. If myocardial recovery is unlikely but other factors have been controlled and improved (including renal and hepatic function, lactate and resolution of pulmonary edema), durable VAD or heart transplantation should be taken into consideration, as longer duration on VA-ECMO can reduce the likelihood of survival to discharge or success towards a bridging option. In a small observational study, survival to discharge was higher for those transitioned within 14 days from VA-ECMO support to a VAD compared to those transitioned longer than 14 days (92 vs. 25%, $p < 0.05$) [34].

6. Weaning strategies

6.1 Pharmacological agents

The pharmacologic agents that have been used to assist with weaning trials have primarily been inotropic agents including dobutamine, epinephrine, dopamine, milrinone and levosimendan. Epinephrine, dopamine and dobutamine are catecholamines, with epinephrine and dopamine having alpha-1 activity and thus some crossover with norepinephrine as vasoconstrictors. Dobutamine acts predominantly on beta-1 and beta-2 receptors. Milrinone and levosimendan on the other hand are inotropes without direct adrenergic receptor targets. Milrinone is a type-3 phosphodiesterase inhibitor and augments myocardial contraction by increasing intracellular concentrations of cAMP and calcium. Levosimendan on the other hand is a calcium sensitizer and is postulated to augment myocardial contractility without increasing intracellular calcium and myocardial oxygen consumption. Current evidence supports the use of both milrinone and levosimendan to assist with VA-ECMO weaning [35, 36].

6.2 Weaning trials

Protocols for weaning VA-ECMO include:

1. A stepwise reduction in VA-ECMO flows either by percent of support or by 0.5–1.0 L/min.

2. A pre-specified time interval in which the VA-ECMO flow is reduced for which can range from 10–15 min to 24 h.

3. Baseline parameter thresholds and subsequent measurements assessing for hemodynamic tolerance and myocardial adaptation to changes in preload and afterload as flows decrease.

4. Using continuous or intermittent transthoracic or transesophageal echocardiogram.

5. Frequency of weaning trials may occur daily, but typically occur 24–72 hours after VA-ECMO institution to allow for reversal and recovery from the inciting injury [29, 37–40].

In addition to requiring full anticoagulation during weaning trials, flows cannot be turned down below 1–1.5 L/min because of concerns for thrombus formation within the VA-ECMO circuit. Thus, clinicians must monitor changes in hemodynamic and echocardiographic parameters as VA-ECMO flows are decreased and terminate weaning if evidence of hemodynamic compromise or intolerance to preload changes such as loss of pulsatility, ventricular dysfunction or increases in filling pressures are seen. Hemodynamic tolerance during the weaning trial is extrapolated to imply myocardial recovery has occurred and that decannulation will be tolerated by the patient. In order to allow clinical assessments off VA-ECMO support entirely, some centers are using arteriovenous cannula bridging strategies that form a circuit that bypasses the patient [41], or a separate technique pioneered in neonates that reduces pump flow until the circuit runs retrograde [42, 43].

7. Proposed weaning protocol

Assessing the readiness for VA-ECMO weaning involves withdrawal or reversal of the inciting injury, maintenance or recovery of extracardiac organ function, and lastly myocardial recovery. Prior to weaning attempts, hemodynamic stability and adequate tissue perfusion defined as a MAP $\geq$ 60–65 mmHg while on minimal pressor support, arterial pulsatility and lactate levels < 2 mmol/L should be achieved. VA-ECMO flow should be reduced by 0.5–1.0 L/min in 5–10-min intervals with continuous invasive hemodynamic and echocardiographic monitoring. In instances where adequate transthoracic windows cannot be achieved, transesophageal echocardiogram should be performed, and biventricular size and function monitored. Because some parameters of left ventricular function including aortic VTI and TDSa are not easily obtained by both transthoracic and transesophageal echocardiography, we recommend measuring changes in ventricular size and visual assessments of ventricular function and valvular regurgitation. In instances where CVP rises to greater than 1518 mmHg (depending on ventilator settings) and the RV dilates with worsening function and tricuspid regurgitation, the weaning trial should be aborted. Left sided function and loading conditions may vary depending on venting strategies, however, in cases where PCWP rises above 20 mmHg and arterial line pulsatility is lost due to LV dysfunction, isolated LV mechanical support should be considered. Prior to final decannulation in the operating room, the VA-ECMO speed should be left at 1.5 L/minutes for an hour to assess stability of hemodynamic, echocardiographic and tissue perfusion parameters.

8. Conclusion

VA-ECMO can rapidly stabilize patients and provide organ perfusion to those with refractory cardiogenic shock or cardiac arrest. Albeit associated with multiple complications that increase with longer duration of support, in the right patient it can improve the survival. Weaning strategies should be implemented as soon as the underlying condition has been corrected and improvement in metabolic, hepatic, pulmonary and renal function has occurred. Use of hemodynamic, echocardiographic and serological markers of recovery should be taken into account prior and during each weaning trial to assess success of weaning or if need of VAD or heart transplantation should be considered.

Author details

Jorge Silva Enciso* and Kimberly N. Hong
Cardiovascular Medicine Institute, University of California San Diego, San Diego, CA, US

*Address all correspondence to: jsilvaenciso@ucsd.edu

References

[1] Hochman JS, Sleeper LA, Webb JG, Sanborn TA, White HD, Talley JD, et al. Early revascularization in acute myocardial infarction complicated by cardiogenic shock. SHOCK investigators. Should we emergently revascularize occluded coronaries for cardiogenic shock. The New England Journal of Medicine. 1999;**341**(9):625-634

[2] Stretch R, Sauer CM, Yuh DD, Bonde P. National trends in the utilization of short-term mechanical circulatory support: Incidence, outcomes and cost analysis. Journal of the American College of Cardiology. 2014;**64**(14):1407-1415

[3] Rihal CS, Naidu SS, Givertz MM, Szeto WY, Burke JA, Kapur NK, et al. SCAI/ACC/HFSA/STS clinical expert consensus statement on the use of percutaneous mechanical circulatory support devices in cardiovascular care: Endorsed by the American Heart Assocation, the cardiological society of India, and sociedad latino Americana de Cardiologia Intervencion; Affirmation of value by the Canadian Association of Interventional Cardiology-Association Canadienne de Cardiologie d'intervention. Journal of the American College of Cardiology. 2015, 2015;**65**(19):e7-e26

[4] Xie A, Phan K, Tsai YC, Yan TD, Forrest P. Venoarterial extracorporeal membrane oxygenation for cardiogenic shock and cardiac arrest: A meta-analysis. Journal of Cardiothoracic and Vascular Anesthesia. 2015;**29**(3):637-645

[5] Affronti A, di Bella I, Carino D, Ragni T. Levosimendan may improve weaning outcomes in venoarterial ECMO patients. ASAIO Journal. 2013;**59**(6):554-557

[6] Cheng R, Hachamovitch R, Kittleson M, Patel J, Arabia F, Moriguchi J, et al. Complications of extracorporeal membrane oxygenation for treatment of cardiogenic shock and cardiac arrest: A meta-analysis of 1,866 adult patients. The Annals of Thoracic Surgery. 2014;**97**(2):610-616

[7] Rastan AJ, Dege A, Mohr M, Doll N, Falk V, Walther T, et al. Early and late outcomes of 517 consecutive adult patients treated with extracorporeal membrane oxygenation for refractory postcardiotomy cardiogenic shock. The Journal of Thoracic and Cardiovascular Surgery. 2010;**139**(2):302-311

[8] Carroll BJ, Shah RV, Murthy V, McCullough SA, Reza N, Thomas SS, et al. Clinical features and outcomes in adults with cardiogenic shock supported by extracorporeal membrane oxygenation. The American Journal of Cardiology. 2015;**116**(10):1624-1630

[9] Sheu JJ, Tsai TH, Lee FY, Fang HY, Sun CK, Leu S, et al. Early extracorporeal membrane oxygenator-assisted primary percutaneous coronary intervention improved 30-day clinical outcomes in patients with ST-segment elevation myocardial infarction complicated with profound cardiogenic shock. Critical Care Medicine. 2010;**38**(9):1810-1817

[10] Cheng R, Hachamovitch R, Kittleson M, Patel J, Arabia F, Moriguchi J, et al. Clinical outcomes in fulminant myocarditis requiring extracorporeal membrane oxygenation: A weighted meta-analysis of 170 patients. Journal of Cardiac Failure. 2014;**20**(6):400-406

[11] Bermudez CA, Rocha RV, Toyoda Y, Zaldonis D, Sappington PL, Mulukutla S, et al. Extracorporeal membrane oxygenation for advanced refractory shock in acute and chronic cardiomyopathy. The Annals of Thoracic Surgery. 2011;**92**(6):2125-2131

[12] Garan AR, Malick WA, Habal M, Topkara VK, Fried J, Masoumi A, et al. Predictors of survival for patients with acute decompensated heart failure requiring extra-corporeal membrane oxygenation therapy. ASAIO J. 9 Oct 2018. DOI: 10.1097/MAT.0000000000000898. https://www.ncbi.nlm.nih.gov/pubmed/30312208 [Epub ahead of print]

[13] Takayama H, Truby L, Koekort M, Uriel N, Colombo P, Mancini DM, et al. Clinical outcome of mechanical circulatory support for refractory cardiogenic shock in the current era. The Journal of Heart and Lung Transplantation. 2013;**32**(1):106-111

[14] Tanaka D, Hirose H, Cavarocchi N, Entwistle JW. The impact of vascular complications on survival of patients on venoarterial extracorporeal membrane oxygenation. The Annals of Thoracic Surgery. 2016;**101**(5):1729-1734

[15] Yeo HJ, Yoon SH, Jeon D, Kim YS, Cho WH, Kim D, et al. The utility of preemptive distal perfusion cannulation during peripheral venoarterial extracorporeal membrane oxygenation support. Journal of Interventional Cardiology. 2016;**29**(4):431-436

[16] Aubron C, Cheng AC, Pilcher D, Leong T, Magrin G, Cooper DJ, et al. Factors associated with outcomes of patients on extracorporeal membrane oxygenation support: A 5-year cohort study. Critical Care. 2013;**17**(2):R73

[17] Mazzeffi M, Greenwood J, Tanaka K, Menaker J, Rector R, Herr D, et al. Bleeding, transfusion, and mortality on extracorporeal life support: ECLS working group on thrombosis and Hemostasis. The Annals of Thoracic Surgery. 2016;**101**(2):682-689

[18] Rousse N, Juthier F, Pincon C, Hysi I, Banfi C, Robin E, et al. ECMO as a bridge to decision: Recovery, VAD, or heart transplantation? International Journal of Cardiology. 2015;**187**:620-627

[19] Truby LK, Takeda K, Mauro C, Yuzefpolskaya M, Garan AR, Kirtane AJ, et al. Incidence and implications of left ventricular distention during venoarterial extracorporeal membrane oxygenation support. ASAIO Journal. 2017;**63**(3):257-265

[20] Schmidt M, Burrell A, Roberts L, Bailey M, Sheldrake J, Rycus PT, et al. Predicting survival after ECMO for refractory cardiogenic shock: The survival after veno-arterial-ECMO (SAVE)-score. European Heart Journal. 2015;**36**(33):2246-2256

[21] Muller G, Flecher E, Lebreton G, Luyt CE, Trouillet JL, Brechot N, et al. The ENCOURAGE mortality risk score and analysis of long-term outcomes after VA-ECMO for acute myocardial infarction with cardiogenic shock. Intensive Care Medicine. 2016;**42**(3):370-378

[22] Smedira NG, Moazami N, Golding CM, McCarthy PM, Apperson-Hansen C, Blackstone EH, et al. Clinical experience with 202 adults receiving extracorporeal membrane oxygenation for cardiac failure: Survival at five years. The Journal of Thoracic and Cardiovascular Surgery. 2001;**122**(1):92-102

[23] Russo JJ, Aleksova N, Pitcher I, Couture E, Parlow S, Faraz M, et al. Left ventricular unloading during extracorporeal membrane oxygenation in patients with cardiogenic shock. Journal of the American College of Cardiology. 2019;**73**(6):654-662

[24] Leick J, Liebetrau C, Szardien S, Fischer-Rasokat U, Willmer M, van Linden A, et al. Door-to-implantation time of extracorporeal life support systems predicts mortality in patients with out-of-hospital cardiac arrest. Clinical Research in Cardiology. 2013;**102**(9):661-669

[25] Aissaoui N, Luyt CE, Leprince P, Trouillet JL, Leger P, Pavie A, et al. Predictors of successful extracorporeal membrane oxygenation (ECMO) weaning after assistance for refractory cardiogenic shock. Intensive Care Medicine. 2011;**37**(11):1738-1745

[26] Huang KC, Lin LY, Chen YS, Lai CH, Hwang JJ, Lin LC. Three-dimensional echocardiography-derived right ventricular ejection fraction correlates with success of decannulation and prognosis in patients stabilized by venoarterial extracorporeal life support. Journal of the American Society of Echocardiography. 2018;**31**(2):169-179

[27] Pappalardo F, Pieri M, Arnaez Corada B, Ajello S, Melisurgo G, De Bonis M, et al. Timing and strategy for weaning from venoarterial ECMO are complex issues. Journal of Cardiothoracic and Vascular Anesthesia. 2015;**29**(4):906-911

[28] Sugiura A, Abe R, Nakayama T, Hattori N, Fujimoto Y, Himi T, et al. Predictors of successful weaning from veno-arterial extracorporeal membrane oxygenation after coronary revascularization for acute myocardial infarction complicated by cardiac arrest: A retrospective multicenter study. Shock C. 3 Aug 2018. DOI: 10.1097/SHK.0000000000001220. https://www.ncbi.nlm.nih.gov/pubmed/30080744 [Epub ahead of print]

[29] Loforte A, Marinelli G, Musumeci F, Folesani G, Pilato E, Martin Suarez S, et al. Extracorporeal membrane oxygenation support in refractory cardiogenic shock: Treatment strategies and analysis of risk factors. Artificial Organs. 2014;**38**(7):E129-E141

[30] Jung C, Ferrari M, Rodiger C, Fritzenwanger M, Goebel B, Lauten A, et al. Evaluation of the sublingual microcirculation in cardiogenic shock. Clinical Hemorheology and Microcirculation. 2009;**42**(2):141-148

[31] Ince C. Hemodynamic coherence and the rationale for monitoring the microcirculation. Critical Care. 2015;**19**(Suppl 3):S8

[32] Akin S, Dos Reis Miranda D, Caliskan K, Soliman OI, Guven G, Struijs A, et al. Functional evaluation of sublingual microcirculation indicates successful weaning from VA-ECMO in cardiogenic shock. Critical Care 2017;**21**(1):265

[33] Yeh YC, Lee CT, Wang CH, Tu YK, Lai CH, Wang YC, et al. Investigation of microcirculation in patients with venoarterial extracorporeal membrane oxygenation life support. Critical Care. 2018;**22**(1):200

[34] Durinka JB, Bogar LJ, Hirose H, Brehm C, Koerner MM, Pae WE, et al. End-organ recovery is key to success for extracorporeal membrane oxygenation as a bridge to implantable left ventricular assist device. ASAIO Journal. 2014;**60**(2):189-192

[35] Cui WW, Ramsay JG. Pharmacologic approaches to weaning from cardiopulmonary bypass and extracorporeal membrane oxygenation. Best Practice & Research. Clinical Anaesthesiology. 2015;**29**(2):257-270

[36] Jacky A, Rudiger A, Kruger B, Wilhelm MJ, Paal S, Seifert B, et al. Comparison of levosimendan and milrinone for ECLS weaning in patients after cardiac surgery—A retrospective before-and-after study. Journal of Cardiothoracic and Vascular Anesthesia. 2018;**32**(5):2112-2119

[37] Aissaoui N, El-Banayosy A, Combes A. How to wean a patient from veno-arterial extracorporeal membrane oxygenation. Intensive Care Medicine. 2015;**41**(5):902-905

[38] Cavarocchi NC, Pitcher HT, Yang Q, Karbowski P, Miessau J, Hastings HM, et al. Weaning of extracorporeal membrane oxygenation using continuous hemodynamic transesophageal echocardiography. The Journal of Thoracic and Cardiovascular Surgery. 2013;**146**(6):1474-1479

[39] Guglin M, Zucker MJ, Bazan VM, Bozkurt B, El Banayosy A, Estep JD, et al. Venoarterial ECMO for adults: JACC Scientific Expert Panel. Journal of the American College of Cardiology. 2019;**73**(6):698-716

[40] Garcia-Gigorro R, Renes-Carreno E, Perez-Vela JL, Marin-Mateos H, Gutierrez J, Corres-Peiretti MA, et al. Mechanical support with venoarterial extracorporeal membrane oxygenation (ECMO-VA): Short-term and long-term prognosis after a successful weaning. Medicina Intensiva. 2017;**41**(9):513-522

[41] Babar ZU, Sharma AS, Ganushchak YM, Delnoij TS, Donker DW, Maessen JG, et al. An arterio-venous bridge for gradual weaning from adult veno-arterial extracorporeal life support. Perfusion. 2015;**30**(8):683-688

[42] Ling L, Chan KM. Weaning adult patients with cardiogenic shock on veno-arterial extracorporeal membrane oxygenation by pump-controlled retrograde trial off. Perfusion. 2018;**33**(5):339-345

[43] Westrope C, Harvey C, Robinson S, Speggiorin S, Faulkner G, Peek GJ. Pump controlled retrograde trial off from VA-ECMO. ASAIO Journal. 2013;**59**(5):517-519

Section 4

Organ System Management

Chapter 11

Isn't Limb as Precious as Life?

Prashant N. Mohite and André R. Simon

Abstract

As utilisation of peripheral extra-corporeal life support (ECLS) is becoming clinical routine, its associated complications become more frequent. Distal limb perfusion in femoral cannulation remains one of the Achille's heels in patients with peripheral ECLS. Unless detected early, limb ischemia may result in loss of limb and sometimes life. A protocol-based approach, precautions during ECLS implantation and explantation procedures and continuous monitoring of the limb during ECLS support are key elements in preventing this complication. Utilisation of a distal limb perfusion cannula helps in prevention as well as management of limb ischemia; however, it may sometimes cause more damage than help. Management and consequence of limb ischemia essentially depends on its severity at the time of detection as well as time of intervention. This chapter offers a brief review of the burden of limb ischemia, means to prevent and approaches to manage it.

Keywords: extra-corporeal life support, limb ischemia, complications, distal limb perfusion

1. Introduction

Extra-corporeal life support (ECLS) for the last 2–3 decades has become an indispensable tool in the armamentarium of physicians and surgeons dealing with patients suffering severe cardio-pulmonary failure [1]. Over the period of time, its utilisation has seen a broadening in terms of indications, age limits and condition of patients [2–9]. Familiarisation with technique, continuous improvement of equipment and changes in strategy in favour of early intervention have helped to improve the survival of patients supported on the ECLS [10, 11]. However, unfortunately, a significant number of patients still suffer and succumb to complications instigated by the ECLS. In fact, not very uncommonly, ECLS related complications play a decisive role in the clinical outcome of the patient. For the purpose of this discussion, we use the term ECLS as a synonym for extra corporeal veno-arterial membrane oxygenation. Alternative technologies such Impella® or short term left ventricular assist (VAD) are not discussed. Initial ECLS in the acutely presenting patients is often implemented via femoral cannulation. Alternative approaches such as via the subclavian, axillary or carotid artery are used less commonly in adults and the incidence of limb ischemia in these scenarios is negligible compared to femoral artery. Therefore, for all practical purposes we will discuss lower extremity limb ischemia in this chapter. Late or chronic limb ischemia, sometimes occurring months after de-cannulation although symptomatic, seldom threatens limb survival and will not be discussed either.

Limb ischemia in patients supported on peripheral ECLS is one of the most dreaded complications and presents with a wide spectrum of clinical symptoms and outcomes.

Interestingly enough, this specific complication can be almost totally avoided with a protocol-based approach and precautions taken during the ECLS support; and if it occurs, it can be managed without significant consequences if detected and addressed immediately.

1.1 Indications

ECLS, although offered by specialised units only, is becoming more and more adopted for treatment of patients presenting with a variety of problems. Recent developments in technology have resulted in easier implantation and maintenance, ability to implement directly at the bedside, complete cardiopulmonary support and cost-effectiveness when compared to other mechanical circulatory support devices.

In surgery, ECLS is utilised as a rescue in post-cardiotomy cardiogenic shock (PCCS) or as a temporary prolongation of cardiopulmonary bypass (CPB) to allow for an extensive weaning. Historically, the ECLS circuit was connected to the central CPB cannulation following unsuccessful weaning attempts of CPB. Recent years have seen a paradigm shift in preference to peripheral access. It is because peripheral cannulation allows for chest closure and avoids bleeding from high pressure aortic and thin-walled right atrial cannulation site and thus, multiple re-explorations for bleeding-temponade. Furthermore, the risk of formation of a positional thrombus on the intraluminal part of the aortic cannula, which may be dislodged at the time of decannulation and result in a catastrophic embolic event is avoided. And lastly, peripheral access obviates reopening of chest at the time of explantation of ECLS [2, 3]. Cannulation is either performed percutaneously or open, depending on the situation and the presenting patient.

A second group experiencing a significant increase in the utilisation of ECLS are patients during primary coronary intervention (PCI) [4, 5], although recent developments may lead to a shift in the technology used, such as Impella®. In this particular clinical setting, the expertise of interventional cardiologists and availability of fluoroscopy obviously lends itself to direct percutaneous implementation of ECLS. Bed-side, emergency direct ECLS implantation in intensive care units is a last and only resort to resuscitate patients after cardiopulmonary arrest undergoing prolonged efforts to re-establish life sustaining cardiac and pulmonary function (e-CPR) [6, 7]. In this situation, percutaneous peripheral access to the groin vessels is the preferable approach in view of the continuation of chest compressions and limited equipment available (e.g. fluoroscopy, surgical set).

In patients with advanced cardiac failure ECLS may be used as a bridge to decision, recovery or heart transplantation. In some of these patients, particularly those awaiting transplantation or long-term VAD implantation it is used in a 'semi-elective emergency situation' where patients are destabilising and showing signs of rapidly deteriorating end-organ function and impending cardiogenic shock. In this particular scenario ECLS is used to re-perfuse and stabilise end-organ function such as liver and kidney to allow for a non-emergency long-term VAD implantation at significantly less perioperative risk in a more stable patient. In this complex group of patients, peripheral access is favoured as it does not necessitate a sternotomy or thoracotomy leaving the chest 'virgin' or which may be complex due to previous, often multiple, surgical interventions. At the time of subsequent surgery ECLS can then easily be converted to CPB and continuation of ECLS post-surgery, if required [8, 9], can be achieved simply by switching back to an ECLS circuit.

In essence, peripheral access for the ECLS has become popular due to its flexibility of implantation outside operation theatre, reduced cannula site bleeding, the option of chest closure, avoidance of chest re-exploration and explantation without chest intervention. With the overall increase in the utilisation of ECLS in PCCS, post-PCI, e-CPR and as a bridge to transplant or ventricular assist devices and even as a bridge-to-lower risk surgery as a preparational tool, ECLS related complications including limb ischemia are being seen more often than ever before.

1.2 Incidence of limb ischemia

ECLS, essentially being temporary mechanical circulatory support requires an exit strategy with a sustainable solution, namely short or long-term ventricular assist device or transplant. Until then, an uninterrupted and uncomplicated distal limb perfusion is essential for the continuation of peripheral ECLS for more than a few hours. Any complications during the period on ECLS support potentially hinder patients' progress to recovery or long-term solutions. Of these, limb ischemia is one of the notorious and unfortunately- most commonly encountered complications in patients supported. As with other complications, limb ischemia remains underreported in institutional audits and the literature and reported incidence of ECLS related limb ischemia vary significantly. The Extra-corporeal Life Support Organisation (ELSO) in its latest report shows 1% incidence of limb ischemia [12]. Whereas, a recent metanalysis reviewing 20 studies comprising 1886 patients revealed a pooled estimate of rate of limb ischemia as high as 16.9% (12.5–22.6%); compartment syndrome at 10.3% (7.3–14.5%) and amputation at 4.7% (2.3–9.3%) [13]. Other contemporary, smaller reviews report limb ischemia in range of 4.4–19% and 11–52% [14, 15]. The variation among published literature in incidence of limb ischemia and related complications may be due to difference in inclusion criteria of patients, difference in definition of limb ischemia and publication bias.

1.3 Causes and presentation spectrum of limb ischemia

Limb ischemia has a broad spectrum of presentation ranging from hypothermia to muscle necrosis. In patients on ECLS it may occur for a number of reasons. Of these, the first and foremost is, of course, the simple complete obstruction of the femoral artery by the systemic perfusion cannula, which is inserted in a retrograde fashion, either percutaneously or open. The second is the requirement of extensive vasoconstrictor and inotropic support, which may restrict the 'residual' flow to the limb to the point of induction of clinically relevant ischemia. The third is the result of a deterioration of remaining cardiac output and loss of pulse wave, as the limb may be perfused—adequately—during the systolic ejection and be completely ischemic should pulse-wave be lost. Finally, insertion of the venous cannula on the ipsilateral side may result in clinically relevant venous congestion by itself and thus exacerbate any arterial perfusion deficit. Thus, careful monitoring and adjustment of several variables is essential in the prevention of ischemia and the treatment must be aimed at not only correcting the underlying causation but also to mitigate the resulting effects as in necrosis or reperfusion induced injury.

The signs and symptoms of acute limb ischemia are classically described with the 6 Ps- **P**ain, **P**allor, **P**ulselessness, **P**araesthesia, **P**oikilothermia, and **P**aralysis [16]. In this context, Rutherford's grading of acute limb ischemia depending upon the clinical examination namely viable, threatened (salvageable if promptly treated) and irreversible (major tissue loss or permanent nerve damage inevitable) is helpful to determine the timing and type of intervention. The onset of fixed mottling of the skin usually implies irreversible changes but does not allow for an estimation as to the extent. Compartment syndrome results from increased pressure (greater than 30–45 mmHg) in the muscle compartments often due to ischemia or reperfusion related swelling which further decreases blood supply leading to a vicious cycle of swelling-ischemia-swelling, rapidly progressing to irreversible necrosis of the affected muscles. Diagnosis is essentially clinical with findings of swelling, stiffness, pain, and loss of pulse. It is a limb and life-threatening emergency and is usually fatal unless immediate action is undertaken, almost always including four compartment fasciotomies [17].

Limb ischemia compromises survival not only of the involved limb but also the patient. The ischemic process, multiple procedures, and transfusions exacerbate the systemic inflammatory response related to ECLS, resulting in increased risk of death [18]. Tanaka *et al.* report a higher number of procedures per patient and an increased frequency of disseminated intravascular coagulation in patients with vascular complications [19]. They also found the rate of survival to discharge as 18 vs. 49% in patients with and without vascular complications, respectively, demonstrating vascular complications as an independent factor of survival in patients on VA ECLS [19]. While some authors did not find any correlation between limb ischemia and patient mortality [20–22], it is widely accepted that apart from severity of the underlying condition, neurological uncertainty, and eligibility for substantive therapy, the limb ischemia plays a seminal role in deciding fate of the patient supported on ECLS.

2. Prevention of limb ischemia

2.1 Prophylactic distal perfusion cannula

Several authors highlight the role of concurrent, prophylactic, selective distal limb perfusion from the time of femoral arterial cannulation for systemic perfusion in the prevention of limb ischemia. In one series, the authors claim no occurrence of limb ischemia in patients with prophylactic distal perfusion via selective cannulation (DPC) compared to a 21% incidence of ischemia in patients without DPC [21]. Tanaka *et al.* demonstrated that the absence of DPC was a significant predisposing factor for vascular complications, while other factors including medical history or risk factors like peripheral vascular disease and severity of baseline condition were not significantly associated with vascular complications [19]. However, from the review of published literature it is difficult to ascertain whether the elective avoidance of DPC or the presence of factors preventing its use (e.g. peripheral artery disease, vessel spasm, vessel injury due to attempted cannulation) are the underlying cause of the vascular complication.

In a comparative study, no limb ischemia was encountered in patients undergoing pro-active DPC in contrast to 9.3% incidence of limb ischemia in patients who underwent re-active DPC as a rescue strategy. They concluded that the delayed distal cannulation not only increased the extent of cannulation site bleeding, but also failed as a rescue therapy as it failed to improve the ischemia [23] whereas pro-active DPC prevented its occurrence. In addition, patients in the pro-active group demonstrated a significantly better weaning rate as well as survival.

However, despite extensive literature advocating DPC as being preventive to limb ischemia, there is no class I evidence about its efficacy. Understandably, it is difficult to design a randomised trial to identify actual protection offered by prophylactic DPC given the multiple factors responsible for mortality and morbidity and grave condition of patients supported on VA-ECMO.

Although DPC offers incessant perfusion to the distal limb, its insertion and maintenance are not always smooth, and it is not devoid of complications. The DPC due to their small calibre, slow and low flow, acute angles, multiple connections are prone to bending, thrombogenesis, and peripheral embolization. It is important to note that DPC blockage due to thrombosis may go unnoticed in absence of continuous monitoring of its flow and result in complete thrombo-embolism and obstruction of the femoral artery. In order to avoid this scenario and assess whether limb perfusion remains adequate in the absence of DCP, Huang *et al.* measured the pressure in the superficial femoral artery distal to the systemic cannula and introduced the DPC only when this pressure was less than 50 mmHg [24]. In their cohort of 26 patients, only 9 patients fulfilling this criterion required the DPC and authors report no limb ischemia in any patients, with or without DPC. These findings are interesting and warrant further evaluation of their technique and confirmation by other study groups.

Compared to open cut-down DPC related complications are more common after percutaneous cannulation, often due to multiple cannulation attempts causing vessel injury, extravasation, hematoma and inadvertent cannulation of the *profunda femoris*. In contrast, while not ubiquitously feasible, technically more challenging and more time consuming, the open cut-down allows visualisation of the artery to ensure an adequate size of the cannula, proper placement, good haemostasis and the abandonment of the site without failed attempts in case of arterial calcifications [15]. Not surprisingly, a significantly higher incidence of limb ischemia was found in patients with a percutaneous DPC compared to patients with no DPC and open cut-down DPC in a series published by the Philadelphia group [25]. In this context, it is worth mentioning the 'chimney graft construction' approach on the femoral artery in which a small vascular graft is placed end-to side onto the main femoral artery, thus allowing for bi-directional perfusion without obstruction of the vessel. This avoids the more complex V-A-DPC-ECLS circuit, the DPC itself and its complications [26]. However, while avoiding ischemia and advocated for small femoral arteries, in bigger vessels it may lead to distal limb hyper-perfusion [15] (**Table 1**).

A generalised and enthusiastic approach for prophylactic DPC should be carefully reviewed and implemented only in cases with high risk for limb ischemia. These include patients with a history and signs of peripheral vascular disease, atherosclerosis, previous utilisation of groin vessels for access and female gender due to smaller vessel size as they are more prone to develop limb ischemia. In addition, young age may be an independent risk factor due to the absence of collateral vascularisation [21]. Also, there are several variables influencing the of risk of development of limb ischemia which can be addressed separately. These include low or no cardiac output resulting in loss of the pulse wave, although in patients with failure to oxygenate blood via the lung a low or absent biological output may be intended to prevent a watershed phenomenon and ensure cerebral oxygenation. High vasopressor support, peripheral shut-down and big calibre flow-occlusive systemic femoral cannulation are other factors influencing perfusion to distal limb and the development of limb ischemia.

As the principal role of the ECLS is temporary cardio-pulmonary support and preservation of organ perfusion, sufficient 'biomechanical' output can be provided often at a reasonable mechanical flow rate without complete replacement of the biological cardiac output. Cannulation with a small calibre systemic cannula may therefore provide enough flow and preserve a pulse wave allowing for sufficient perfusion of the distal limb. A 17F systemic cannula easily provides 4–5 L/min flow with a driving pressure of around 100 mmHg. Takayama *et al.* compared outcome in patients based on the size of the systemic cannula and showed that a 15F size cannula, while allowing for significantly less blood flow when compared to bigger (17–24F) cannulas, resulted in no difference in use of vasoactive medication, hemodynamic parameters or laboratory values measured [27]. On the other hand, significantly less cannulation-related adverse events were observed in the 15F group.

Patients on ECLS support may develop severe vasoplegia requiring high dose vasopressor support to sustain arterial blood pressure for satisfactory end-organ perfusion. Efforts to maintain a negative fluid balance to reabsorb peripheral and pulmonary oedema in a bid to wean ECLS may intensify vasopressor requirement

Prevention of limb ischemia
Implantation
Cut down and under vision cannulation whenever feasible
Percutaneous cannulation only with USG/Fluoroscopy
Use of small calibre systemic arterial cannula
Use of Prophylactic distal arterial perfusion cannula
Use of Prophylactic distal venous drainage cannula
Utilise contralateral limb for venous drainage cannula
Maintenance
Bear high suspicion for ischemia
Accept low ECLS flow when possible to reduce cannula size
Maintain left ventricular ejection
Maintain pulsatile flow
Wean vasopressors as soon as possible
Selective infusion of prostacyclin via distal perfusion cannula
Keep patient awake- can complain of limb pain (ischemia)
Suspect limb ischemia if serum Lactate levels high
Achieve and maintain good anticoagulation
Monitoring
Near infra-red spectroscopy in distal limb
Continuous measurement of DPC flow
Doppler Ultrasound of distal limb arteries
Temperature
Explantation
Prefer open cut-down and repair of vessels
Perform balloon thrombo-embolectomy
Avoid groin compression

Table 1.
Prevention of limb ischemia.

further. While maintaining central blood pressure levels, capillary perfusion of end organs, specifically the intestine as well as the limbs may be significantly reduced in such a scenario. Therefore, it is important to strike a balance between vasopressor delivery dependent blood pressure management, maintenance of fluid balance, arterio-venous perfusion pressure delta and capillary delivery, prioritising vasopressor weaning over 'drying up the lungs'. Maintenance of good intravascular volume also allows better ECLS flow and cardiac output along with pulsatility.

In essence, utilisation of a small calibre systemic femoral cannula, when possible, acceptance a biomechanical output with low ECLS flow, continued pulsatile flow and avoidance of high dose vasopressors obviate the need for prophylactic DPC insertion in patients, potentially protecting them from DPC related complications. With this conservative management and a protocol of continuous, diligent monitoring, patients that develop limb ischemia can then be detected at an early stage and treated with subsequent DPC, if necessary.

2.2 ECLS and DPC implantation strategies

The individual approach of ECLS implantation heavily depends upon the place (out of the hospital, floor, bedside or operation theatre), urgency (elective or emergency), and aetiology (PCCS, post-PCI, primary graft failure or bridge to transplant) of the cardio-respiratory failure. In patients with cardiopulmonary arrest under resuscitation or peri-arrest patients, quick introduction of ECLS through is of utmost importance in order to sustain the patient's life. In this situation, the primary goal is the insertion of systemic arterial and venous cannulas and there may not be time for simultaneous DPC insertion. Such emergency bedside ECLS implantation in the intensive therapy unit is a scenario that usually does not offer facilities of an operation theatre making percutaneous insertion of peripheral cannulas necessary (**Figure 1**), often without availability of sonography to appropriately size for the smallest cannulae or fluoroscopy for intravascular positioning. In this context, it is important to note that percutaneous insertion of the DPC can be challenging in the presence of a systemic arterial cannula already in place, either due to the reduction or even absence of blood flow distal to the cannulation site or vasospasm and vessel injury during primary cannulation. Nevertheless, if it is attempted, ultrasound guidance during insertion is helpful and angiographic confirmation of DPC tip position in the superficial femoral artery should be obtained [25, 28].

PCCS is a scenario usually encountered after complex and long operations and has an extreme mortality. While ECLS is the only treatment option for these patients, it is important to make the decision to use it as early as possible and avoid repeated and prolonged attempts to wean the patient of CPB as these cause considerable collateral damage. ECLS should not be viewed as a last resort after all else has failed and the patient is in a catastrophic state but rather as a tool to be proactively used to ensure protection of organ function, continuous, uninterrupted sufficient perfusion and maintenance of a functioning coagulation system, thus preventing the well-known ICU exsanguination of these patients and offering both the heart as well as the patient a reasonable chance to recover.

For this, CPB can be converted directly to central ECLS, using the established cannulation or to peripheral ECLS. Peripheral ECLS allows the chest to be fully closed and no re-opening is needed for explantation of the ECLS system or for cannula-site bleeding especially in these patients on anti-coagulation therapy. With the patient stable on CPB it is safe and easy to perform a cut down to the groin vessels and placement of the cannulas under direct vision (**Figure 2**). If necessary, DPC can be introduced simultaneously. If the myocardial function is somewhat preserved, ECLS flows should be kept at a level allowing for blood flow through the heart to maintain left ventricular ejection in order to prevent its dilatation, stasis of

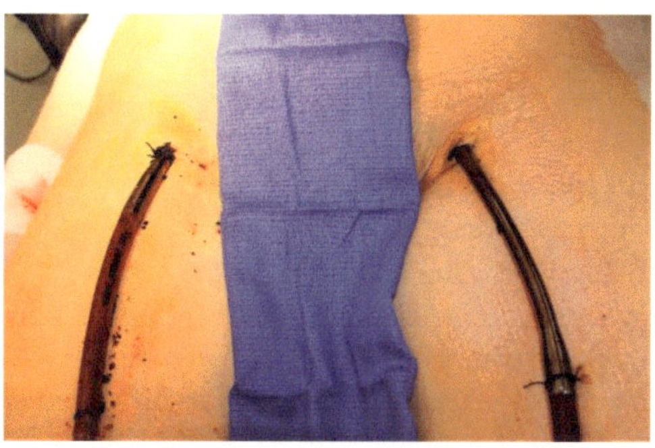

Figure 1.
Percutaneous cannulation.

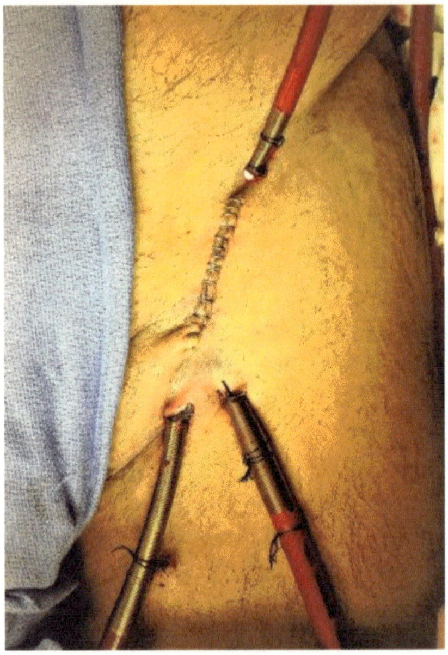

Figure 2.
Open cut-down cannulation.

blood and possible atrial and ventricular thrombus formation. In severe myocardial injury, the heart can be rested with full ECLS flow without ejection. In this case, the need for ventricular decompression should be discussed. With biological no-flow, a case of high vasopressor requirement or expected longer duration of support, the DPC can introduced at the same time.

Peri or post-PCI, with fluoroscopy readily available, all ECLS cannulas can be introduced percutaneously and their position be confirmed before the patient leaves the cath-lab. ECLS as a bridge to transplant in awake patients is a recent trend that offers early ambulation and avoids ventilator-associated complications [29]. However, bedside ECLS can be challenging as a cut down is not comfortable in such patients and difficult outside the environment of the operating theatre. In these patients, the systemic arterial and venous cannulae are introduced percutaneously under local anaesthesia or the patient undergoes a short analgo-sedation as full sedation may be too high risk. As a general principal, contralateral femoral arterial and venous cannulation should be encouraged, as the venous stasis and possible limb oedema caused by the venous cannula may intensify any ipsilateral arterial cannula related compromised distal limb perfusion [15].

2.3 Expectant monitoring of limb

2.3.1 Continuous monitoring

Continuous diligent monitoring of the limb for any signs of ischemia is a key to allow for timely and appropriate intervention. One elegant and inexpensive method of continuous monitoring is placing an additional pulse-oximetry probe on the toes of the cannulated limb. Its reading and waveform can be compared with the probe placed on the normal limb. However, hypothermia and non-pulsatile flow may not offer reliable pulse-oximetry reading. Near infra-red spectroscopy (NIRS), routinely used and established in transcranial cerebral oximetry can be helpful in such cases and is an alternative method for continuous monitoring. It involves application of sensor pads on the legs that detects regional oxygen saturation (rSO_2)

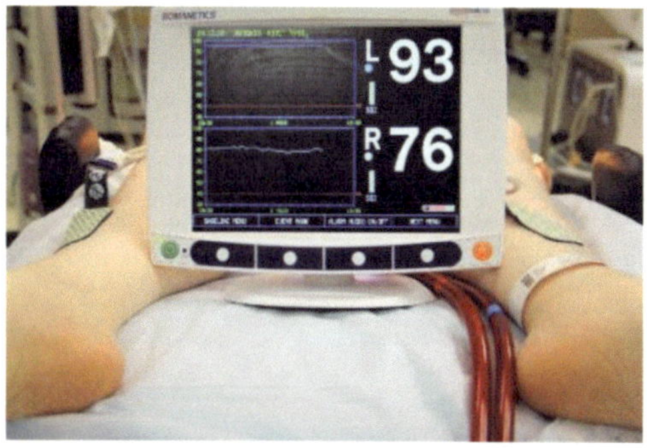

Figure 3.
NIRS continuous monitoring.

continuously, representing adequacy of tissue oxygenation. It should be applied as soon as ECLS is started. The rSO2 of the cannulated limb is compared with that of the opposite limb as well as with the baseline rSO2 providing live evidence of a drop in limb perfusion (**Figure 3**). A reduction in rSO_2 values in the cannulated limb to less than 40 or more than 25% from baseline suggest inadequate limb perfusion and mandates urgent intervention [30, 31]. Technical glitches, however, like improper sensor pads attachments should be addressed before attempting to improve distal limb perfusion. Dong and colleagues utilised the NIRS successfully in a group of ECLS patients to detect and successfully treat limb ischemia with DPC in all patients having NIRS whereas 13.9% of the cohort not monitored required a fasciotomy [31]. Indeed, NIRS may reliably detect limb ischemia before it becomes clinically evident [31, 32]. Lamb *et al.* suggest continuous monitoring of limb utilising NIRS and evaluation of pedal doppler signals in case of a drop in baseline NIRS values to ensure adequate distal limb perfusion [33]. If available, we suggest that NIRS should be part of the protocol for peripheral ECLS.

In presence of DPC, continuous monitoring of its trans-canullar flow is the gold standard in monitoring distal limb perfusion (**Figure 4**). The DPC flow is dependent on a variety of factors, namely total ECLS flow, mean arterial pressure and systemic and peripheral vascular resistance, and possible thrombo-embolic occlusion in the DPC or distal artery. Therefore, any drop in the DPC flow must be correlated with these factors before any intervention. A drop in the DPC flow should also be cross-checked with the clinical signs of limb ischemia and drop in NIRS rSO_2. An hourly record of the DPC flow along with other ECLS parameters should be maintained and perfusionists should be alerted if there is a significant change. Cannula or connecting line bending, thrombosis and dislocation are common non patient related reasons for decreased DPC flow. Both antegrade and retrograde blood flow should be checked by clamps on either side of DPC side-port [10]. In the absence of a side-port, the DPC may have to be disconnected to assess for backflow through the cannula and appropriate flow in the proximal line. Thrombosis in the DPC is usually accompanied by embolization into the distal femoral artery and mandates embolectomy and DPC replacement. Only in the minority of cases it can be addressed by aspiration of the thrombotic material.

2.3.2 Hourly monitoring

Despite continuous monitoring of limb perfusion by means of NIRS and DPC flow, hourly inspection for skin colour change, palpation for temperature, capillary return at toe tips, calf palpation and calf girth measurement for compartment syndrome is of paramount importance. Pedal pulses should be checked in the *dorsalis pedis* and

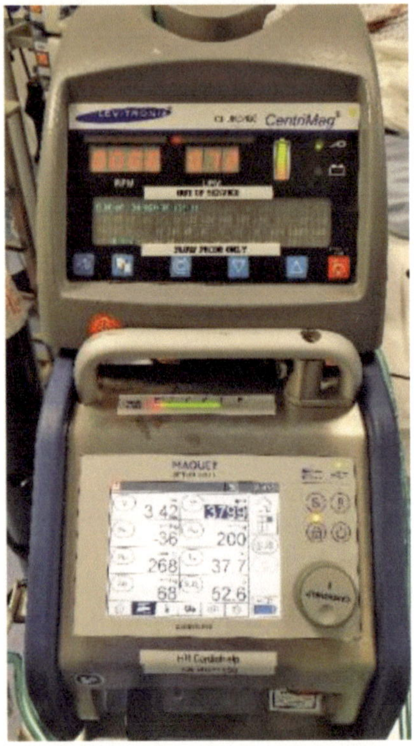

Figure 4.
Continuous DPC flow monitoring.

posterior tibial artery and when not palpable a hand-held ultrasound Doppler should be utilised to confirm the flow. The flow may be graded for documentation as palpable-strong pulsatile, palpable- weak pulsatile, doppler- pulsatile, doppler- continuous flow and absent flow. Hourly recording of continuously monitored variables namely DPC flow, NIRS rSO_2 are necessary to establish trends and detect limb ischemia before it is clinically apparent. Numbers and signs that may be missed during continuous monitoring can be caught in a vigilant hourly survey. Ischemia in toes is seen not uncommon, even in the presence of well-maintained DPC flow due to peripheral micro thrombo-embolization and/or vasospasm due to peripheral shut down or high dose vasopressors.

2.4 Early detection of limb ischemia

Early detection of inadequate limb perfusion allows for immediate intervention to avoid its catastrophic consequences. In absence of the DPC, continuous NIRS monitoring supplemented by an hourly survey by means of clinical examination and Doppler ultrasound flow check in the distal arteries is usually adequate to detect limb ischemia at an early stage. NIRS rSO_2, clinical signs and ultrasound Doppler flow in the cannulated limb should be compared with opposite limb, not to confuse ischemia with peripheral shut down and peripheral vasospasm. In patients with a prophylactic or therapeutic introduction of DPC, it is important to remember that the DPC does not guarantee adequate perfusion. Thus, continuous measurement of DPC flow, maintenance of adequate anticoagulation and monitoring of actual limb perfusion remains essential. Awake non-intubated, non-sedated patients supported on ECLS may complain of pain, tingling- numbness or stiffness with the onset of limb ischemia. An increase in lactate levels without an attributable source and acute kidney failure may be signs of subclinical rhabdomyolysis and should immediately raise suspicion of ischemia. Finally, signs of ischemia may be seen only in the toes, even with a good DPC flow due to peripheral embolization through DPC.

2.5 Explantation

ECLS is a lifesaver for patients with compromised cardiopulmonary function; however, it may instigate life-threatening complications and the incidence of complications increases with increase in duration of the ECLS. Yoe *et al.* found the duration of ECLS more than 7 days is a factor associated with the development of limb ischemia [23]. Therefore, weaning of ECLS should begin with recovery of vital organ function with the aim of its explantation as soon as possible. Extra caution is mandated during weaning of patients with the DPC, as the decrease in total ECLS flow decreases DPC flow that may lead to inadequate limb perfusion as well as thrombosis of the DPC. In this situation, the DPC flow should be maintained around at least 300 ml/min by applying a gate clamp on the retrograde arterial cannula. Explantation of ECLS at the end of successful weaning should be performed as an elective case in the operation theatre. The vessels are exposed and controlled with slings before removal of cannulas. Embolectomy is attempted multiple times with balloon tip catheters till satisfactory retro and antegrade blood flow is achieved. The artery is then repaired with or without a patch or an interposition graft to maintain its original calibre without flow limitation. The limb is monitored for at least 48 hours following ECLS explantation for any signs of residual or fresh ischemia.

3. Treatment of limb ischemia

Traditionally, 6 hours are recommended as a golden period for intervention in limb ischemia. In a series analysing limb ischemia in ECLS patients an additional retrograde reperfusion within 6 hours of onset of symptoms avoided amputations completely, whereas the same procedure after that period was burdened with a 20% amputation rate or permanent neurological deficit [34]. Therefore, every attempt should be made to re-establish adequate blood supply in the ischemic limb as soon as possible to avoid catastrophic consequences and residual damage (**Table 2**).

3.1 Therapeutic insertion of distal perfusion cannula

Limb ischemia due to inadequate flow in the distal artery detected at early stage ideally should be treated with the introduction of the DPC if not placed at ECLS implantation. Apart from conscious avoidance, reasons for not introducing

Management of established limb ischemia
Introduce distal perfusion cannula (DPC)- cut down
Percutaneous DPC- Check position with fluoroscopy
Continuous Epoprostenol in DPC
Thrombo-embolectomy
Change of cannulation site
Decompression compartment fasciotomy
Amputation

Table 2.
Management of limb ischemia.

prophylactic DPC are among others: failed percutaneous insertion, atherosclerotic plaque palpated in open cut-down and need to return to the intensive care unit for patient stabilisation. In a metanalysis reviewing 22 retrospective studies comparing peripheral ECLS with or without DPC, the presence of a DPC was associated with at least a 15.7% absolute reduction in the incidence of limb ischemia; although without any impact on the patient survival [35].

Several cannulas from an introducer sheath up to a paediatric arterial cannula are recommended in the literature for this purpose. An ideal is the one that is resistant to bending and thrombosis and offering a least resistance to flow. We found the incidences of limb ischemia and limb ischemia requiring surgical intervention were significantly higher for the introducer sheath compared with the 10–12F Bio-Medicus® paediatric seldinger cannula utilised for distal limb perfusion (30.6 vs. 15.6% and 15.4 vs. 6.25%, respectively) [11].

To introduce the DPC percutaneously, the superficial femoral artery may be visualised distal to the systemic cannula via Ultrasound. If this is not possible, a cut-down insertion should be performed. If introduced bedside, especially percutaneously, the position of the DPC should be confirmed via x-ray.

3.2 Continuous infusion of anticoagulants and vasodilator drugs

Any ECLS circuit exposes blood to non-biological surfaces and is in itself thrombogenic. Therefore, adequate anticoagulation, usually achieved by continuous intravenous delivery of unfractionated heparin is essential to prevent complications such as thrombus formation and clotting of the circuit and stroke, limb and bowel ischemia. Conventionally heparin is delivered via a central venous catheter. As the small arteries of the distal limb are specifically at risk of micro-thrombotic clotting complications a targeted delivery of anticoagulants may offer a strategy to prevent distal ischemia. Continuous heparin delivery in the ECLS circuit before oxygenator at beginning of ECLS should be considered in any institutional protocol.

Due to the discrepancy in size of the aorta and distal superficial femoral artery as well as resistance between the systemic cannula and the DPC, there is a significant discrepancy in the flow rate between them, sometimes resulting in very little or almost no flow through the for DPC. In these cases, a gate clamp on the systemic arm can be helpful; however, it may cause flow turbulence, is potentially thrombogenic and increases driving pressure in the system.

Alternatively, and already mentioned above, Epoprostenol, a potent vasodilator, which is established in the treatment of peripheral vascular disease, can be delivered directly into the limb via DPC side-port in order to induce peripheral vasodilatation and increase perfusion. Some paediatric aortic cannulas have a side-port that can be readily used for this purpose [10]. Otherwise, a 3/8–3/8″ connector with a side-port can be inserted into the arm feeding the DPC. In some patients this may result in an increased requirement of vasopressors to maintain central arterial pressure. As a word of caution, selective infusion of vasodilators may also result in hyper-perfusion and clinically relevant oedema, especially in presence of an *ipsilateral* venous cannula.

3.3 Change of cannulation site

Peripheral access for ECLS seek mainly due to urgency or bedside scenario is converted to central access once patient is stabilised or develops complication due to peripheral cannulation. One of the strategies in suspected or established limb involves shifting the arterial cannulation site followed by embolectomy and, if necessary, repair of the vessel. In many cases this may be the ascending aorta, as this offers certain advantages such as oxygenated blood supply to coronaries and avoidance of any watershed phenomenon, even in patients with compromised lung function. Also, the opposite superficial femoral artery or axillary artery may be utilised if the treating physician wants to avoid sternotomy or cannulation of the aorta is difficult. In patients with acceptable lung function and compromised cardiac function, ECLS can be converted into a uni- or bi-ventricular short-term ventricular assist device at this time avoiding the further use of the oxygenator and thus allowing for a less stringent anticoagulation regime and easier mobilisation of the patient.

3.4 Management of advanced limb ischemia

Fasciotomy is a decompression manoeuvre performed on the limb with acute compartment syndrome, a surgical emergency. Release of pressure allows reperfusion of the ischemic muscles potentially avoiding amputation. A recent metanalysis consisting 1886 patients found 10% incidence of compartment syndrome requiring fasciotomy [13].

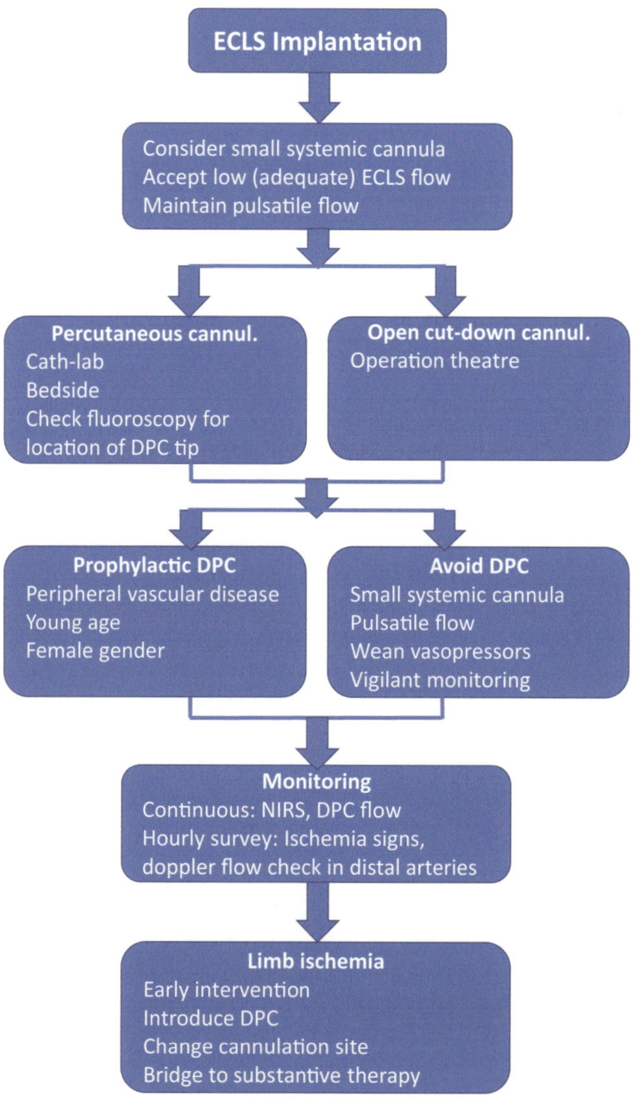

Figure 5.
Protocol for management of limb ischemia.

Several authors confirm that the procedure is effective provided it is performed as soon as the diagnosis of compartment syndrome is established. It can be performed bedside under local anaesthesia [36, 37]. Four chamber fasciotomies essentially involve decompression of anterior and posterior compartment of the thigh and anterolateral and posteromedial compartments of lower leg. Primary closure of these wounds can be performed following explantation of ECLS and decrease of limb swelling.

A last and unfortunate resort in the management of advanced limb ischemia to save a life is to give up a limb. Irreversible ischemic damage to skin and muscles causes rhabdomyolysis, acute kidney injury, and metabolic acidosis. In such cases, amputation of the limb remains the only option to save the patient's life. Contemporary retrospective observational studies report incidence of lower limb amputation in patients supported with ECLS between 1 to 10% [11, 13, 15, 20, 21, 38]. However, some prospective studies with utilisation of newer technology and ideas such as NIRS for early detection of ischemia and distal arterial pressure based or pre-emptive introduction of DPC reported no amputations [23, 24, 31]. However, apart from the obvious benefit of these newer techniques, patients in studies focusing on limb ischemia may have received significant additional attention and care to prevent and treat limb ischemia at early stage. This in itself may have had a profound effect, further corroborating that early detection of limb ischemia with expectant monitoring and protocol-based prompt intervention may avoid its catastrophic consequences (**Figure 5**).

4. Conclusions

Care of the cannulated limb with maintenance of adequate perfusion to avoid ischemia is as important as the preservation of vital organ function. Limb ischemia plays a seminal role in the fate of a patient supported on ECLS. Vascular complications, particularly limb ischemia negatively affect survival in patients on ECLS. Expectant continuous monitoring utilising NIRS, if used, a flow monitored distal perfusion cannula and hourly surveys of flow in distal arteries and signs of ischemia are key in timely detection of limb ischemia. A prophylactic distal perfusion cannula should always be used in patients with risk factors for development of limb ischemia and can most likely be avoided in others if a small calibre systemic cannula is used. Acceptance of lower ECLS flow, maintenance of pulsatility and avoidance of vasopressors are additional important elements. Prompt intervention to re-establish adequate blood supply after suspicion of limb ischemia is essential to avoid its catastrophic consequences. The safest method of prophylactic or therapeutic introduction of a distal perfusion cannula remains the open cut-down and exposure. Percutaneously inserted distal perfusion cannulas should be checked for their position by fluoroscopy. Also, change of cannulation site and bridging ECLS to a substantive therapy should be part of any strategy for patients on ECLS. If properly integrated into an institutional protocol and adhered to, these strategies allow for successful treatment of patients in need of extracorporeal life support with low complication and high success rates.

Acknowledgements

Authors are not funded for preparation of this manuscript. Authors thank Olaf Maunz for helping with manuscript editing.

Conflict of interest

Authors do not have any conflicts of interest.

Author details

Prashant N. Mohite* and André R. Simon
Royal Brompton and Harefield NHS Foundation Trust, Harefield Hospital, United Kingdom

*Address all correspondence to: p.mohite@rbht.nhs.uk

References

[1] Thiagarajan RR, Barbaro RP, Rycus PT, Mcmullan DM, Conrad SA, Fortenberry JD, et al. Extracorporeal life support organization registry international report 2016. ASAIO Journal. 2017;**63**(1):60-67

[2] Khorsandi M, Dougherty S, Bouamra O, Pai V, Curry P, Tsui S, et al. Extra-corporeal membrane oxygenation for refractory cardiogenic shock after adult cardiac surgery: A systematic review and meta-analysis. Journal of Cardiothoracic Surgery. 2017;**12**(1):55

[3] Pappalardo F, Montisci A. Veno-arterial extracorporeal membrane oxygenation (VA ECMO) in postcardiotomy cardiogenic shock: How much pump flow is enough? Journal of Thoracic Disease. 2016;**8**(10):E1444-E1448

[4] Sung PH, Wu CJ, Yip HK. Is extracorporeal membrane oxygenator a new weapon to improve prognosis in patients with profound cardiogenic shock undergoing primary percutaneous coronary intervention? Circulation Journal. 2016;**80**:572-578

[5] Tsao NW, Shih CM, Yeh JS, et al. Extracorporeal membrane oxygenation-assisted primary percutaneous coronary intervention may improve survival of patients with acute myocardial infarction complicated by profound cardiogenic shock. Journal of Critical Care. 2012;**27**:530. e1-530.e11

[6] Ortega-Deballon I, Hornby L, Shemie SD, Bhanji F, Guadagno E. Extracorporeal resuscitation for refractory out-of-hospital cardiac arrest in adults: A systematic review of international practices and outcomes. Resuscitation. 2016;**101**:12-20

[7] Tonna JE, Johnson NJ, Greenwood J, Gaieski DF, Shinar Z, Bellezo JM, et al. Extracorporeal REsuscitation ConsorTium (ERECT) Research Group. Practice characteristics of Emergency Department extracorporeal cardiopulmonary resuscitation (eCPR) programs in the United States: The current state of the art of Emergency Department extracorporeal membrane oxygenation (ED ECMO). Resuscitation. 2016;**107**:38-46

[8] Durinka JB, Bogar LJ, Hirose H, Brehm C, Koerner MM, Pae WE, et al. End-organ recovery is key to success for extracorporeal membrane oxygenation as a bridge to implantable left ventricular assist device. ASAIO Journal. 2014;**60**(2):189-192

[9] Chung JC, Tsai PR, Chou NK, Chi NH, Wang SS, Ko WJ. Extracorporeal membrane oxygenation bridge to adult heart transplantation. Clinical Transplantation. 2010;**24**(3):375-380

[10] Mohite PN, Maunz O, Simon AR. Pearls and pitfalls in short-term mechanical circulatory assist: How to avoid and manage complications. Artificial Organs. 2014;**38**(10):829-837

[11] Mohite PN, Fatullayev J, Maunz O, Kaul S, Sabashnikov A, Weymann A, et al. Distal limb perfusion: Achilles' heel in peripheral venoarterial extracorporeal membrane oxygenation. Artificial Organs. 2014;**38**(11):940-944

[12] Extracorporeal Life Support Organisation. ECLS Registry Report. Ann Arbor. 2017. Downloaded Nov 2017

[13] Cheng R, Hachamovitch R, Kittleson M, Patel J, Arabia F, Moriguchi J, et al. Complications of extracorporeal membrane oxygenation for treatment of cardiogenic shock and cardiac arrest: A meta-analysis of 1,866 adult patients. The Annals of Thoracic Surgery. 2014;**97**(2):610-616

[14] von Segesser L, Marinakis S, Berdajs D, Ferrari E, Wilhelm M, Maisano F. Prevention and therapy of leg ischaemia in extracorporeal life support and extracorporeal membrane oxygenation with peripheral cannulation. Swiss Medical Weekly. 2016;**146**:w14304

[15] Roussel A, Al-Attar N, Khaliel F, Alkhoder S, Raffoul R, Alfayyadh F, et al. Arterial vascular complications in peripheral extracorporeal membrane oxygenation support: A review of techniques and outcomes. Future Cardiology. 2013;**9**(4):489-495

[16] Brearley S. Acute leg ischaemia. BMJ. 2013;**346**:f2681

[17] Tiwari A, Haq AI, Myint F, Hamilton G. Acute compartment syndromes. The British Journal of Surgery. 2002;**89**(4):397-412. Review

[18] Levi M. Current understanding of disseminated intravascular coagulation. British Journal of Haematology. 2004;**124**:567-576

[19] Tanaka D, Hirose H, Cavarocchi N, Entwistle JW. The impact of vascular complications on survival of patients on venoarterial extracorporeal membrane oxygenation. The Annals of Thoracic Surgery. 2016;**101**(5):1729-1734

[20] Bisdas T, Beutel G, Warnecke G, et al. Vascular complicationsin patients undergoing femoral cannulation for extracorporeal membrane oxygenation support. The Annals of Thoracic Surgery. 2011;**92**:626-631

[21] Foley PJ, Morris RJ, Woo EY, Acker MA, Wang GJ, Fairman RM, et al. Limb ischemia during femoral cannulation for cardiopulmonary support. Journal of Vascular Surgery. 2010 Oct;**52**(4):850-853

[22] Avalli L, Sangalli F, Migliari M, Maggioni E, Gallieri S, Segramora V, et al. Early vascular complications after percutaneous cannulation for extracorporeal membrane oxygenation for cardiac assist. Minerva Anestesiologica. 2016;**82**(1):36-43

[23] Yeo HJ, Yoon SH, Jeon D, Kim YS, Cho WH, Kim D, et al. The utility of preemptive distal perfusion cannulation during peripheral venoarterial extracorporeal membrane oxygenation support. Journal of Interventional Cardiology. 2016;**29**(4):431-436

[24] Huang SC, Yu HY, Ko WJ, Chen YS. Pressure criterion for placement of distal perfusion catheter to prevent limb ischemia during adult extracorporeal life support. The Journal of Thoracic and Cardiovascular Surgery. 2004;**128**(5):776-777

[25] Vallabhajosyula P, Kramer M, Lazar S, McCarthy F, Rame E, Wald J, et al. Lower-extremity complications with femoral extracorporeal life support. The Journal of Thoracic and Cardiovascular Surgery. 2016;**151**(6):1738-1744

[26] Jackson KW, Timpa J, McIlwain RB, et al. Side-arm grafts for femoral extracorporeal membrane oxygenation cannulation. The Annals of Thoracic Surgery. 2012;**94**:111-112

[27] Takayama H, Landes E, Truby L, Fujita K, Kirtane AJ, Mongero L, et al. Feasibility of smaller arterial cannulas in venoarterial extracorporeal membrane oxygenation. The Journal of Thoracic and Cardiovascular Surgery. 2015;**149**(5):1428-1433

[28] Black MC, Slaughter MS. Proactive or reactive? Best approach to limb ischemia in peripheral venoarterial extracorporeal life support. The Journal of Thoracic and Cardiovascular Surgery. 2016;**151**(6):1745-1746

[29] Mohite PN, Sabashnikov A, Reed A, Saez DG, Patil NP, Popov AF, et al.

Extracorporeal life support in "Awake" patients as a bridge to lung transplant. The Thoracic and Cardiovascular Surgeon. 2015;**63**(8):699-705

[30] Wong JK, Smith TN, Pitcher HT, Hirose H, Cavarocchi NC. Cerebral and lower limb near-infrared spectroscopy in adults on extracorporeal membrane oxygenation. Artificial Organs. 2012;**36**:659-667

[31] Kim DJ, Cho YJ, Park SH, Lim C, Park KH, Jheon S, et al. Near-infrared spectroscopy monitoring for early detection of limb ischemia in patients on veno-arterial extracorporeal membrane oxygenation. ASAIO Journal. 2017;**63**(5):613-617

[32] Prkic I, Stuth EA. Near-infrared spectroscopy provides continuous monitoring of compromised lower extremity perfusion during cardiac surgery. Journal of Clinical Anesthesia. 2016;**31**:38-41

[33] Lamb KM, DiMuzio PJ, Johnson A, Batista P, Moudgill N, McCullough M, et al. Arterial protocol including prophylactic distal perfusion catheter decreases limb ischemia complications in patients undergoing extracorporeal membrane oxygenation. Journal of Vascular Surgery. 2017;**65**(4):1074-1079

[34] Spurlock DJ, Toomasian JM, Romano MA, Cooley E, Bartlett RH, Haft JW. A simple technique to prevent limb ischemia during veno-arterial ECMO using the femoral artery: The posterior tibial approach. Perfusion. 2012;**27**:141-145

[35] Juo YY, Skancke M, Sanaiha Y, Mantha A, Jimenez JC, Benharash P. Efficacy of distal perfusion cannulae in preventing limb ischemia during extracorporeal membrane oxygenation: A systematic review and meta-analysis. Artificial Organs. 2017;**41**(11):E263-E273

[36] Go JY, Min YS, Jung TD. Delayed onset of acute limb compartment syndrome with neuropathy after venoarterial extracorporeal membrane oxygenation therapy. Annals of Rehabilitation Medicine. 2014;**38**(4):575-580

[37] Wall CJ, Santamaria J. Extracorporeal membrane oxygenation: An unusual cause of acute limb compartment syndrome. Anaesthesia and Intensive Care. 2010;**38**:5602

[38] Gander JW, Fisher JC, Reichstein AR, Gross ER, Aspelund G, Middlesworth W, et al. Limb ischemia after common femoral artery cannulation for venoarterial extracorporeal membrane oxygenation: An unresolved problem. Journal of Pediatric Surgery. 2010;**45**:2136-2140

Chapter 12

Normothermic Regional Perfusion in Solid Organ Transplantation

Amelia J. Hessheimer and Constantino Fondevila

Abstract

Normothermic regional perfusion (NRP) is used to restore the flow of oxygenated blood following cardiac arrest and reverse warm ischemic injury in donation after circulatory death (DCD) organ transplantation. The use of NRP in this setting has typically been limited to the abdominal cavity, though its use has recently been expanded to chest to help recover DCD hearts, as well. This chapter evaluates the principles behind the use of NRP in DCD organ transplantation as well as not only technical but also ethical and legal aspects associated with its application and the clinical results that have been achieved to date when it has been used to recover various solid organs through the DCD process.

Keywords: controlled donation after circulatory death, kidney transplantation, liver transplantation, uncontrolled donation after circulatory death, warm ischemia

1. Introduction

Donation after circulatory death (DCD) donors, which are declared dead following cardiorespiratory arrest, are an increasingly more common source of organs for transplantation. They may be classified among four categories depending on events and conditions surrounding arrest: category I, dead on arrival (no attempt at resuscitation); category II, sudden cardiac arrest followed by unsuccessful resuscitation; category III, arrest following intentional withdrawal of life support in ventilated patient not meeting brain death criteria; and category IV, cardiac arrest while brain dead. Categories 1, 2 and 4 are classified as uncontrolled DCD (uDCD) and category 3 as controlled DCD (cDCD) [1]. In practice, category III cDCD and, to a lesser extent, category II uDCD donors comprise essentially all DCD donors that are used for transplantation globally. The period of warm ischemia surrounding arrest, however, provokes organ injury, and DCD in general yields fewer organs per donor and ones of inferior quality when compared with donation after brain death (DBD) [2]. For this reason, there has been increasing interest in forgoing rapid cold preservation and recovery following the declaration of death (still the "gold standard" for DCD organ recovery in most transplant centers) and instead using normothermic regional perfusion (NRP) to temporarily restore oxygenated blood flow the abdominal and more recently thoracic organs prior to recovery.

2. Principles behind the use of normothermic regional perfusion in donation after circulatory death

During warm ischemia, ATP degradation leads to the progressive accumulation of xanthine and hypoxanthine, important sources of superoxide radical at organ reperfusion [3]. A period of post-ischemic NRP in DCD donors is useful to restore cellular energy substrates [4], reduce levels of nucleotide degradation products [5], improve the concentrations of endogenous antioxidants [6], and even stimulate processes of cellular repair prior to graft recovery [7] (**Figure 1**). An experimental study demonstrates that by blocking the A2 receptors of adenosine, the beneficial effects of NRP are abolished, indicating that NRP mediates its effect, at least in part, through adenosine as a form of ischemic preconditioning [8]. Post-ischemic NRP may also be useful to reduce the vasoconstrictive effects of cold graft washout with the static cold storage solution [9] and offers an opportunity to assess organ viability prior to recovery [10, 11].

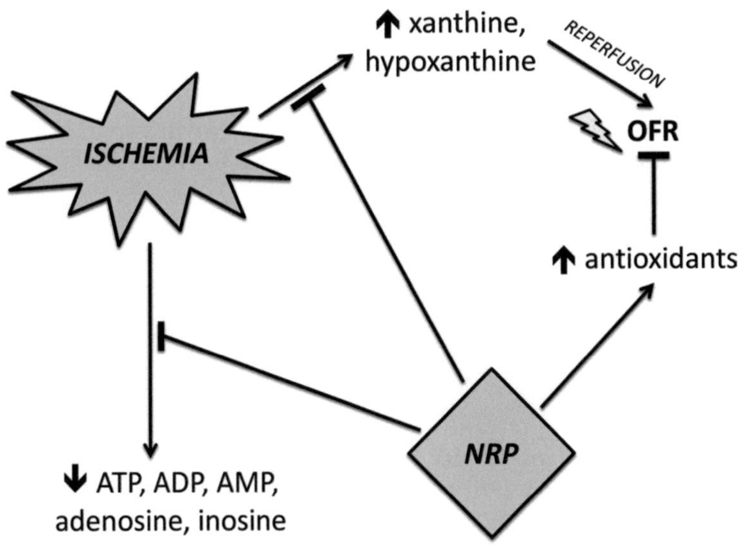

Figure 1.
During ischemia, the concentrations of adenine nucleotides (ATP, ADP, AMP) and nucleosides (adenosine, inosine) progressively decline. Also, the concentrations of nucleotide breakdown products (xanthine, hypoxanthine) increase, thereby leading to the production of oxygen free radicals upon reperfusion. Normothermic regional perfusion is capable of reversing these processes and increases the concentrations of endogenous antioxidants, effectively recharging and reconditioning organs in the abdomen and chest prior to recovery for transplantation.

3. Techniques for establishing normothermic regional perfusion in donation after circulatory death

While NRP relies on extracorporeal membrane oxygenation (ECMO) technology, its clinical application is, in general, less complex than that of therapeutic ECMO. A venous cannula is placed to derive blood from the donor inferior vena cava or right atrium, which is then pumped through a membrane oxygenator and a heat exchanger before returning to the donor arterial bed (aorta or iliac or femoral artery). An in-line reservoir may be included in the circuit, as well, to allow for replacement of volume prior to circuit failure in the event of volume loss or inadequate venous return due to severe vasoplegia (particularly relevant in the setting of uDCD). The precise positioning of occlusion balloon catheters or clamps used to exclude other vascular beds is what determines whether NRP is either thoracoabdominal or abdominal only.

3.1 Abdominal normothermic regional perfusion

In uDCD, cannulation for the establishment of abdominal NRP is performed post-mortem after death is declared, typically in the emergency department. In cDCD, in contrast, cannulation for abdominal NRP may be performed either prior to the withdrawal of life support (pre-mortem) or following the declaration of death. Pre-mortem cannulation may be performed either percutaneously or via femoral cut-down in a variety of settings (intensive care unit, radiology suite, operating room). Post-mortem cannulation, on the other hand, is most often done in open abdomen in the operating room, though some centers have used femoral artery and vein catheters or guidewires placed prior to withdrawal of care to access and thereby cannulate the femoral vasculature following the declaration of death [12].

For uDCD donors and cDCD donors with pre-mortem cannulation, a bolus of heparin is administered, and cannulation of unilateral femoral vessels is performed either via open femoral cutdown and isolation of the femoral artery and vein or percutaneously using Seldinger technique [11]. Cannulae are left clamped and connected to the tubing of the primed NRP circuit. The contralateral femoral artery is also cannulated with an aortic occlusion balloon catheter, which is left deflated in the case of cDCD and advanced into the supraceliac aorta under radiographic control. Following the withdrawal of life support and the declaration of death in cDCD, the aortic occlusion balloon is inflated, and the abdominal NRP circuit is initiated (**Figure 2**). Proper positioning of the balloon excluding the aortic arch vessels is confirmed by chest radiograph and absence of flow measured in a left radial arterial catheter.

For cDCD donors undergoing open post-mortem cannulation, once death has been declared, the surgical team performs midline laparotomy to cannulate the abdominal aorta immediately proximal to and the infrarenal inferior vena cava immediately distal to their respective bifurcations. Cannulae are connected to the tubing of the primed NRP circuit, the supraceliac aorta is clamped, and NRP is initiated.

Blood is sampled at baseline and every 30 minutes during abdominal NRP to determine biochemical, hematological, and acid-base parameters. In general, pump flow is maintained >1.7 L/min/m^2, temperature 35–37°C, PaO_2 100–150 mmHg, and hemoglobin >7 g/dL. Hepatic transaminases should remain stable throughout NRP; levels >3× the upper limit of normal at baseline and/or >4× the upper limit of normal at the end of NRP may be considered relative contraindications for recovery of the liver and pancreas [10, 11]. In general, NRP is run for a minimum of 1 hour and a maximum of 4 hours to allow adequate reconditioning of the abdominal organs and recovery of energy substrates without provoking additional end-organ injury [4, 5, 7, 8, 13, 14].

3.2 Thoracoabdominal normothermic regional perfusion

While the circuit for abdominal NRP may be established pre-mortem, cannulation to establish a complete thoracoabdominal NRP circuit is done post-mortem in the operating room. After the declaration of death, the chest is entered through a midline sternotomy, and the pericardium is opened. A bolus of heparin is injected into the heart directly, an arterial cannula is inserted into the distal ascending aorta/aortic arch, and a venous cannula is inserted into the right atrium. Cannulae are connected to the tubing of the primed NRP circuit, the aortic arch vessels are clamped, and NRP is initiated.

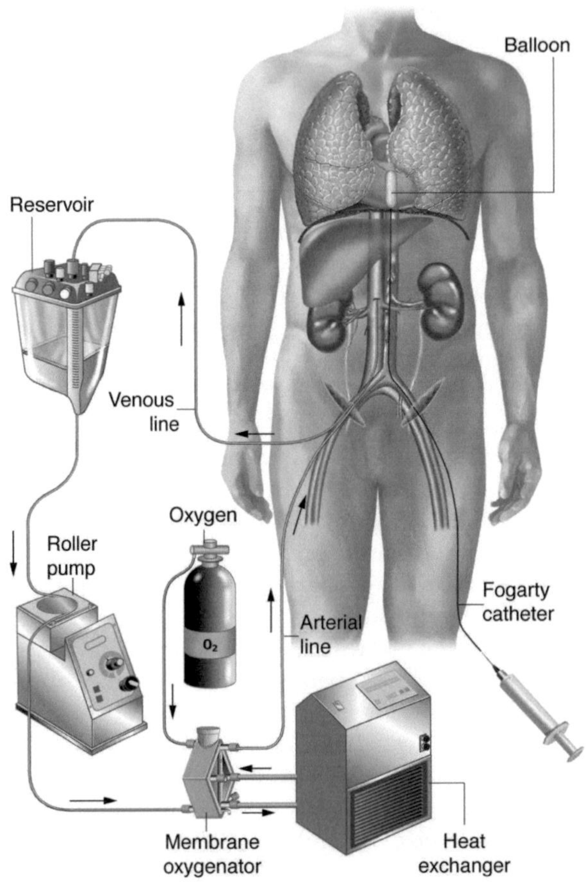

Figure 2.
Abdominal normothermic regional perfusion. Cannulae are placed in the femoral artery and vein in the groin region. A Fogarty balloon catheter is introduced through the contralateral femoral artery and positioned in the supraceliac abdominal or thoracic aorta.

During thoracoabdominal NRP, pump flow is maintained ≥2.5 L/min/m^2, temperature 35°C, and hemoglobin >10 g/dL. Prompt laparotomy is performed to assess hepatic and intestinal perfusion and to exclude the lower extremities from the perfusion circuit. Once cardiac contractility has been restored, weaning from NRP is attempted. If the heart is able to take over circulation, functional assessment is performed using transesophageal echocardiography and pulmonary artery flotation catheter (Swan-Ganz) monitoring. In general, acceptance criteria for a cDCD heart recovered with NRP include central venous pressure ≤12 mmHg, pulmonary capillary wedge pressure ≤12 mmHg, cardiac index ≥2.5 L/min/m^2, and left ventricular ejection fraction ≥50% [15–17].

4. Clinical outcomes using normothermic regional perfusion in donation after circulatory death

To date, the great majority of human transplants performed using organs recovered with NRP have been donor using DCD kidneys and livers. In more recent years, the use of DCD pancreata and even hearts recovered with NRP has also been reported.

4.1 Kidney transplantation

When compared with other solid organs for transplantation, the kidney is relatively resilient and withstands the ischemic insult inherent to the DCD process relatively well. Nonetheless, kidneys from DCD donors recovered with NRP as opposed to rapid *in situ* cold preservation or hypothermic perfusion/"total body cooling" (TBC) have demonstrated significantly better immediate as well as ongoing graft function [18–20]. Reports from different groups in Europe, the United States, and Asia have described the use of NRP in both uDCD and cDCD kidney transplantation, with rates of delayed graft function (DGF) around 50–70% and 30–40%, respectively; negligible (if any) primary non-function (PNF); and excellent 1-, 5-, and even 10-year graft survival rates [19–27]. While reported rates of DGF may still seem to be high even among DCD kidneys recovered with NRP (especially those arising through uDCD), the pathogenesis and, consequentially, implications of DGF seem to be less severe than those associated with DGF arising in the context of DBD kidney transplantation. Ischemic injury appears to be implicated to a greater extent in the development of DGF among DCD kidneys, whereas, in DBD, alloimmune phenomena prevail [28]. A recent large single-center study reported 73% DGF among 237 uDCD kidneys recovered with NRP versus 46% among a contemporary cohort of matched DBD kidneys, but 10-year graft survival rates did not vary at all between the two groups and were excellent in both (82 and 80%, respectively). The authors also noted that while donor age >50 years was significantly associated with graft loss among uDCD kidneys, the development of DGF in the immediate post-transplant period was not [27].

4.2 Liver transplantation

The cells of the liver, in particular those lining the biliary tree, are particularly sensitive to warm ischemia, and initial experiences with DCD liver transplantation described high rates of graft dysfunction and non-function and non-anastomotic biliary strictures/ischemic type biliary lesions (ITBL) in up to 50% of cases [29]. While complication rates have improved with experience, the rate of post-transplant ITBL remains higher among recipients of DCD versus DBD grafts: 16 versus 3%, according to two meta-analyses [30, 31]. The clinical relevance of ITBL lies in the fact that up to 70% of patients with ITBL require re-transplantation or die [32].

After an initial period where different donor maintenance techniques were used, including rapid *in situ* cold preservation, simultaneous chest and abdominal compressions, and TBC, NRP has come to be the "gold standard" and primary means by which uDCD livers are recovered for transplantation. Using NRP, even livers with extensive pre-recovery warm ischemic periods of up to 2.5 hours have been successfully transplanted, with biliary complication and graft survival rates comparable to those seen using cDCD livers that have suffer considerably less warm ischemia [10, 11, 33–35].

In spite of its relative success in the setting of uDCD, the application of NRP in cDCD liver transplantation remains more limited. The great majority of cDCD livers that are transplanted in the world today are still recovered with rapid *in situ* cold preservation, and reports on the use of NRP in cDCD liver transplantation have been, until recently, anecdotal [12, 24–26, 36, 37]. In the past year, however, two larger multicenter studies have come out describing the benefits that may be achieved with post-mortem NRP in cDCD liver transplantation. First, a Spanish national study compared the results of 95 cDCD liver transplants performed with post-mortem NRP with those of 117 cDCD liver transplants performed with super rapid recovery (SRR). Median donor age in the study was relatively high (57 years [25-75% interquartile range, IQR 45–65] NRP, 56 years [25-75% IQR, 47–64] SRR). With a median follow-up of 20 months, the use of post-mortem NRP appeared to significantly reduce rates of postoperative biliary complications (overall 8% NRP vs. 31% SRR, $p < 0.001$; ischemic type biliary lesions 2% NRP vs. 13% SRR, $p = 0.008$) and graft loss (12% NRP vs. 24% SRR, $p = 0.008$) [38]. Similarly, a combined experience from centers in Cambridge and Edinburgh in the United Kingdom compared the results of 43 cDCD liver transplants performed with post-mortem NRP with those of a contemporary cohort of 187 cDCD liver transplants performed with SRR. Median donor age was less for cDCD livers with NRP versus those with SRR: 41 years (25-75% IQR 33–57) vs. 54 years (25-75% IQR 38–63), respectively. Reported rates of anastomotic biliary strictures were 7% NRP vs. 27% SRR ($p = 0.004$), ITBL 0 NRP vs. 27% SRR ($p < 0.001$), and 90-day graft loss 2% NRP vs. 10% SRR ($p = 0.102$) [39].

4.3 Pancreas transplantation

The Michigan Group described one cDCD pancreas transplant in which the donor was maintained with NRP, though the outcome of the graft was not mentioned [24]. In another multicenter report from the United Kingdom, two SPK were described (again, outcomes not mentioned), and two more pancreata were sent for isolation of islets, one with good yield [25]. In Spain, where NRP is now routinely used to recover abdominal organs when cDCD liver and/or pancreas transplantation is contemplated, a total of five cDCD pancreas transplants were performed between 2015 and 2017, and all these grafts remain functional at the time of this writing [40].

4.4 Heart transplantation

The application of thoracoabdominal NRP has been described in clinical series on cDCD heart transplantation; however, no report has been published to date describing the transplantation of the lungs from these same cDCD donors. (Transplantation of DCD lungs recovered with "dual temperature" *in situ* cold flushing in the chest with abdominal NRP running simultaneously, on the other hand, has been described and is performed routinely in some settings.) The fact remains that DCD donor lungs tolerate warm ischemia and the process of DCD donation and recovery relatively well, and post-DCD lung transplantation outcomes without NRP appear to be comparable to those of DBD lung transplantation [41].

The cDCD heart, on the other hand, is more susceptible to warm ischemic injury, and cDCD hearts recovered and transplanted after *in situ* cold preservation followed by static *ex situ* cold storage can offer suboptimal outcomes. A recent report on pediatric cDCD heart transplantation describes 61% 1-year graft survival as opposed to 91% for DBD hearts of similar baseline characteristics [42]. Performing thoracic NRP, on the other hand, allows for restoration of contractile function and performance of a standard functional assessment in ischemically injured cDCD cardiac allografts prior to recovery. Clinical application of thoracoabdominal NRP in cDCD heart transplantation has been described by the Papworth Hospital Group from the United Kingdom. In combination with subsequent *ex situ* normothermic machine perfusion (NMP), the use of thoracoabdominal NRP has allowed 100% utilization of organs subsequently undergoing NMP and lower early allograft dysfunction versus cDCD hearts undergoing NMP only (8% vs. 17%, respectively) [16, 17]. Thoracoabdominal NRP followed by static cold storage has even been used to successfully transplant a cDCD heart procured at the same center [17]. If broader application of this last strategy is shown to be just as efficacious, it has the potential to significantly reduce the costs associated with cDCD heart transplantation by obviating the need for *ex situ* NMP, which is a very expensive modality costing approximately $45,000 for each heart perfusion unit.

5. Ethical and legal concerns surrounding the use of normothermic regional perfusion in donation after circulatory death

There are some ethical concerns surrounding the use of NRP in donation after circulatory death, and laws vary from one country to another regarding whether or not NRP may be applied in DCD and, if so, how and when.

5.1 Uncontrolled donation after circulatory death

In uDCD, cardiac arrest is sudden and unexpected, and death is declared based on the irreversible loss of cardio-respiratory function (demonstrated after prolonged efforts to reverse it have failed). Death is usually declared in the emergency room by a team entirely independent of that responsible for organ recovery and preservation. More often than not, potential uDCD donors are declared dead prior to the arrival of next-of-kin. Based on a consequentialist ethical standpoint and the principles of utility and donor autonomy, certain countries, including Spain and France, allow cannulation maneuvers to commence in this setting, even in cases where first-person consent may not have yet been obtained [43, 44]. The will of the patient regarding donation is always subsequently investigated in the context a family interview, where information regarding the circumstances of the arrest, the outcome of resuscitation maneuvers, and the measures taken related to the donation process is relayed. Next-of-kin then decide, taking into consideration the potential donor's wishes, whether to proceed with donation or abort the process.

It should be clear that NRP is organ maintenance and not therapy. While the technology employed is similar, terms such as "extracorporeal membrane oxygenation/ECMO" and "extracorporeal life support/ECLS" should not be used in relation to organ donation. Such terminology is confusing, especially considering the fact that it is used to describe therapeutic maneuvers that may be used to recover patients suffering sudden cardiac arrest more commonly occurring inside the hospital itself.

5.2 Controlled donation after circulatory death

In cDCD, the usual stand-down period of 2–5 min of asystole that is used to declare death does not necessarily reflect an irreversible loss of cardiac function, evidenced by the fact that cDCD hearts have been recovered and successfully transplanted [17, 45]. The "irreversibility" of death in cDCD is therefore predicated on the concept of permanence—the fact that loss of cardiac function will eventually become irreversible because it will not be reversed (and eventually lead to the loss of all brain and brain stem functions, as well). As it re-establishes circulation to some parts of the body, however, the use of NRP in this context remains controversial. At the least, clear and effective measures need to be put in place to ensure that cerebral reperfusion does not occur when NRP is established. Through the use of NRP, circulation is only restored to a limited region of the body, and a critical aspect of NRP in cDCD is ensuring lack of flow to the aortic arch vessels, thereby maintaining the permanence of circulatory arrest in the brain and brainstem. With pre-mortem cannulation, positioning of the aortic occlusion balloon in the supradiaphragmatic aorta distal to the left subclavian artery is confirmed radiographically prior to withdrawal of care. As additional measure, the aortic occlusion balloon may be briefly inflated for a few seconds prior to ventilatory withdrawal, in order to ensure disappearance of femoral arterial pressure and simultaneous maintenance of a normal pressure waveform in the left radial arterial line. In doing so, the minimum filling volume needed to entirely blocks the supradiaphragmatic aorta may be recorded [46]. Once NRP is initiated, adequate occlusion is confirmed through the use of a left radial artery catheter demonstrating absence of flow.

The timing of when cannulation for abdominal NRP may be performed in potential cDCD donors varies by country. In certain countries, such as Spain and the United States, pre-withdrawal heparinization and cannulation are permitted [24, 43]. In the United Kingdom, on the other hand, a potential cDCD donor may only be cannulated once death has been declared [25]. Pre-mortem cannulation is advantageous in that it is performed in a less stressful and more orderly fashion, and regional perfusion may be commenced immediately after the death declaration, thereby limiting the length of warm ischemia suffered. Ideally, pre-mortem cannulation should be performed in the least invasive manner possible (e.g., percutaneously).

6. Summary and future directions

Table 1 summarizes the current state of NRP in the various fields of clinical DCD organ transplantation. The application of post-mortem NRP appears particularly relevant and advantageous in DCD kidney, liver, and heart transplantation, and the future will tell if it can have impact the fields of DCD pancreas and lung transplantation, as well. Some ethical concerns remain surrounding its use, primarily in the context of cDCD, and clear and effective steps need to always be taken to ensure lack of reperfusion of the brain and brainstem once NRP has been initiated. Through these measures and continued dialog with both intensive care as well as extra- and intrahospitalary emergency medical professionals, the hope is that the use of NRP and, thereby, DCD organ transplantation in general may be expanded to offer more organs and ones of better quality to a greater number of patients with end-stage organ disease.

Kidney	Lower rates of immediate post-transplantation delayed graft function and primary non-function and improved ongoing graft function among both uDCD and cDCD allograft recipients.
Liver	Lower rates of post-transplantation biliary complications, including ischemic type biliary lesions, and less graft loss among cDCD livers; considered essential for the evaluation and recovery of uDCD livers
Pancreas	Feasible, though more experience is required to determine its true impact
Lung	No reports to date
Heart	Less early allograft dysfunction; allows for *in situ* functional assessment that can not only help avoid subsequent costly and potentially unsuccessful *ex situ* normothermic machine perfusion functional assessment but perhaps even the use of NMP altogether

Table 1.
Clinical results observed to date with application of normothermic regional perfusion in donation after circulatory death organ transplantation.

Conflict of interest

None to declare.

Author details

Amelia J. Hessheimer and Constantino Fondevila*
General and Digestive Surgery, Digestive and Metabolic Disease Institute (ICMDM), Hospital Clínic, CIBERehd, IDIBAPS, University of Barcelona, Spain

*Address all correspondence to: cfonde@clinic.cat

References

[1] Thuong M, Ruiz A, Evrard P, Kuiper M, Boffa C, Akhtar MZ, et al. New classification of donation after circulatory death donors definitions and terminology. Transplant International. 2016;**29**(7):749-759

[2] Tuttle-Newhall JE, Krishnan SM, Levy MF, McBride V, Orlowski JP, Sung RS. Organ donation and utilization in the United States: 1998-2007. American Journal of Transplantation. 2009;**9** (4 Pt 2):879-893

[3] Harvey PR, Iu S, McKeown CM, Petrunka CN, Ilson RG, Strasberg SM. Adenine nucleotide tissue concentrations and liver allograft viability after cold preservation and warm ischemia. Transplantation. 1988;**45**(6):1016-1020

[4] Gonzalez FX, Garcia-Valdecasas JC, Lopez-Boado MA, Tabet J, Net M, Grande L, et al. Adenine nucleotide liver tissue concentrations from non-heart-beating donor pigs and organ viability after liver transplantation. Transplantation Proceedings. 1997;**29**(8):3480-3481

[5] Net M, Valero R, Almenara R, Rull R, Gonzalez FJ, Taura P, et al. Hepatic xanthine levels as viability predictor of livers procured from non-heart-beating donor pigs. Transplantation. 2001;**71**(9):1232-1237

[6] Aguilar A, varez-Vijande R, Capdevila S, Alcoberro J, Alcaraz A. Antioxidant patterns (superoxide dismutase, glutathione reductase, and glutathione peroxidase) in kidneys from non-heart-beating-donors: Experimental study. Transplantation Proceedings. 2007;**39**(1):249-252

[7] Kerforne T, Allain G, Giraud S, Bon D, Ameteau V, Couturier P, et al. Defining the optimal duration for normothermic regional perfusion in the kidney donor: A porcine preclinical study. American Journal of Transplantation. 2018

[8] Net M, Valero R, Almenara R, Barros P, Capdevila L, Lopez-Boado MA, et al. The effect of normothermic recirculation is mediated by ischemic preconditioning in NHBD liver transplantation. American Journal of Transplantation. 2005;**5**(10):2385-2392

[9] Das S, Maggio AJ, Sacks SA, Smith RB, Kaufman JJ. Effects of preliminary normothermic flushing on hypothermic renal preservation. Urology. 1979;**14**(5):505-508

[10] Fondevila C, Hessheimer AJ, Ruiz A, Calatayud D, Ferrer J, Charco R, et al. Liver transplant using donors after unexpected cardiac death: Novel preservation protocol and acceptance criteria. American Journal of Transplantation. 2007;**7**(7):1849-1855

[11] Fondevila C, Hessheimer AJ, Flores E, Ruiz A, Mestres N, Calatayud D, et al. Applicability and results of Maastricht type 2 donation after cardiac death liver transplantation. American Journal of Transplantation. 2012;**12**(1):162-170

[12] Foss S, Nordheim E, Sorensen DW, Syversen TB, Midtvedt K, Asberg A, et al. First scandinavian protocol for controlled donation after circulatory death using normothermic regional perfusion. Transplantation direct. 2018;**4**(7):e366

[13] Garcia-Valdecasas JC, Tabet J, Valero R, Taura P, Rull R, Garcia F, et al. Liver conditioning after cardiac arrest: The use of normothermic recirculation in an experimental animal model. Transplant International. 1998;**11**(6):424-432

[14] Net M, Valero R, Almenara R, Deulofeu R, Lopez-Boado MA, Capdevila L, et al. Hepatic

preconditioning after prolonged warm ischemia by means of S-adenosyl-L-methionine administration in pig liver transplantation from non-heart-beating donors. Transplantation. 2003;**75**(12):1970-1977

[15] Messer S, Page A, Axell R, Berman M, Hernandez-Sanchez J, Colah S, et al. Outcome after heart transplantation from donation after circulatory-determined death donors. The Journal of Heart and Lung Transplantation. 2017;**36**(12):1311-1318

[16] Tsui SSL, Oniscu GC. Extending normothermic regional perfusion to the thorax in donors after circulatory death. Current Opinion in Organ Transplantation. 2017;**22**(3):245-250

[17] Messer S, Page A, Colah S, Axell R, Parizkova B, Tsui S, et al. Human heart transplantation from donation after circulatory-determined death donors using normothermic regional perfusion and cold storage. The Journal of Heart and Lung Transplantation. 2018;**37**(7):865-869

[18] Valero R, Cabrer C, Oppenheimer F, Trias E, Sanchez-Ibanez J, De Cabo FM, et al. Normothermic recirculation reduces primary graft dysfunction of kidneys obtained from non-heart-beating donors. Transplant International. 2000;**13**(4):303-310

[19] Barrou B, Billault C, Nicolas-Robin A. The use of extracorporeal membranous oxygenation in donors after cardiac death. Current Opinion in Organ Transplantation. 2013;**18**(2):148-153

[20] Demiselle J, Augusto JF, Videcoq M, Legeard E, Dube L, Templier F, et al. Transplantation of kidneys from uncontrolled donation after circulatory determination of death: Comparison with brain death donors with or without extended criteria and impact of normothermic regional perfusion. Transplant International. 2016;**29**(4):432-442

[21] Abboud I, Viglietti D, Antoine C, Gaudez F, Meria P, Tariel E, et al. Preliminary results of transplantation with kidneys donated after cardiocirculatory determination of death: A French single-centre experience. Nephrology, Dialysis, Transplantation. 2011;**27**(6):2583-2587

[22] Lee JH, Hong SY, Oh CK, Hong YS, Yim H. Kidney transplantation from a donor following cardiac death supported with extracorporeal membrane oxygenation. Journal of Korean Medical Science. 2012;**27**(2):115-119

[23] Reznik ON, Skvortsov AE, Reznik AO, Ananyev AN, Tutin AP, Kuzmin DO, et al. Uncontrolled donors with controlled reperfusion after sixty minutes of asystole: A novel reliable resource for kidney transplantation. PLoS One. 2013;**8**(5):e64209

[24] Rojas-Pena A, Sall LE, Gravel MT, Cooley EG, Pelletier SJ, Bartlett RH, et al. Donation after circulatory determination of death: The university of michigan experience with extracorporeal support. Transplantation. 2014;**98**(3):328-334

[25] Oniscu GC, Randle LV, Muiesan P, Butler AJ, Currie IS, Perera MT, et al. In situ normothermic regional perfusion for controlled donation after circulatory death—The United Kingdom experience. American Journal of Transplantation. 2014;**14**(12):2846-2854

[26] Minambres E, Suberviola B, Dominguez-Gil B, Rodrigo E, Ruiz-San Millan JC, Rodriguez-San Juan JC, et al. Improving the outcomes of organs obtained from controlled donation after circulatory death donors using abdominal normothermic regional perfusion. American Journal of Transplantation. 2017;**17**(8):2165-2172

[27] Molina M, Guerrero-Ramos F, Fernandez-Ruiz M, Gonzalez E, Cabrera J, Morales E, et al. Kidney transplant from uncontrolled donation after circulatory death donors maintained by nECMO has long-term outcomes comparable to standard criteria donation after brain death. American Journal of Transplantation. 2018;**19**(2):434-447

[28] Brook NR, White SA, Waller JR, Veitch PS, Nicholson ML. Non-heart beating donor kidneys with delayed graft function have superior graft survival compared with conventional heart-beating donor kidneys that develop delayed graft function. American Journal of Transplantation. 2003;**3**(5):614-618

[29] Maheshwari A, Maley W, Li Z, Thuluvath PJ. Biliary complications and outcomes of liver transplantation from donors after cardiac death. Liver Transpl 2007 Dec;**13**(12):1645-1653

[30] Jay CL, Lyuksemburg V, Ladner DP, Wang E, Caicedo JC, Holl JL, et al. Ischemic cholangiopathy after controlled donation after cardiac death liver transplantation: A meta-analysis. Annals of Surgery. 2011;**253**(2):259-264

[31] O'Neill S, Roebuck A, Khoo E, Wigmore SJ, Harrison EM. A meta-analysis and meta-regression of outcomes including biliary complications in donation after cardiac death liver transplantation. Transplant International. 2014;**27**(11):1159-1174

[32] Foley DP, Fernandez LA, Leverson G, Anderson M, Mezrich J, Sollinger HW, et al. Biliary complications after liver transplantation from donation after cardiac death donors: An analysis of risk factors and long-term outcomes from a single center. Annals of Surgery. 2011;**253**(4):817-825

[33] Savier E, Dondero F, Vibert E, Eyraud D, Brisson H, Riou B, et al. First experience of liver transplantation with type 2 donation after cardiac death in France. Liver Transplantation. 2015;**21**(5):631-643

[34] Schlegel A, Scalera I, Perera MTPR, Kalisvaart M, Mergental H, Mirza DF, et al. Impact of donor age in donation after circulatory death liver transplantation: Is the cutoff "60" still of relevance? Liver Transplantation. 2018;**24**(3):352-362

[35] Croome KP, Mathur AK, Lee DD, Moss AA, Rosen CB, Heimbach JK, et al. Outcomes of donation after cardiac death liver grafts from donors >/= 50 years of age: A multi-center analysis. Transplantation. 2018;**102**(7):1108-1114

[36] De CR, Di SS, Lauterio A, Botta F, Ferla F, Andorno E, et al. Liver grafts from donors after cardiac death on regional perfusion with extended warm ischemia compared with donors after brain death. Liver Transplantation. 2018;**24**(11):1523-1535

[37] Ruiz P, Gastaca M, Bustamante FJ, Ventoso A, Palomares I, Prieto M, et al. Favorable outcomes after liver transplantation with normothermic regional perfusion from donors after circulatory death: A single-center experience. Transplantation. 2018

[38] Hessheimer AJ, Coll E, Torres F, Ruíz P, Gastaca M, Rivas JI, et al. Normothermic regional perfusion versus super rapid recovery in controlled donation after circulatory death liver transplantation. Journal of Hepatology. 2019

[39] Watson C, Hunt F, Messer S, Currie I, Large S, Sutherland A, et al. In situ normothermic perfusion of livers in controlled circulatory death donation may prevent ischemic cholangiopathy and improve graft survival. American Journal of Transplantation. 2019

[40] Organización Nacional de Trasplantes. Informe de Actividad de

Donación y Trasplante de Donantes en Asistolia. 2017

[41] Cypel M, Levvey B, van Raemdonck D, Erasmus M, Dark J, Love R, et al. International Society for Heart and Lung Transplantation Donation After Circulatory Death Registry Report. The Journal of Heart and Lung Transplantation. 2015;**34**(10):1278-1282

[42] Kleinmahon JA, Patel SS, Auerbach SR, Rossano J, Everitt MD. Hearts transplanted after circulatory death in children: Analysis of the international society for heart and lung transplantation registry. Pediatric Transplantation. 2017;**21**(8):e13064

[43] Royal Decree 1723/2012. 28 December 2012, Annex I, Section 3: Diagnosis of death based on circulatory and respiratory criteria. Available from: noticias.juridicas.com/base_datos/Admin/rd1723-2012.html#n3

[44] Organización Nacional de Trasplantes. Donación en Asistolia en España: Situación Actual y Recomendaciones. 2012

[45] Boucek MM, Mashburn C, Dunn SM, Frizell R, Edwards L, Pietra B, et al. Pediatric heart transplantation after declaration of cardiocirculatory death. The New England Journal of Medicine. 2008;**359**(7):709-714

[46] Perez-Villares JM, Rubio JJ, Del RF, Minambres E. Validation of a new proposal to avoid donor resuscitation in controlled donation after circulatory death with normothermic regional perfusion. Resuscitation. 2017;**117**:46-49

Chapter 13

Neurologic Complications and Neuromonitoring on ECMO

Venessa Lynn Pinto

Abstract

Extracorporeal membrane oxygenation is challenged by several potential complications. Adverse neurologic events such as intracranial hemorrhages, strokes, seizures, and brain death are among the most detrimental and even catastrophic of ECMO complications. There are several risk factors related to the patients, their underlying conditions and the therapy itself that predispose these patients to neurologic injuries. In this chapter, we review different types of neurological complications, the identification and management of which can be difficult. We will also discuss some of the currently available technologies for multimodal neurological monitoring as a complement to clinical exam.

Keywords: stroke, hemorrhage, MRI, neuromonitoring, neuroimaging, ECMO

1. Introduction

ECMO is a cardiopulmonary bypass circuit to support patients in severe cardiac and/or respiratory failure. It is an advanced life support therapy for patients at high risk of dying from their respiratory or cardiac disease. Extracorporeal life support, while life-saving in many instances, can pose serious risks and is associated with several neurologic complications. In this chapter, we will review some of the more common neurologic adverse events seen in patients on extracorporeal membrane oxygenation (ECMO), as well as review some of the neuromonitoring modalities available for early recognition of neurologic morbidity. Based on a recent report from the Extracorporeal Life Support Organization (ELSO), the current survival to discharge after ECMO ranges from 28% for adult ECPR patients to 73% for neonatal respiratory ECMO [1]. As survival after ECMO improves with advances in technologies and patient care, there is ever increasing emphasis placed on reducing morbidity experience by survivors.

Majority of the literature on neurologic injuries come from analyses of the ELSO Registry and single center experiences. The ELSO registry currently collects limited information on presence of seizures (clinical or EEG confirmed), central nervous system (CNS) hemorrhages (intraventricular or parenchymal) as determined by ultrasound (US), Computed tomography (CT) or Magnetic Resonance Imaging (MRI); diffuse ischemia or CNS infarction; need for neurosurgical intervention, and brain death on ECMO [2]. In spite of advances in ECMO circuitry, anticoagulation, and clinical management, the rate of occurrence of neurologic injury has not changed in recent times [3].

ECMO was first trialed on a neonate and the success with that patient gradually spread its popularity among the neonatal and eventually pediatric patient populations [4]. The H1N1 influenza pandemic in 2009 is primarily credited for the adoption of ECMO in many adult centers and its use in adults has grown exponentially since. While most of the early data came from neonates, more recent studies on neurologic injuries in adults are informing care of the ECMO patient. As ECMO is becoming more ubiquitously used, this chapter discusses neurologic complications noted across the age spectrum. However risk factors, types of complications and management often vary by patient population, from neonates to adults. Effort has been made to specify if certain descriptions are only applicable to a certain age group, and information may not be relevant for all ages.

2. Epidemiology

Quantification of the burden of neurologic complications has been difficult due to voluntary and retrospective nature of reporting, variability and lack of consensus on neuromonitoring and heterogeneous populations.

An ELSO registry analysis of neonates on ECMO from 2005 to 2010 showed that 20% had some neurologic complications [5]. Non hemorrhagic complications such as cerebral infarction, brain death and seizures were far less common than intracranial hemorrhage. A look at the subgroup of neonates with congenital heart disease failed to show an association between type of cardiac lesion and CNS injury [6]. The pediatric patient population is more heterogeneous than the neonatal group. A study by Hervey-Jumper et al. looked at children on ECMO from 1990 to 2009 and found that intracranial hemorrhage occurred in 7.4%, cerebral infarction in 5.7% and clinical seizures in 8.4% of all patients [7].

A systematic review of studies from 1990 to 2017 found that intracranial hemorrhage was the most common type of neurologic injury in adults, followed by acute ischemic stroke [8]. Incidence reported varies widely with a range of 2–21% for intracranial hemorrhage and 1–33% for acute ischemic stroke, with a median proportion of 5% of patients experiencing hemorrhages and another 5% with stroke. Seizures had the lowest incidence of about 2%. The study did find that neurologic injury was overall more commonly reported in VA ECMO than VV ECMO. The occurrence of neurologic injury significantly increases the in-hospital mortality with median mortality of 96% for hemorrhages, 84% for ischemic strokes 84, and 40% for seizures.

An analysis of the ELSO registry of almost 5000 adult patients on VV ECMO found an overall incidence of neurologic complications in 7.1% of patients [3]. Injuries included hemorrhage in 42.5%, brain death in 23.5%, stroke in 19.9%, and seizures in 14.1%. This study also found that in-hospital mortality was much higher (75.8% versus 37.8%) for patients with neurological injuries. An analysis of the ELSO registry for adult patients on VA ECMO, by the same group, found similar findings in the venoarterial cohort [9]. A decade's review of the Nationwide Inpatient Sample, that included over 23,000 patients, found that adult patients with acute ischemic stroke and intracranial hemorrhage on ECMO had higher rates of discharge to a long term facility and longer length of stay when compared to patients without neurologic injury [10].

A recent international randomized controlled trial, comparing ECMO to conventional mechanical ventilation for severe ARDS, showed a very low rate of ischemic stroke in the ECMO population [11]. Out of 124 patients randomized to receive ECMO, none had ischemic strokes compared to 5% of the patients initially randomized to conventional therapy, although there was the option of crossover to ECMO for refractory ARDS. It is unclear if this is due to a restrictive inclusion criteria of less than 7 days of mechanical ventilation combined with less severe hypoxemia and acidosis from early ECMO cannulation. However, the rates of hemorrhagic stroke were similar in the two groups.

3. Cerebral blood flow and oxygenation on ECMO

Cerebral autoregulation is the term used to describe the ability of cerebral arterioles to maintain steady cerebral blood flow across a wide range of cerebral blood pressure. This is achieved through dilation and constriction of cerebral blood vessels in response to fluctuations in mean arterial pressure. This is a complex process mediated through neurogenic regulation, involving sympathetic and cholinergic mechanisms, myogenic regulation involving smooth muscle tone, and metabolic regulation influenced by local concentration of metabolites [12]. Cerebral autoregulation can become disrupted focally or globally in pathological conditions leading to cerebral ischemia, hemorrhage or edema. These conditions associated with ECMO include vasospasm, severe acidosis, low cardiac output states, hypotension and hypertension, reperfusion injury and absence of pulsatile flow in VA ECMO. Hypercapnia is associated with cerebral vasodilation while hypocapnia causes cerebral vasoconstriction. A rapid decline in paCO2 after initiation of VV ECMO has been associated with central nervous system (CNS) injury [13].

A study by O'Brien using transcranial Doppler (TCD) showed that in patients that did not have neurologic injury, cerebral blood flow velocities on ECMO were much lower than predicted and returned closer to baseline after decannulation. However in patients that did have cerebral hemorrhage on ECMO, supranormal flows were noted in the days preceding the event [14]. A more recent multicenter study by the same author confirmed lower flow velocities on ECMO but did not show a difference in flow velocities in children with cerebral ischemia compared to those without. No patients in this study had cerebral hemorrhage [15].

Cannulation of cervical vessels relies on a competent Circle of Willis to allow for cerebral perfusion of both hemispheres. Occlusion of vessels can cause ipsilateral venous stasis and this venous congestion can lead to venous hypertension and decreased cerebral perfusion. Changes in cerebral blood flow rate and volume can contribute to altered cerebral oxygenation as demonstrated by cerebral oximetry [12]. Impairments in cerebral autoregulation, based on wavelet transform coherence, are associated with findings on neuroimaging and neurologic outcomes [16].

4. Risk factors for neurologic injury

These can be divided into factors prior to initiation of ECMO and factors inherent to ECMO therapy [17]. There are also risk factors for neurological injury after ECMO such as ligation or anastomosis of cervical blood vessels. Because CNS injury is often multifactorial, and lesions are often detected retrospectively on imaging after ECMO, the exact timing of injury can be difficult to determine.

4.1 Pre-ECMO

The underlying physiologic conditions that necessitate ECMO cannulation, such as labile hemodynamics, severe hypoxemia and acidosis, refractory hypotension, etc., leave the patient vulnerable to neurologic insults. These can alter the mechanisms responsible for maintaining cerebral autoregulation and make the vasculature more susceptible to alterations in systemic blood pressure. Prematurity is associated with an increase in intraventricular and intracranial hemorrhage and can be a contraindication for ECMO cannulation. A prior history of neurologic injury puts one at further risk of adverse cerebrovascular events.

4.2 ECMO-related

Animal models have demonstrated the effects of carotid artery and jugular vein cannulation and ligation on cerebral blood flow [18, 19]. Adults with atherosclerosis may develop emboli during arterial cannulation. ECMO cannulae and circuits expose a patient to prothrombotic surfaces and the foreign materials often incite an inflammatory response. Platelets are consumed in the circuit components leading to thrombocytopenia, putting a patient at increased risk of bleeding. Maintaining patency of the circuits requires the use of anticoagulation, which needs to be closely monitored to avoid complications such as bleeding, or thrombosis and embolism. Reperfusion injury is another risk factor after adequate oxygenation and blood flow delivery have been ensured following a period of severe hypoxemia. VA ECMO cannulation for cardiogenic shock is also associated with non-pulsatile flow which is not physiologic. Neurologic exams are often limited for patients on ECMO, confounded by sedation and limited mobility, which can lead to delayed diagnosis and recognition. A precannulation lactate greater than 10 mmol/L was found to be associated with increased odds for ischemic strokes in adults [8]. A history of pre ECMO cardiac arrest, need for renal replacement therapy and elevated bilirubin levels were associated with increased odds of neurologic injury [3]. A study of neonates found that birth weight less than 3 kg, gestational age less than 34 weeks, a history of prior ECMO cannulation and severe acidosis were risk factors for neurologic injury [5].

4.3 Veno-arterial (VA) versus veno-venous (VV)

VA ECMO carries with it the increased risk of embolization as blood is directly pumped into the arterial system, unlike in VV ECMO where the oxygenated blood is returned to the venous system where the lungs can filter thrombi. However, a study by Zahraa found that there was no difference in central nervous system complications between pediatric respiratory failure patients supported on VA versus VV ECMO [20]. Differential hypoxia, where the arterial oxygen tension is lower in the upper half of the body than in the lower half, is a phenomenon occasionally seen in patients supported on peripheral VA ECMO that causes cerebral ischemia [21]. For pediatric patients on VA ECMO, the incidence of stroke was much lower for transthoracic or central cannulation compared to peripheral cannulation [22]. VA ECMO is also unique in that poor cardiac function results in absence of pulsatile flow, with potential implications for cerebral autoregulation and vascular reactivity.

4.4 Carotid repair

The right carotid artery and internal jugular vein are commonly sacrificed during ECMO cannulation. Taylor et al. showed the feasibility of vascular repair with antegrade flow, without increasing the incidence of embolic phenomenon [23]. A larger, more recent study of neonates on VA ECMO, showed over 84% patency of repaired vessels. While 43% of all patients had a severe brain lesion after ECMO, there was no difference in early neurologic outcomes between the groups that underwent carotid repair versus carotid ligation [24].

4.5 Extracorporeal cardiopulmonary resuscitation (ECPR)

ECPR is the rapid deployment of VA ECMO for a patient in cardiac arrest, with ongoing CPR, prior to the return of spontaneous circulation. A systematic review of adult ECPR data showed that a shockable rhythm and duration of CPR were significantly associated with a favorable neurologic outcome [25]. A study of the

ELSO registry looking at pediatric patients that received ECPR found an overall incidence of acute neurologic injury in 22% of patients [26]. The in-hospital mortality was high for these patients at 89%. An analysis of neonatal and pediatric ECPR events from a multicenter, national registry showed that while only 43.7% of patients survived to hospital discharge, the majority of survivors had favorable neurologic outcomes [27]. Another study comparing survivors of ECPR and those with return of circulation after conventional CPR found comparable neurologic outcomes between the two groups, with total duration of cardiac arrest being the only predictor of survival [28].

5. Types of neurological complications and their management

There is a wide variety of neurological injuries that are noted after ECMO including embolic strokes, hypoxic-ischemic encephalopathy, cerebral infarction, intracranial and subarachnoid hemorrhages, seizures, cerebral edema and even brain death. Other complications, such as critical illness myopathy, neuropathies, delirium, hearing loss, vocal cord paralysis etc. are related to prolonged hospitalization and ICU stays, need for prolonged mechanical ventilation or tracheostomy, prolonged exposure to sedation, and limited mobility that often accompany ECMO runs. In this section of the chapter, we will look at some of the more common neurologic complications experienced by patients treated with ECMO.

5.1 Hemorrhagic complications

Intracranial hemorrhage (ICH) is one of the most common adverse neurologic events on ECMO, carrying a high mortality rate. It can occur as intraparenchymal, intraventricular or subarachnoid hemorrhages. Gestational age at time of ECMO cannulation, severe acidosis needing correction, sepsis, need for epinephrine, therapeutic hypothermia and need for cardiopulmonary resuscitation (CPR) have been associated with intracranial hemorrhage in neonates [29–31]. A longer duration of ECMO, higher activated clotting times (ACTs), presence of bleeding at other sites, pre-admission antithrombotic therapy, and low platelet counts were associated with hemorrhage in adults [32, 33]. Rapid $PaCO_2$ decrease/correction of hypercapnia and renal failure at ICU admission were associated with increased intracranial hemorrhage in one adult study [13]. In order to detect intracranial hemorrhage while on ECMO, cranial ultrasounds are used in neonates while CT imaging is used in children and adults. In one observational study, 42% of the cohort underwent withdrawal of life sustaining therapy, 18% did not require any intervention and 40% were treated. Treatments included hemostatic interventions, ICP management and surgical interventions with 14% of the cohort uneventfully decannulated [34]. Patients that have clinically significant bleeds, with progression of brain injury and little to no improvement on ECMO ultimately end up with withdrawal of life sustaining therapies due to poor prognosis and risk of progression of the bleed. Patients with very small or clinically insignificant hemorrhages can continue their ECMO courses with close neurological monitoring, decannulation at the earliest feasible time and possibly lowering of anticoagulation parameters while balancing thrombotic risks. Platelets and anti-fibrinolytics may need to be administered. Occasionally ECMO circuits can be trialed without any anticoagulation keeping a close eye on the circuit for clots and fibrin deposition. Life-threatening hemorrhage can be severe enough to warrant a craniotomy [7, 35]. Hematoma evacuation on ECMO is high risk and carries a high mortality although there are reports of patients who survived [34]. There is heterogeneity in practice with drugs used for anticoagulation (heparin versus bivalirudin), tests to assess for anticoagulation (TEG,

ROTEM, activated clotting time, PT/PTT, heparin assays) and therapeutic targets for titration. Further research is needed to help develop guidelines and consensus on best practice to minimize and treat bleeding complications on ECMO.

5.2 Ischemic complications

It occurs in about 5–6% of children and adults [8, 36], and is best identified on MR imaging. Due to multifactorial etiology for ischemic strokes such as hypotension, large vessel occlusion, thromboembolism, septic embolism, etc. it is difficult to characterize lesions anatomically or to prognosticate based on imaging. Timing of injury is also difficult to ascertain. There are conflicting reports on laterality of lesions [37] but seem to occur in the middle cerebral artery vascular territory. A single center pediatric study found that majority of strokes were bilateral, a few were unilateral right sided lesions and no patients had unilateral left sided strokes; majority of the lesions were in the anterior cerebral circulation distribution [22]. Ischemic lesions are associated with electrographic seizures and decreased survival [38]. Asymmetry in regional cerebral saturation or on continuous EEG monitoring might be suggestive of focal ischemia. Once detected, hemodynamics should be optimized through adequate pump flows on VA ECMO, vasoactives can be used if needed, and further neurologic injury should be minimized by avoiding hyperoxia and treating seizures.

5.3 Seizures

Although less common than intracranial hemorrhage and stroke, seizures can be difficult to recognize if they are nonconvulsive or subclinical. A study of children and neonates undergoing ECMO revealed that 18% of patients had electrographic seizures, with 61% of those patients having electrographic status epilepticus and 83% having exclusively electrographic seizures [39]. Another recent study of neonatal and pediatric patients found electrographic seizures in 23% of their patients, especially within the first 24 hours of ECMO [40]. Patients with seizures had decreased survival to discharge (44% versus 74%). Older studies that reported lower incidence of seizures may have missed patients if only clinical seizures were reported, as the routine use of continuous EEG monitoring for patients is not yet a widespread practice, although recent recommendations advocate for its use in ECMO. Given that patients on ECMO are a high risk population, seizures should be treated with the help of neurologists.

5.4 Sensorineural hearing loss

Sensorineural hearing loss has been reported in neonatal ECMO graduates with a frequency of 3–21% [41]. Diagnosis of congenital diaphragmatic hernia, duration of ECMO, and aminoglycoside antibiotic use were associated with hearing loss [42]. A follow-up study found that even children diagnosed with hearing loss after ECMO can go on to have normal language development [43].

5.5 Myopathy

Prolonged immobilization, sedation and paralytics, hemodynamic instability, all contribute to neuromuscular weakness in ECMO patients. Studies have proved that active physiotherapy, with early mobilization, is feasible and safe in ECMO patients when performed with an experienced, multidisciplinary team [44, 45]. It may also shorten hospital duration and improve functional outcomes for patients [46].

5.6 Delirium

A small study of pediatric cardiac ECMO patients diagnosed delirium in all their patients, in 21% of coma-free ECMO days [47]. Use of validated delirium screening tools can aid in early recognition and management of delirium. The move to liberate ICU patients should include patients on ECMO whenever feasible, with an emphasis on delirium prevention.

5.7 Brain death on ECMO

Progressive cerebral edema and large hemorrhages, whether from insults prior to cannulation or secondary to complications from ECMO, can ultimately lead to brain death in patients supported on ECMO. Diagnosis of brain death can be challenging on ECMO, but is important to determine as it is medically and ethically unreasonable to continue ECMO for a patient who has met criteria for brain death.

5.7.1 Determination of brain death

The American Academy of Neurology issued guidelines on the determination of brain death in adults, most recently revised in 2010 [48]. Similarly the Society of Critical care Medicine, American Academy of pediatrics and the Child Neurology Society jointly published guidelines for the determination of brain death in children and infants in 2011 [49]. The following general criteria apply to all patients undergoing brain death testing, although the specifics may vary by institutional policies. Patients should be relatively normothermic, and electrolytes and glucose should be within acceptable ranges. Any medications that may interfere with respiratory drive and neurologic function must be discontinued, with drug levels obtained if needed. The patient must demonstrate absence of all motor function and lack of responsiveness to stimuli, except spinal reflexes. Cranial nerve testing should reveal absence of pupillary reflexes, corneal reflexes, oculovestibular and oculocephalic reflexes, absence of cough and gag reflexes and absent brain stem reflexes.

The apnea test is an important component of brain death testing without which ancillary studies such as cerebral angiography, nuclear scanning for cerebral blood flow, electroencephalography, transcranial Doppler etc. are required to demonstrate absence of blood flow to the brain. The apnea test is performed to demonstrate absence of spontaneous respiratory drive in the presence of rising $paCO_2$ levels in the blood. The patient is pre-oxygenated with 100% FiO_2 and ventilated to achieve normocarbia, if possible. A baseline blood gas analysis is obtained. The patient is then disconnected from the ventilator and oxygenated via a T-piece or flow-inflating anesthesia bag. The patient is closely observed for signs of spontaneous respiration or chest rise. Serial blood gases are obtained at every few minute intervals. A rise in $paCO_2 > 60$ mmHg and > 20 mmHg above baseline is conclusive of absence of respiratory drive. If the patient were to become hypoxic or hemodynamically unstable the apnea test should be discontinued and ancillary studies obtained.

5.7.2 Apnea testing on ECMO

While clinical criteria of absence of cortical function and brain stem reflexes can be assessed in the usual manner, apnea testing can be difficult on ECMO. A proposed method for apnea testing is oxygenating the patient by use of continuous positive airway pressure (CPAP) or T-piece or by placing the patient on a self-inflating anesthesia bag with a PEEP valve, while watching for spontaneous respirations. The oxygenator on the circuit can then be capped. Alternatively, the sweep gas is decreased to 0.5 –1 L/minute and oxygen increased to 100% FiO2 through the circuit, without any changes to extracorporeal blood flow [50, 51]. In-line gas monitoring on the ECMO circuit can be used to trend venous paCO2, but serial arterial blood gas analysis should be used to confirm the lack of ventilation secondary to central apnea. For patients on VA ECMO, hemodynamics should be maintained through circuit flows and use of vasoactive medications as needed. Patients found to be brain dead on ECMO can be considered as candidates for organ donation.

6. Neurological monitoring

There are currently no consensus guidelines for neuromonitoring on ECMO, with variations in practice at different institutions. Neuromonitoring may include assessment of brain structure or morphology via imaging, assessment of brain function via EEG or SSEPs, assessment of cerebral perfusion via cerebral oximetry or transcranial doppler, and assessment for neurological injury via biomarkers. Bembea and colleagues performed a systematic review of the literature; 39 observational and case-control studies met inclusion criteria, with most of the literature coming from neonatal studies [52]. There was very little data in pediatric and adult cohorts, and the study found limited data on the use and effectiveness of monitoring technologies. A recent review by Lin et al. discusses neuromonitoring in the neonatal ECMO patient [53].

6.1 Exam

Neuromonitoring of the ECMO patient should begin with daily neurologic assessments that are documented in the patients chart. These are limited by reliability when performed by multiple providers from different disciplines, however are useful for obtaining a daily baseline that can be suggestive of injury when a change is noted. This would also require daily sedation holidays for accurate assessments as well as using the least amount of sedation to keep the patient safe and comfortable. Use of neuromuscular blockade should be reserved for extremely ill patients and those whose movement limits ECMO flows. A change in neurologic exam is often the trigger for seeking additional information such as through neuroimaging.

6.2 Neuroimaging

Cranial or head ultrasound (HUS) is a mode of imaging limited to neonates and infants with open fontanelles. Ultrasound uses high frequency sound waves transmitted via a probe that are reflected back based on the tissue's composition as well as distance from the probe. Changes in tissue density from hemorrhage or ischemia will reflect back sound waves differently from surrounding tissue. Cranial ultrasounds are portable, easy to use, relatively inexpensive, and do not carry radiation risks. Most neonatal ECMO programs will obtain a HUS prior to ECMO cannulation as well as daily HUS for the 1st few days on ECMO. While it is best for detecting hemorrhages, ischemic changes are harder to interpret on HUS [54]. HUS can also give information on changes in ventricular size that would be seen in hydrocephalus. It is not as sensitive as other imaging techniques and a study showed that MRI was significantly more sensitive for detection of CNS lesions than HUS alone [55, 56]. The quality of images depends on the skill level of the ultrasound technician and interpretation of acquired images can be subjective and variable. HUS findings have not consistently correlated with neurodevelopmental outcomes and should not be used for predicting outcomes in neonatal ECMO survivors [37, 56].

Computed tomography (CT) is a diagnostic imaging modality that utilizes X-Rays directed at the patient that are picked up by a detector and sent to a computer to create thin 2D image slices, at different tissue depths. Multiple images can then be stacked to create a 3D picture. It is the most frequently used imaging modality for diagnosis of acute intracranial injury for patients on ECMO. A CT scan can be quickly obtained and has better sensitivity and specificity for detecting intracranial hemorrhage that might lead to clinical changes in management [53]. A disadvantage is exposure to radiation and its associated risks. Transporting a patient on ECMO to a CT scanner in the radiology department can be challenging in the absence of a portable scanner that can be brought to bedside. ELSO currently recommends a CT scan prior to hospital discharge for patients less than 4 years of age and if there is an abnormal neurologic exam for patients older than 4 years of age as part of post-ECMO follow up [57].

Magnetic Resonance Imaging (MRI) is a non-invasive technology that creates 3D anatomic images without exposing the patient to radiation. A strong magnetic field is used to force protons in the body into alignment. Then a brief radiofrequency pulse stimulates protons causing a change in alignment. The scanner can detect electromagnetic energy transmitted as the protons realign. It is reserved for patients after decannulation from ECMO, due to MRI incompatible materials in the cannulae and circuits. MRI is the most sensitive and specific imaging technique available. However it takes much longer time to obtain the study compared to a CT and is more expensive. While diffusion-restriction can be seen up to 10 days after acute ischemic injury, the optimal timing for obtaining an MRI after ECMO remains unclear [53].

6.3 Electroencephalography (EEG)

While neuroimaging provides information on the structure of the brain, EEG provides real-time information on the electrical activity of the brain. Information is obtained via electrodes placed on the scalp, connected to a monitor, with very little burden to the patient that would include scalp abrasions. Continuous EEG (cEEG) monitoring requires technicians to set up the electrodes as well as neurologists to read the EEGs, which can be time consuming. Amplitude-integrated EEG (aEEG) compresses the raw EEG data from 1 to 2 leads, is easier to set up and interpret, but due to lower sensitivity, can be used as a screening tool or in resource limited settings [53]. Ischemic and hemorrhagic injuries can predispose a patient to seizures that require prompt treatment. Continuous EEG monitoring is important for early identification and treatment of subclinical seizures or electrical status epilepticus that may not be otherwise detected, although studies are needed to show its benefit in improving long term outcomes. EEG monitoring is especially useful in paralyzed patients in whom a neurological exam cannot be elicited. EEG can be used to detect early cerebral ischemia through loss of fast alpha and beta frequencies to slowing and even suppression of all electrical activity as might be seen in an infarct. In 2011, the American Clinical Neurophysiology Society deemed ECMO as a high risk clinical scenario in neonates that would warrant long term EEG monitoring due to cardiac or pulmonary risks for acute brain injury and clinical encephalopathy [58]. This recommendation is supported by ELSO in their guidelines for management of neonatal respiratory failure [59]. In their 2015 consensus statement on continuous EEG in critically ill adults and children, the American Clinical Neurophysiology Society recommended continuous EEG monitoring for patients treated with pharmacologic paralysis, including patients on ECMO [60].

6.4 Transcranial doppler ultrasound (TCD)

This is a non-invasive, portable test that is based on the Doppler effect. A Doppler probe is used to emit high frequency sound waves through the cranium that are reflected back by moving red blood cells in the blood vessels. The difference in frequencies of emitted and reflected waves is proportional to the cerebral blood flow. Studies have found that TCD velocities (TCDV) are much lower for pediatric patients on ECMO when compared to normative values for healthy and critically-ill children [15, 61]. While there was no significant association between global TCDV (systolic flow velocity, diastolic flow velocity, mean flow velocity) and neurologic injury, increased pulsatility index and regional increases in velocities or asymmetries might be predictive of neurologic injury.

6.5 Cerebral near infra-red spectroscopy (NIRS)

NIRS monitoring is a non-invasive technology that uses near-infrared wavelength of light that penetrates brain tissue via a scalp electrode. It provides a continuous measurement of regional tissue oxygen saturation (rSO2), which is a marker of the balance between oxygen delivery and demand in the tissues. When the probe is placed on the forehead, it measures cerebral oximetry. An analysis of adult patients on VA ECMO showed that cerebral desaturation was common and mortality higher for patients with cerebral desaturation compared to those without [21]. A sudden decrease in cerebral saturation can be associated with an acute neurological event, prompting further investigation. It can also serve as an early predictor of inadequate oxygenation and cardiac output especially peri-cannulation [62]. It can influence management by prompting a need for increased flows in VA ECMO or alternate cannulation strategies if there is differential hypoxia. A very high rSO2 could also be suggestive of very poor oxygen extraction and poor neurologic outcomes.

6.6 Biomarkers

Several plasma proteins have been evaluated as potential markers for brain injury [63]. These biomarkers include substances associated with glial injury (glial fibrillary acidic protein and s-100b), neuronal injury (neuron-specific enolase and brain-derived neurotrophic factor) and neuro-inflammation (intercellular adhesion molecue-5). Unfavorable neurologic outcomes have been associated with higher biomarker concentrations [64], with combinations of biomarkers providing higher sensitivities and specificities for detection of neurologic injury. These tests are more expensive and require laboratory equipment and processing availability. While not currently a routine component of neuromonitoring on ECMO in most institutions, there is potential for further research and applicability if these results can be obtained in real time to influence management.

6.7 Somato-sensory evoked potentials (SSEPs)

SSEPs measure electrical signals in the somatosensory cortex after a peripheral stimulus, assessing the pathway of neuronal conduction from the peripheral nerve to the cortex. They are assessed as normal, abnormal (increased latency) or absent. ECMO cannulation is not thought to alter the ability to assess SSEPs from the hemispheres [65]. Small studies have shown an association between abnormal SSEPs and poor neurologic outcome after ECMO [66], but the predictive value of evoked potentials remains to be determined. In one study, absence of bilateral SSEPs was associated with progression to brain death for patients treated with ECPR [67].

6.8 Optic nerve sheath diameter (ONSD)

It is a simple bedside test used to detect elevated intracranial pressure. A cut-off of 5.2 mm is sensitive and specific for intracranial hypertension [68]. Its use in

ECMO management is still in its infancy, although a study showed that higher ONSD was associated with poor neurological outcome after ECPR [69].

7. Therapeutic hypothermia

Therapeutic hypothermia has been shown to be neuroprotective for term neonates at risk of hypoxic ischemic encephalopathy secondary to perinatal asphyxia. However a randomized controlled study out of the United Kingdom did not show an improvement in outcomes for neonates on ECMO treated with mild hypothermia [70]. On the other hand, therapeutic hypothermia has been associated as a risk factor for intracranial hemorrhage and should be avoided [30]. In 2015, the American Heart Association recommended targeted temperature management of 32–36°C for comatose patients with return of spontaneous circulation after cardiac arrest [71]. This was also applied to patients who suffered in- hospital cardiac arrest leading to ECPR. A more recent large, multicenter, randomized control trial failed to show a benefit in survival with favorable neurological outcome for children with in-hospital cardiac arrest. There is no data to support routine therapeutic hypothermia for children undergoing ECPR although maintaining normothermia is still encouraged.

8. Conclusion

Neurologic complications contribute to significant morbidity and mortality for patients on ECMO, who constitute a high risk population. There are many modalities currently available for neuromonitoring, and as we gain more experience and information through more frequent use, we will be able to develop consensus guidelines and protocols to provide better care. A multimodal approach to active surveillance, early recognition and prompt management of neurologic injuries as they arise, may improve outcomes for patients on ECMO.

Conflict of interest

The author has no "conflict of interest" to disclose.

Author details

Venessa Lynn Pinto
Texas Children's Hospital and Baylor College of Medicine, Houston, Texas, USA

*Address all correspondence to: vlpinto@bcm.edu

References

[1] ECLS Registry Report. Extracorporeal Life Support Organization. 2017. Available from: https://www.elso.org/Portals/0/Files/Reports/2017/International%20Summary%20January%202017.pdf [Accessed: 30-01-2019]

[2] ECLS Registry Form. ELSO. 2018. Available from: https://www.elso.org/Portals/0/ELSOECLSRegistryForm5_0%202018-03-01.pdf [Accessed: 05-12-2018]

[3] Lorusso R, Gelsomino S, Parise O, Di Mauro M, Barili F, Geskes G, et al. Neurologic injury in adults supported with veno-venous extracorporeal membrane oxygenation for respiratory failure: Findings from the extracorporeal life support organization database. Critical Care Medicine. 2017;**45**(8):1389-1397

[4] Bartlett RH. Esperanza: The first neonatal ECMO patient. American Society for Artificial Internal Organs: 1992. 2017;**63**(6):832-843

[5] Polito A, Barrett CS, Wypij D, Rycus PT, Netto R, Cogo PE, et al. Neurologic complications in neonates supported with extracorporeal membrane oxygenation. An analysis of ELSO registry data. Intensive Care Medicine. 2013;**39**(9):1594-1601

[6] Polito A, Barrett CS, Rycus PT, Favia I, Cogo PE, Thiagarajan RR. Neurologic injury in neonates with congenital heart disease during extracorporeal membrane oxygenation: An analysis of extracorporeal life support organization registry data. American Society for Artificial Internal Organs: 1992. 2015;**61**(1):43-48

[7] Hervey-Jumper SL, Annich GM, Yancon AR, Garton HJL, Muraszko KM, Maher CO. Neurological complications of extracorporeal membrane oxygenation in children. Journal of Neurosurgery. Pediatrics. 2011;**7**(4):338-344

[8] Sutter R, Tisljar K, Marsch S. Acute neurologic complications during extracorporeal membrane oxygenation: A systematic review. Critical Care Medicine. 2018;**46**(9):1506-1513

[9] Lorusso R, Barili F, Mauro MD, Gelsomino S, Parise O, Rycus PT, et al. In-hospital neurologic complications in adult patients undergoing venoarterial extracorporeal membrane oxygenation: Results from the extracorporeal life support organization registry. Critical Care Medicine. 2016;**44**(10):e964-e972

[10] Nasr DM, Rabinstein AA. Neurologic complications of extracorporeal membrane oxygenation. Journal of Clinical Neurology. 2015;**11**(4):383-389

[11] Combes A, Hajage D, Capellier G, Demoule A, Lavoué S, Guervilly C, et al. Extracorporeal membrane oxygenation for severe acute respiratory distress syndrome. The New England Journal of Medicine. 2018;**378**(21):1965-1975

[12] Kazmi SO, Sivakumar S, Karakitsos D, Alharthy A, Lazaridis C. Cerebral pathophysiology in extracorporeal membrane oxygenation: Pitfalls in daily clinical management. Critical Care Research and Practice. 2018;**2018**:3237810

[13] Luyt C-E, Bréchot N, Demondion P, Jovanovic T, Hékimian G, Lebreton G, et al. Brain injury during venovenous extracorporeal membrane oxygenation. Intensive Care Medicine. 2016;**42**(5):897-907

[14] O'Brien NF, Hall MW. Extracorporeal membrane oxygenation and cerebral blood flow velocity in children. Pediatric Critical Care Medicine. 2013;**14**(3):e126-e134

[15] O'Brien NF, Buttram SDW, Maa T, Lovett ME, Reuter-Rice K, LaRovere KL, et al. Cerebrovascular physiology during pediatric extracorporeal membrane oxygenation: A multicenter study using transcranial doppler ultrasonography. Pediatric Critical Care Medicine. 2018;**20**(2):178-186

[16] Tian F, Morriss MC, Chalak L, Venkataraman R, Ahn C, Liu H, et al. Impairment of cerebral autoregulation in pediatric extracorporeal membrane oxygenation associated with neuroimaging abnormalities. Neurophotonics. 2017;**4**(4):041410

[17] Xie A, Lo P, Yan TD, Forrest P. Neurologic Complications of Extracorporeal Membrane Oxygenation: A Review. Journal of Cardiothoracic and Vascular Anesthesia. 2017;**31**(5):1836-1846

[18] Short BL. The effect of extracorporeal life support on the brain: A focus on ECMO. Seminars in Perinatology. 2005;**29**(1):45-50

[19] Graziani LJ, Gringlas M, Baumgart S. Cerebrovascular complications and neurodevelopmental sequelae of neonatal ECMO. Clinics in Perinatology. 1997;**24**(3):655-675

[20] Zahraa JN, Moler FW, Annich GM, Maxvold NJ, Bartlett RH, Custer JR. Venovenous versus venoarterial extracorporeal life support for pediatric respiratory failure: Are there differences in survival and acute complications? Critical Care Medicine. 2000;**28**(2):521-525

[21] Pozzebon S, Blandino Ortiz A, Franchi F, Cristallini S, Belliato M, Lheureux O, et al. Cerebral near-infrared spectroscopy in adult patients undergoing veno-arterial extracorporeal membrane oxygenation. Neurocritical Care. 2018;**29**(1):94-104

[22] Pinto VL, Pruthi S, Westrick AC, Shannon CN, Bridges BC, Le TM. Brain magnetic resonance imaging findings in pediatric patients post extracorporeal membrane oxygenation. American Society for Artificial Internal Organs: 1992. 2017;**63**(6):810-814

[23] Taylor GA, Short BL, Glass P, Ichord R. Cerebral hemodynamics in infants undergoing extracorporeal membrane oxygenation: Further observations. Radiology. 1988 Jul;**168**(1):163-167

[24] Duggan EM, Maitre N, Zhai A, Krishnamoorthi H, Voskresensky I, Hardison D, et al. Neonatal carotid repair at ECMO decannulation: Patency rates and early neurologic outcomes. Journal of Pediatric Surgery. 2015;**50**(1):64-68

[25] Wang J, Ma Q, Zhang H, Liu S, Zheng Y. Predictors of survival and neurologic outcome for adults with extracorporeal cardiopulmonary resuscitation: A systemic review and meta-analysis. Medicine (Baltimore). 2018;**97**(48):e13257

[26] Barrett CS, Bratton SL, Salvin JW, Laussen PC, Rycus PT, Thiagarajan RR. Neurological injury after extracorporeal membrane oxygenation use to aid pediatric cardiopulmonary resuscitation. Pediatric Critical Care Medicine. 2009;**10**(4):445-451

[27] Raymond TT, Cunnyngham CB, Thompson MT, Thomas JA, Dalton HJ, Nadkarni VM, et al. Outcomes among neonates, infants, and children after extracorporeal cardiopulmonary resuscitation for refractory inhospital pediatric cardiac arrest: A report from the National Registry of Cardiopulmonary Resuscitation. Pediatric Critical Care Medicine. 2010;**11**(3):362-371

[28] Cesana F, Avalli L, Garatti L, Coppo A, Righetti S, Calchera I, et al. Effects of extracorporeal cardiopulmonary resuscitation on neurological and cardiac

outcome after ischaemic refractory cardiac arrest. European Heart Journal Acute Cardiovascular Care. 2018;7(5):432-441

[29] Dela Cruz TV, Stewart DL, Winston SJ, Weatherman KS, Phelps JL, Mendoza JC. Risk factors for intracranial hemorrhage in the extracorporeal membrane oxygenation patient. Journal of Perinatology. 1997;**17**(1):18-23

[30] Cashen K, Reeder RW, Shanti C, Dalton HJ, Dean JM, Meert KL, et al. Is therapeutic hypothermia during neonatal extracorporeal membrane oxygenation associated with intracranial hemorrhage? Perfusion. 2018;**33**(5):354-362

[31] Hardart GE, Fackler JC. Predictors of intracranial hemorrhage during neonatal extracorporeal membrane oxygenation. The Journal of Pediatrics. 1999;**134**(2):156-159

[32] Omar HR, Mirsaeidi M, Mangar D, Camporesi EM. Duration of ECMO is an independent predictor of intracranial hemorrhage occurring during ECMO support. American Society for Artificial Internal Organs: 1992. 2016;**62**(5):634-636

[33] Fletcher Sandersjöö A, Bartek J, Thelin EP, Eriksson A, Elmi-Terander A, Broman M, et al. Predictors of intracranial hemorrhage in adult patients on extracorporeal membrane oxygenation: An observational cohort study. Journal of Intensive Care. 2017;**5**:27

[34] Fletcher-Sandersjöö A, Thelin EP, Bartek J, Elmi-Terander A, Broman M, Bellander B-M. Management of intracranial hemorrhage in adult patients on extracorporeal membrane oxygenation (ECMO): An observational cohort study. PLoS One. 2017;**12**(12):e0190365

[35] Fletcher-Sandersjöö A, Thelin EP, Bartek J, Broman M, Sallisalmi M, Elmi-Terander A, et al. Incidence, outcome, and predictors of intracranial hemorrhage in adult patients on extracorporeal membrane oxygenation: A systematic and narrative review. Frontiers in Neurology. 2018;**9**:548

[36] Wien MA, Whitehead MT, Bulas D, Ridore M, Melbourne L, Oldenburg G, et al. Patterns of brain injury in newborns treated with extracorporeal membrane oxygenation. AJNR. American Journal of Neuroradiology. 2017;**38**(4):820-826

[37] Bulas D, Glass P. Neonatal ECMO: Neuroimaging and neurodevelopmental outcome. Seminars in Perinatology. 2005;**29**(1):58-65

[38] LaRovere KL, Vonberg FW, Prabhu SP, Kapur K, Harini C, Garcia-Jacques R, et al. Patterns of head computed tomography abnormalities during pediatric extracorporeal membrane oxygenation and association with outcomes. Pediatric Neurology. 2017;**73**:64-70

[39] Lin J-J, Banwell BL, Berg RA, Dlugos DJ, Ichord RN, Kilbaugh TJ, et al. Electrographic seizures in children and neonates undergoing extracorporeal membrane oxygenation. Pediatric Critical Care Medicine. 2017;**18**(3):249-257

[40] Okochi S, Shakoor A, Barton S, Zenilman AR, Street C, Streltsova S, et al. Prevalence of seizures in pediatric extracorporeal membrane oxygenation patients as measured by continuous electroencephalography. Pediatric Critical Care Medicine. 2018;**19**:1162-1167

[41] Cheung PY, Robertson CM. Sensorineural hearing loss in survivors of neonatal extracorporeal membrane oxygenation. Pediatric Rehabilitation. 1997;**1**(2):127-130

[42] Fligor BJ, Neault MW, Mullen CH, Feldman HA, Jones DT. Factors associated with sensorineural hearing loss among survivors of extracorporeal

membrane oxygenation therapy. Pediatrics. 2005;**115**(6):1519-1528

[43] van den Hondel D, Madderom MJ, Goedegebure A, Gischler SJ, Mazer P, Tibboel D, et al. Sensorineural hearing loss and language development following neonatal extracorporeal membrane oxygenation. Pediatric Critical Care Medicine. 2013;**14**(1):62-69

[44] Abrams D, Javidfar J, Farrand E, Mongero LB, Agerstrand CL, Ryan P, et al. Early mobilization of patients receiving extracorporeal membrane oxygenation: A retrospective cohort study. Critical Care (London, England). 2014;**18**(1):R38

[45] Munshi L, Kobayashi T, DeBacker J, Doobay R, Telesnicki T, Lo V, et al. Intensive care physiotherapy during extracorporeal membrane oxygenation for acute respiratory distress syndrome. Annals of the American Thoracic Society. 2017;**14**(2):246-253

[46] Thiagarajan RR, Teele SA, Teele KP, Beke DM. Physical therapy and rehabilitation issues for patients supported with extracorporeal membrane oxygenation. Journal of Pediatric Rehabilitation Medicine. 2012;**5**(1):47-52

[47] Patel AK, Biagas KV, Clark EC, Traube C. Delirium in the pediatric cardiac extracorporeal membrane oxygenation patient population: A case series. Pediatric Critical Care Medicine. 2017;**18**(12):e621-e624

[48] Wijdicks EFM, Varelas PN, Gronseth GS, Greer DM. American Academy of Neurology. Evidence-based guideline update: Determining brain death in adults: Report of the Quality Standards Subcommittee of the American Academy of Neurology. Neurology. 2010 8;**74**(23):1911-1918

[49] Nakagawa TA, Ashwal S, Mathur M, Mysore M. Society of critical care medicine, section on critical care and section on neurology of American Academy of Pediatrics, Child Neurology Society. Clinical report—guidelines for the determination of brain death in infants and children: An update of the 1987 task force recommendations. Pediatrics. 2011;**128**(3):e720-e740

[50] Giani M, Scaravilli V, Colombo SM, Confalonieri A, Leo R, Maggioni E, et al. Apnea test during brain death assessment in mechanically ventilated and ECMO patients. Intensive Care Medicine. 2016;**42**(1):72-81

[51] Muralidharan R, Mateen FJ, Shinohara RT, Schears GJ, Wijdicks EFM. The challenges with brain death determination in adult patients on extracorporeal membrane oxygenation. Neurocritical Care. 2011;**14**(3):423-426

[52] Bembea MM, Felling R, Anton B, Salorio CF, Johnston MV. Neuromonitoring during extracorporeal membrane oxygenation: A systematic review of the literature. Pediatric Critical Care Medicine. 2015;**16**(6):558-564

[53] Lin N, Flibotte J, Licht DJ. Neuromonitoring in the neonatal ECMO patient. Seminars in Perinatology. 2018;**42**(2):111-121

[54] van Heijst AFJ, de Mol AC, Ijsselstijn H. ECMO in neonates: Neuroimaging findings and outcome. Seminars in Perinatology. 2014;**38**(2):104-113

[55] Rollins MD, Yoder BA, Moore KR, Barnhart DC, Jones C, Null DM, et al. Utility of neuroradiographic imaging in predicting outcomes after neonatal extracorporeal membrane oxygenation. Journal of Pediatric Surgery. 2012;**47**(1):76-80

[56] Lazar EL, Abramson SJ, Weinstein S, Stolar CJ. Neuroimaging of brain injury in neonates treated with extracorporeal membrane oxygenation: Lessons learned from

serial examinations. Journal of Pediatric Surgery. 1994;**29**(2):186-190; discussion 190-191

[57] ELSO Recommendations for Follow-up for ECMO Patients. 1997. Available from: https://www.elso.org/Portals/0/IGD/Archive/FileManager/2440a82ecdcusersshyerdocuments elsorecommendationsforneonatal pediatricecmopatientfollowup.pdf [Accessed: 07-12-2018]

[58] Shellhaas RA, Chang T, Tsuchida T, Scher MS, Riviello JJ, Abend NS, et al. The American Clinical Neurophysiology Society's Guideline on continuous electroencephalography monitoring in neonates. Journal of Clinical Neurophysiology. 2011;**28**(6):611-617

[59] ELSO. Guidelines for Neonatal Respiratory Failure. Ann Arbor, MI, USA: ELSO; 2017. Available from: https://www.elso.org/Portals/0/ELSOGuidelinesNeonatalRespiratory Failurev1_4_1.pdf

[60] Herman ST, Abend NS, Bleck TP, Chapman KE, Drislane FW, Emerson RG, et al. Consensus statement on continuous EEG in critically ill adults and children, part I: Indications. Journal of Clinical Neurophysiology. 2015;**32**(2):87-95

[61] Rilinger JF, Smith CM, deRegnier RAO, Goldstein JL, Mills MG, Reynolds M, et al. Transcranial doppler identification of neurologic injury during pediatric extracorporeal membrane oxygenation therapy. Journal of Stroke and Cerebrovascular Diseases. 2017;**26**(10):2336-2345

[62] Maldonado Y, Singh S, Taylor MA. Cerebral near-infrared spectroscopy in perioperative management of left ventricular assist device and extracorporeal membrane oxygenation patients. Current Opinion in Anaesthesiology. 2014;**27**(1):81-88

[63] Bembea MM, Rizkalla N, Freedy J, Barasch N, Vaidya D, Pronovost PJ, et al. Plasma biomarkers of brain injury as diagnostic tools and outcome predictors after extracorporeal membrane oxygenation. Critical Care Medicine. 2015;**43**(10):2202-2211

[64] Nguyen DN, Huyghens L, Wellens F, Schiettecatte J, Smitz J, Vincent J-L. Serum S100B protein could help to detect cerebral complications associated with extracorporeal membrane oxygenation (ECMO). Neurocritical Care. 2014;**20**(3):367-374

[65] Carter BG, Butt WW. Median nerve somatosensory evoked potentials in children receiving ECMO. Pediatric Neurology. 1995;**12**(1):42-46

[66] Amigoni A, Pettenazzo A, Biban P, Suppiej A, Freato F, Zaramella P, et al. Neurologic outcome in children after extracorporeal membrane oxygenation: Prognostic value of diagnostic tests. Pediatric Neurology. 2005;**32**(3):173-179

[67] Casadio MC, Coppo A, Vargiolu A, Villa J, Rota M, Avalli L, et al. Organ donation in cardiac arrest patients treated with extracorporeal CPR: A single centre observational study. Resuscitation. 2017;**118**:133-139

[68] Raffiz M, Abdullah JM. Optic nerve sheath diameter measurement: A means of detecting raised ICP in adult traumatic and non-traumatic neurosurgical patients. The American Journal of Emergency Medicine. 2017;**35**(1):150-153

[69] Ryu J-A, Chung CR, Cho YH, Sung K, Suh GY, Park TK, et al. The association of findings on brain computed tomography with neurologic outcomes following extracorporeal cardiopulmonary resuscitation. Critical Care (London, England). 2017;**21**(1):15

[70] Field D, Juszczak E, Linsell L, Azzopardi D, Cowan F, Marlow N, et al.

Neonatal ECMO study of temperature (NEST): A randomized controlled trial. Pediatrics. 2013;**132**(5):e1247-e1256

[71] Callaway CW, Donnino MW, Fink EL, Geocadin RG, Golan E, Kern KB, et al. Part 8: Post-cardiac arrest care: 2015 American Heart Association Guidelines Update for cardiopulmonary resuscitation and emergency cardiovascular care. Circulation. 2015;**132**(18 Suppl 2):S465-S482

Chapter 14

Anticoagulation in Pediatric Extracorporeal Membrane Oxygenation

Jamie Weller, Lakshmi Raman, Ayesha Zia and Ali McMichael

Abstract

Anticoagulation during extracorporeal membrane oxygenation (ECMO) is necessary to prevent catastrophic circuit clotting, but significant morbidity and mortality continue to be attributed to hemorrhagic and thrombotic complications. Due to the inflammatory response from the extracorporeal circuit and developmental hemostasis, anticoagulation can be challenging particularly for pediatric patients. Unfractionated heparin (UFH) is the gold standard anticoagulant used in ECMO, but there is an expanding area of research evaluating other anticoagulants, such as direct thrombin inhibitors. This chapter provides an overview of anticoagulant options for pediatric patients on ECMO as well as describes the various tests used to monitor and titrate anticoagulation.

Keywords: extracorporeal membrane oxygenation, anticoagulation, unfractionated heparin, bivalirudin

1. Introduction

Anticoagulation during extracorporeal membrane oxygenation (ECMO) is necessary to prevent catastrophic circuit clotting, but it contributes to significant morbidity and mortality. The Extracorporeal Life Support Organization (ELSO) international registry shows a 24% increase in the number of patients placed on ECMO and a 55% growth of centers utilizing ECMO from 2009 to 2015 [1]. Although there has been rapid growth in ECMO around the world, pediatric mortality rates have remained static or even increased depending on the reason for cannulation [1]. In a multicenter study, Dalton et al. showed that 19–70% of patients had a bleeding event and 12–43% of pediatric patients had a thrombotic event while anticoagulated on ECMO [2]. With the increase in centers utilizing ECMO, anticoagulation has become an important area of research.

2. Overview of hemostasis

In order to discuss the intricacies of anticoagulation during ECMO, a basic understanding of the mechanisms required for hemostasis and the coagulation cascade is necessary (**Figure 1**). Hemostasis occurs by vascular constriction, platelet plug creation, and clot formation through fibrin [3]. The vasculature surrounding the damaged tissue constricts limiting blood flow to the area. Platelets adhere to the exposed endothelium

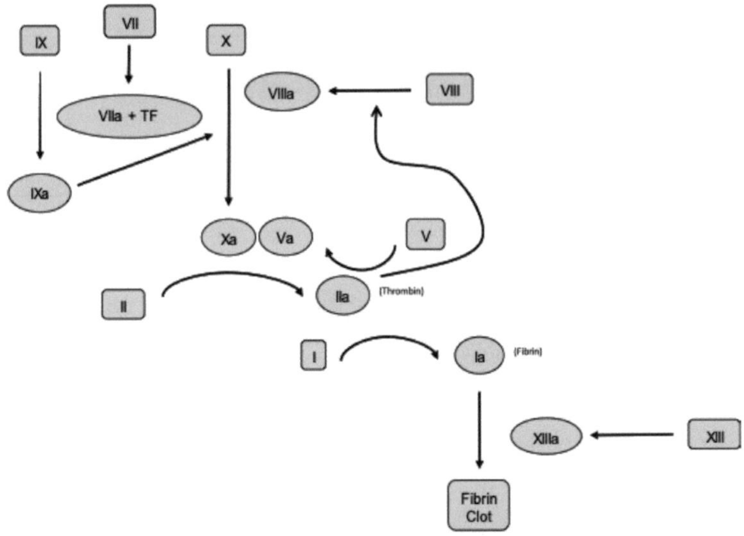

Figure 1.
In vivo concept of coagulation. The clotting system is classified into the initiation, amplification, and propagation phase. TF, tissue factor (thromboplastin); II, prothrombin; I, fibrinogen.

via von Willebrand factor creating a platelet plug to temporize the bleeding. Finally, the clotting cascade is activated by the presence of tissue factor released when blood vessels are damaged [3]. The clotting cascade has been traditionally described as the intrinsic and extrinsic pathways merging to initiate the common pathway, and resulting in the activation of fibrinogen to fibrin to form a stable clot. This classification is pertinent for understanding *in vitro* coagulation tests, but fails to account for the *in vivo* coagulation process [4, 5]. Current evidence suggests that the initial cascade augments the formation of thrombin through multiple feedback loops. The initiation phase is activated with exposure of tissue factor from damaged blood vessels. The initial amount of thrombin produced is insufficient to achieve adequate hemostasis, thus a series of feedback loops prompted by thrombin act to catalyze the factor (F) V and FVIII, eventually accelerating the activity of FXa and FIXa. This second phase is classified as the amplification phase [4]. The propagation phase ensures continued production of thrombin and thus fibrin, by forming sufficient prothrombinase complexes [4].

The hemostatic processes are counterbalanced by antithrombotic factors such as protein C, protein S, thrombomodulin, antithrombin, and tissue factor pathway inhibitor. Clot degradation is initiated by the fibrinolytic factors such as tissue plasminogen activator (tPA), plasminogen, and urokinase plasminogen activator [3]. The extracorporeal circuit interferes with the described mechanisms designed to achieve adequate hemostasis. Immediately upon contact with the foreign ECMO circuit, the coagulation cascade is activated and a complex inflammatory response occurs [6]. Platelets, neutrophils, and leukocytes are activated along with thrombin and plasmin. Platelets adhere to the foreign surface leading to both platelet and factor consumption. Activated neutrophils contribute to the inflammatory response by producing cytokines. In addition, thrombin, FXa, and FVIIa cause complement activation further causing an inflammatory state. The end result is a consumptive state with disequilibrium of coagulation [7–10].

3. Anticoagulation with unfractionated heparin in ECMO

Although anticoagulation during ECMO is necessary to prevent circuit thrombosis and subsequent thromboembolic events in the patient, it continues to be a

	ICH N(%)	Surgical site bleeding N(%)	GI hemorrhage N(%)	Cerebral infarct N(%)
Neonatal cardiac	326(11)	739(26)	35(1)	93(3)
Neonatal respiratory	643(11)	386(7)	89(2)	180(3)
Pediatric cardiac	251(6)	974(25)	79(2)	231(6)
Pediatric respiratory	243(5)	332(10)	135(4)	158(7)

Table 1.
Patient-related hemorrhagic and thrombotic complications extrapolated from the ELSO registry, 2009–2015 [1]. ICH, intracranial hemorrhage; GI, gastrointestinal.

significant risk factor for complications in ECMO patients. The most common bleeding complications during ECMO include intracranial hemorrhage (ICH), surgical site bleeding, and gastrointestinal hemorrhage (**Table 1**). Surgical site bleeding is the most frequent complication and occurs in up to 25% of pediatric cardiac and respiratory ECMO patients [1]. Bleeding events are associated with increased mortality [2]. For example, while ICH is not a frequent complication, the effect is significant with a survival rate of 17–40% compared to 45–68% for those who do not have an ICH [1]. In addition to hemorrhage, thrombotic complications can occur. While not as common as bleeding complications, cerebral infarcts accounted for 3–7% of complications described in the ELSO registry report [1]. Unfractionated heparin continues to be the most widely studied and used anticoagulant for anticoagulation in ECMO, but alternative agents are increasingly being used in pediatric and adult ECMO patients.

3.1 Unfractionated heparin

Unfractionated heparin (UFH) is the gold standard anticoagulant during ECMO and is commonly used in ECMO centers worldwide. Heparin acts as a catalyst to potentiate the action of antithrombin III, inhibiting thrombin and activated coagulation factor X, thus inhibiting the conversion of fibrinogen to fibrin [11]. The half-life of heparin is approximately 1–2 hours in healthy adults, but can vary significantly in pediatric patients. Heparin is metabolized by the reticuloendothelial system in the liver and spleen, and is excreted in the urine [11]. In the pediatric population, developmental hemostasis and the patient's age may affect the pharmacokinetics of heparin [12]. For example, the neonatal population frequently requires additional monitoring and higher bolus and infusion rates to obtain effective anticoagulation [6, 12–14]. Another complication due to unfractionated heparin use is heparin-induced thrombocytopenia that is seen in 1–2% of pediatric patients [11].

For patients with preexisting conditions that preclude them from safe anticoagulation, such as trauma patients with intracranial hemorrhage or patients that develop hemorrhagic complications while on ECMO, successful use of heparin-free ECMO management with or without heparin-bonded circuits has been documented [15–17]. However, the published literature is limited primarily to specific populations and for a limited duration of time.

4. Monitoring during heparin anticoagulation

Close monitoring to ensure anticoagulation is therapeutic is necessary to decrease the risk of hemorrhage or thrombosis during ECMO. The common tests used to monitor heparin during ECMO are activated clotting time (ACT), activated partial thromboplastin time (aPTT), and anti-factor Xa. No single test has been found to be superior to monitor heparin during ECMO. ECMO centers worldwide vary in their practices on the type of test or combination of tests used to monitor heparin [2, 18].

4.1 Activated clotting time

The activated clotting time (ACT) is a whole blood test used at the bedside that provides immediate results [3, 6]. The ACT measures the time in seconds to form a fibrin clot after the addition of specific coagulation activators, thus it does not solely measure the effect of unfractionated heparin. It is a relatively inexpensive test that has been widely used to monitor heparin during cardiopulmonary bypass, but coagulation factor deficiencies, hemodilution, platelet function, and hypofibrinogenemia may affect the value [3, 19]. Due to these limitations in ACT, Baird and colleagues retrospectively reviewed 600 pediatric ECMO patients and found only a modest correlation between ACT and UFH dose suggesting that ACT may not be an accurate tool for monitoring UFH anticoagulation [20]. Bembea and colleagues found similar results to Baird with only a 42% correlation between target ACTs and anti-factor Xa [21].

4.2 Activated partial thromboplastin time

Activated partial thromboplastin time (aPTT) is a plasma-based test, instead of a whole blood test, which only measures the initial 5% of thrombin generated and without incorporating platelet function or assessing clot strength. The aPTT measures the time from FXII activation to fibrin formation after addition of the PTT reagent and calcium [3, 19]. The therapeutic range for aPTT in adults has been shown to correlate to 1.5–2.5× the patient's baseline aPTT [22]. However, this range has not been validated in pediatric patients and can vary significantly compared to adults. For example, an aPTT that correlates to anti-factor Xa between 0.35 IU/ml and 0.7 IU/ml in a patient less than 1 year old is between 58 and 105 seconds, but in a patient 6–10 years old the anti-factor Xa correlates to an aPTT between 45 and 251 seconds [23]. The results of aPTT can be affected by fibrinogen level, presence of acute phase reactants, and increased levels of FVIII. These variables are often skewed in critically ill patients, which can lead to a high degree of intra- and inter-patient variability [19].

4.3 Anti-factor Xa assay

The anti-Xa assay is a plasma-based test that measures the ability of UFH to catalyze antithrombin's inhibition of factor Xa. Anti-Xa assay differs from ACT and aPTT as it measures the heparin concentration in the patient's blood [24]. Since the anti-Xa assay only measures one specific action of heparin, the value is used as a surrogate to approximate overall function [19]. The anti-Xa value may be affected in patients with elevated plasma-free hemoglobin, hyperbilirubinemia, hypertriglyceridemia, and antithrombin (depending on test reagants). A point of care anti-Xa test is available, but it is currently not widely used. Anti-factor Xa has been shown to have improved correlation to heparin activity as compared to aPTT and ACT [25]. In addition, a retrospective review of 62 pediatric ECMO patients with a mean anti-factor Xa level >0.2 IU/ml was associated with decreased circuit change [26].

Published literature supports the correlation between anti-factor Xa values and UFH dose. Unfortunately, many studies have shown a poor correlation between anti-factor Xa and ACT and/or aPTT. Multiple cardiac studies evaluating patients requiring cardiopulmonary bypass report disparities between ACT values and anti-Xa as compared to UFH doses [27–30]. ECMO adult studies have shown an improved correlation between aPTT and UFH concentrations, but pediatric studies demonstrate poor correlation to anti-factor Xa levels [31–33].

4.4 Viscoelastic testing

Viscoelastic testing such as thromboelastography (TEG) and rotational thromboelastometry (ROTEM) are whole blood tests that measure the interaction of clotting factors, fibrinogen, and platelets as well as fibrinolysis (**Figure 2**). By measuring more than clotting factors, viscoelastic tests can give a more global picture of the coagulation system and allow for tailored transfusion management [3, 19]. **Figure 2** shows the standard TEG measurements including reaction time (R), kinetics (K), and maximum amplitude (MA). The R value is the time necessary for the initial clot formation. This value can be affected by the presence of anticoagulants, factor deficiencies, and hypercoagulable states. The K value measures the time for the clot to strengthen and can be affected by platelet count, fibrinogen, and coagulation factors. The maximum amplitude quantifies the final strength of the clot. Overall clot strength can be affected by the amount and function of fibrinogen and platelets [3]. In general, viscoelastic tests can be limited by static flow conditions [19]. While there is limited evidence in trauma, obstetrics, liver transplantation, and hemophilia using viscoelastic testing to help define coagulopathy and decrease overall blood product transfusions, studies are needed to confirm these results in ECMO patients [34]. Furthermore, prospective studies should examine the use of TEG and ROTEM in conjunction with aPTT and/or anti-factor Xa.

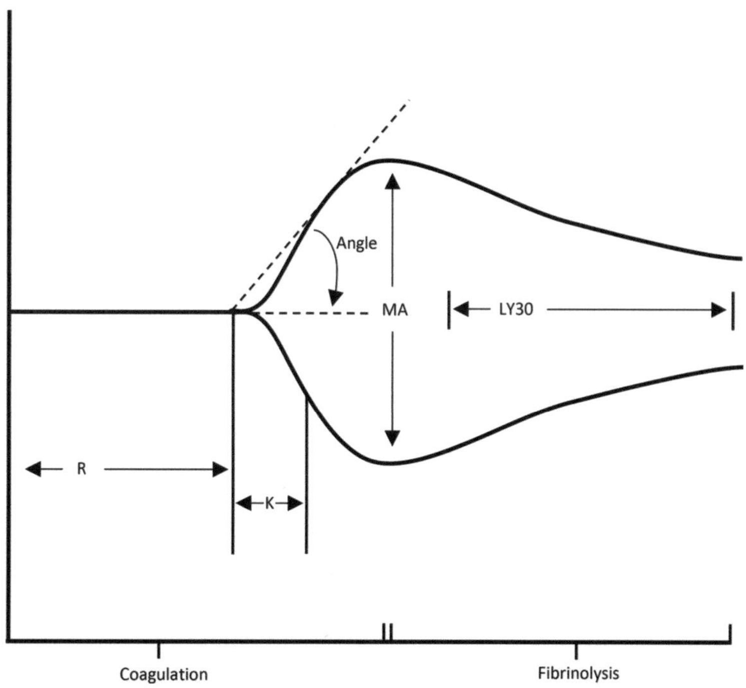

Figure 2.
Thromboelastography (TEG). R, reaction time; K, kinetics; MA, maximum amplitude; LY30, amplitude at 30 minutes.

5. Direct thrombin inhibitors

5.1 Bivalirudin

Alternative agents, such as direct thrombin inhibitors (DTI), have been increasingly used in ECMO centers worldwide. Bivalirudin is a DTI that binds to both circulating and clot-bound thrombin [35]. The basic structure of thrombin consists of the active site, exosite 1, and exosite 2. Exosite 1 is the location where specific substrates, such as fibrin, can bind and orient peptide bonds toward the active site of thrombin [36]. Bivalirudin is a bivalent DTI that blocks thrombin at the active site and exosite 1 [36, 37]. Bivalirudin is primarily metabolized by proteolytic enzymes with 20% renally excreted [36]. With limited evidence to support the safety and therapeutic profile of bivalirudin in patients undergoing ECMO, bivalirudin has primarily been used in patients unresponsive to unfractionated heparin or those who developed heparin-induced thrombocytopenia [38]. In *in vitro* studies, bivalirudin inhibits both soluble and clot-bound thrombin, a unique mechanism of action not known to occur with unfractionated heparin [35]. Two prospective studies assessing clot resolution found that patients anticoagulated with bivalirudin for the treatment of deep vein thrombosis (DVT) had complete or partial clot resolution within 48 hours [39, 40].

5.2 Argatroban

Argatroban is a L-arginine derivative that reversibly binds and inhibits thrombin. Argatroban is a univalent DTI that binds solely to the active site of thrombin. It is metabolized by hepatic CYP3A4/5 oxidases and is excreted primarily in the feces [36, 41, 42]. Menk and colleagues retrospectively reviewed 78 adult patients with acute respiratory distress syndrome (ARDS) on ECMO. The single center study supported that patients anticoagulated with argatroban had no difference in major or minor bleeding and had more goal aPTT values compared to UFH controls [43]. Multiple studies have shown that doses vary widely between adult and pediatric patients anticoagulated with argatroban on ECMO, thus careful monitoring is imperative to ensure optimal anticoagulation [43–45]. A literature analysis reviewed nine articles describing 34 patients anticoagulated with argatroban. Pediatric patients were administered a dose ranging from 0.1 to 12 mcg/kg/min to achieve therapeutic anticoagulation. There was no correlation between the dose of argatroban and the age of the patient [45].

Bivalirudin and argatroban remain the most commonly utilized direct thrombin inhibitors for anticoagulation during ECMO, but small case studies have evaluated the efficacy of lepirudin [46, 47]. Unfortunately, the product is no longer available due to production discontinuation by the manufacturer.

5.3 Direct thrombin inhibitor use in ECMO

Disadvantages of DTIs include limited availability of laboratory monitoring specific to DTIs and lack of antidote. Currently, most centers that use DTIs follow aPTT for monitoring, which as mentioned previously can be affected by several patient variables. Ecarin chromogenic assay and dilute thrombin time are possible superior tests for monitoring, but are currently not widely available [36]. Unlike heparin, which can be reversed with protamine, no antidote exists for DTIs, but recombinant factor VIIa has been shown to be an effective reversal agent [48]. Plasmapheresis has also been shown to be effective in clearing bivalirudin, but limited evidence has been published supporting its use. An advantage of bivalirudin over argatroban is that it can be quickly removed by continuous renal replacement therapy [49].

Evidence of DTIs for ECMO patients is limited to case series or retrospective analyses. To confirm the safety and efficacy of DTIs and superiority (or at least non-inferiority) to heparin, prospective randomized trials of pediatric and adult patients are needed. Two randomized studies are currently enrolling to compare bivalirudin to UFH for pediatric and adult ECMO patients (NCT03318393 and NCT03707418).

6. Nitric oxide

At present, systemic anticoagulation is the primary method to prevent thrombus formation during ECMO, but the use of nitric oxide within the extracorporeal circuit may be used to inhibit platelet adhesion. Nitric oxide (NO) is an endogenous substance released by the endothelial cells. NO temporarily inactivates platelets resulting in decreased function and aggregation [50, 51]. However, the effect of NO only temporarily inhibits platelets and after rapid degradation of NO by hemoproteins, platelets will regain normal function [52]. The utility of NO within ECMO circuits to limit or negate the requirement of systemic anticoagulation remains a promising area of research, but further studies to evaluate the long-term risks of thrombosis are warranted.

7. Conclusion

In summary, while the goal for ECMO anticoagulation is to prevent clinically significant bleeding and clotting, the morbidity and mortality for these complications remain high for pediatric patients. Unfractionated heparin continues to be the most commonly used anticoagulant for ECMO patients in spite of its many disadvantages including altered pharmacokinetics in children and difficulty in lab monitoring. While there is a large variation between lab monitoring of heparin among ECMO centers, combination testing with anti-factor Xa and/or aPTT with viscoelastic tests is potentially superior. DTIs such as bivalirudin and argatroban remain promising alternatives to heparin, but prospective studies are needed to confirm their safety and efficacy.

Author details

Jamie Weller*, Lakshmi Raman, Ayesha Zia and Ali McMichael
Pediatric Critical Care, University of Texas Southwestern Medical Center, Dallas, Texas, United States of America

*Address all correspondence to: jamie.weller@utsouthwestern.edu

References

[1] Barbaro RP, Paden ML, Guner YS, Raman L, Ryerson LM, Alexander P, et al. ELSO member centers. Pediatric extracorporeal life support organization registry international report 2016. ASAIO Journal. 2017;**63**(4):45-463

[2] Dalton HJ, Reeder R, Garcia-Filion P, et al. Factors associated with bleeding and thrombosis in children receiving extracorporeal membrane oxygenation. American Journal of Respiratory and Critical Care Medicine. 2017;**196**(6):762-771

[3] Giglia TM, Witmer C. Bleeding and thrombosis in pediatric cardiac intensive care. Pediatric Critical Care Medicine. 2016;**17**(8):S287-S295

[4] Palta S et al. Overview of the coagulation system. Indian Journal of Anaesthesia. 2014;**58**(5):515-523

[5] Smith S, Travers R, Morrissey J. How it all starts: Initiation of the clotting cascade. Critical Reviews in Biochemistry and Molecular Biology. 2015;**9238**(4):326-336

[6] Oliver WC. Anticoagulation and coagulation management for ECMO. Seminars in Cardiothoracic and Vascular Anesthesia. 2009;**13**(3):154-175

[7] Wan S, LeClerc JL, Vincent JL. Inflammatory response to cardiopulmonary bypass. Chest. 1997;**112**:676-692

[8] Bowen FW, Edmunds HL Jr. Coagulation, anticoagulation and the interaction of blood and artificial surfaces. In: Zwischenberger JB, Steinhorn RH, Bartlett RH, editors. ECMO: Extracorporeal Cardiopul-Monary Support in Critical Care. 2nd ed. Ann Arbor, Michigan: ELSO; 2000. pp. 67-96

[9] Fortenberry JD, Bhardwaj V, Niemer P, et al. Neutrophil and cytokine activation with neonatal extracorporeal membrane oxygenation. The Journal of Pediatrics. 1996;**128**:670-678

[10] Furie B, Furie BC. Molecular and cellular biology of blood coagulation. The New England Journal of Medicine. 1992;**326**:800-806

[11] Heparin: Pediatric and Neonatal Lexi-Drugs. Lexicomp. Riverwoods, IL: Wolters Kluwer Clinical Drug Information Inc. Available from: http://onine.lexi.com [Accessed: December, 2018]

[12] Edmunds LH Jr, Colman RW. Thrombin during cardiopulmonary bypass. The Annals of Thoracic Surgery. 2006;**82**(6):2315-2322

[13] McDonald MM et al. Heparin clearance in the newborn. Pediatric Research. 1981;**15**(7):1015-1018

[14] Andrew M et al. Heparin clearance and ex vivo recovery in newborn piglets and adult pigs. Thrombosis Research. 1988;**52**(6):517-527

[15] Muellenbach RM et al. Prolonged heparin-free extracorporeal membrane oxygenation in multiple injured acute respiratory distress syndrome patients with traumatic brain injury. Journal of Trauma and Acute Care Surgery. 2012;**72**:1444-1447

[16] Perchinsky MJ, Long WB, Hill JG, et al. Extracorporeal cardiopulmonary life support with heparin-bonded circuitry in the resuscitation of massively injured trauma patients. American Journal of Surgery. 1995;**169**:488-491

[17] Reynolds HN, Cottingham C, McCunn M, et al. Extracorporeal lung support in a patient with traumatic brain injury: The benefit of heparin-bonded circuitry. Perfusion. 1999;**14**:489-493

[18] Bembea MM, Annich G, Rycus P, Oldenburg G, Berkowitz I, Pronovost P. Variability in anticoagulation management of patients on extracorporeal membrane oxygenation: An international survey. Pediatric Critical Care Medicine. 2013;**14**:e77-e84

[19] Ryerson LM, Lequier LL. Anticoagulation management and monitoring during pediatric extracorporeal life support: A review of current issues. Frontiers in Pediatrics. 2016;**4**:1-7

[20] Baird CW, Zurakowski D, Robinson B, Gandhi S, Burdis-Koch L, Tamblyn J, et al. Anticoagulation and pediatric extracorporeal membrane oxygenation: Impact of activated clotting time and heparin dose on survival. The Annals of Thoracic Surgery. 2007;**83**:912-919. DOI: 10.1016/j.athoracsur.2006.09.054

[21] Bembea M, Schwartz J, Shah N, et al. Anticoagulation monitoring during pediatric extracorporeal membrane oxygenation. ASAIO Journal. 2013;**59**:63-68

[22] Basu D, Gallus A, Hirsh J, Cade J. A prospective study of the value of monitoring heparin treatment with the activated partial thromboplastin time. The New England Journal of Medicine. 1972;**287**:327-327. DOI: 10.1056/NEJM197208172870703

[23] Ignjatovic V, Summerhayes R, Than J, Gan A, Monagle P. Therapeutic range for unfractionated heparin therapy: Age-related differences in response in children. Journal of Thrombosis and Haemostasis. 2006;**4**:2280-2283

[24] Bates SM, Weitz JI. Coagulation assays. Circulation. 2005;**112**(4):e53-e60

[25] Liveris A, Bello RA, Friedman P, Duffy MA, Manwani D, Killinger JS, et al. Anti-factor Xa assay is a superior correlate of heparin dose than activated partial thromboplastin time or activated clotting time in pediatric extracorporeal membrane oxygenation. Pediatric Critical Care Medicine. 2014;**15**(2):e72-e79

[26] Irby K, Swearingen CJ, Byrnes JW, Bryant J, Prodhan P, Fiser RT. Unfractionated heparin activity measured by anti-factor Xa levels is associated with the need for extracorporeal membrane oxygenation circuit/membrane oxygenator change: A retrospecitve pediatric study. Pediatric Critical Care Medicine. 2014;**15**(4):e175-e182

[27] Gruenwald C, de Souza V, Chan AK, et al. Whole blood heparin concentrations do not correlate with plasma antifactor Xa heparin concentrations in pediatric patients undergoing cardiopulmonary bypass. Perfusion. 2000;**15**:203-209

[28] Guzzetta NA, Monitz HG, Fernandez JD, et al. Correlations between activated clotting time values and heparin concentration measurements in young infants undergoing cardiopulmonary bypass. Anesthesia and Analgesia. 2010;**111**:173-179

[29] Raymond PD, Ray MJ, Callen SN, et al. Heparin monitoring during cardiac surgery. Part 2: Calculating the overestimation of heparin by the activated clotting time. Perfusion. 2003;**18**:277-281

[30] Martindale SJ, Shayevitz JR, D'Errico C. The activated coagulation time: Suitability for monitoring heparin effect and neutralization during pediatric cardiac surgery. Journal of Cardiothoracic and Vascular Anesthesia. 1996;**10**:458-463

[31] Chan AK, Black L, Ing C, et al. Utility of aPTT in monitoring unfractionated heparin in children. Thrombosis Research. 2008;**122**:135-136

[32] Kuhle S, Eulmesekian P, Kavanagh B, et al. Lack of correlation between heparin dose and standard clinical monitoring

tests in treatment with unfractionated heparin in critically ill children. Haematologica. 2007;**92**:554-557

[33] Brill-Edwards P, Ginsberg JS, Johnston M, et al. Establishing a therapeutic range for heparin therapy. Annals of Internal Medicine. 1993;**119**:104-109

[34] Whiting D, DiNardo JA. TEG and ROTEM: Technology and clinical applications. American Journal of Hematology. 2014;**89**(2):228-232

[35] The Medicines Company. Bivalirudin Drug Information; 2016

[36] Di Nisio M, Middeldorp S, Büller HR. Direct thrombin inhibitors. New England Journal of Medicine. 2005;**353**(10):1028-1040

[37] Hunt B. Bleeding and coagulopathies in critical care. The New England Journal of Medicine. 2014;**370**:847-859

[38] Young G, Male C, Heleen van Ommen C. Anticoagulation in children: Making the most of little patients and little evidence. Blood Cells, Molecules, and Diseases. 2017;**67**:48-53

[39] O'Brien SH, Yee DL, Lira J, Goldenberg NA, Young G. UNBLOCK: An open-label, dose finding, pharmacokinetic and safety of bivalirudin in children with deep vein thrombosis. Journal of Thrombosis and Haemostasis. 2015;**13**:1615-1622

[40] Young G, Tarantino MD, Wohrley J, Weber LC, Belvedere M, Nugent DJ. Pilot dose-finding and safety study of bivalirudin in infants <6 months of age with thrombosis. Journal of Thrombosis and Haemostasis. 2007;**5**:1654-1659

[41] Jeske WP et al. Pharmacology of argatroban. Expert Review of Hematology. 2010;**3**(5):527-539

[42] Weller J, Raman L, McMichael A. Anticoagulation and monitoring in pediatric extracorporeal membrane oxygenation. The Egyptian Journal of Critical Care Medicine. 2018;**6**(3):69-71

[43] Menk M et al. Efficacy and safety of argatroban in patients with acute respiratory distress syndrome and extracorporeal lung support. Annals of Intensive Care. 2017;**7**(1):82

[44] Beiderlinden M et al. Argatroban in extracorporeal membrane oxygenation. Artificial Organs. 2007;**31**(6):461-465

[45] Hursting MJ, Dubb J, Verme-Gibboney CN. Argatroban anticoagulation in pediatric patients: A literature analysis. Journal of Pediatric Hematology/Oncology. 2006;**28**(1):4-10

[46] Balasubramanian SK, Tiruvoipati R, Chatterjee S, Sosnowski A, Firmin RK. Extracorporeal membrane oxygenation with lepirudin anticoagulation for Wegener's granulomatosis with heparin-induced thrombocytopenia. ASAIO Journal. 2005;**51**(4):477-479

[47] Dager WE, Gosselin RC, Yoshikawa R, Owings JT. Lepirudin in heparin-induced thrombocytopenia and extracorporeal membranous oxygenation. The Annals of Pharmacotherapy. 2004;**38**(4):598-601

[48] Young G, Yonekawa KE, Nakagawa PA, et al. Recombinant activated factor VII effectively reverses the anticoagulant effects of heparin, enoxaparin, fondaparinux, argatroban and bivalirudin. Blood Coagulation & Fibrinolysis. 2007;**18**:547-553

[49] Koster A et al. An assessment of different filter systems for extracorporeal elimination of bivalirudin: An in vitro study. Anesthesia and Analgesia. 2003;**96**(5):1316-1319

[50] Ontaneda A, Annich G. Novel surfaces in extracorporeal membrane

oxygenation circuits. Frontiers in Medicine. 2018;**5**:321

[51] Annich GM et al. Reduced platelet activation and thrombosis in extracorporeal circuits coated with nitric oxide release polymers. Critical Care Medicine. 2000;**28**(4):915-920

[52] Reynolds MM, Annich GM. The artificial endothelium. Organogenesis. 2014;**7**:42-49